Brighton & Hove
City Council

BRIGHTON & HOVE CITY LIBRAF

24 hour renewal service via

www.citylibraries.info

or tel: 0303 123 0035

To renew please have ready:

- Your library card number
- Your PIN for online, automated and self -service transactions

FOOD CURES

Heal What Ails You with DELICIOUS SUPERFOODS!

Reader's Digest

New York | Montreal

READER'S DIGEST BOOK

Copyright © 2019 Trusted Media Brands, Inc.

The Library of Congress catalogued the previous edition as follows:

Food cures : breakthrough nutritional prescriptions for everything from
Colds to cancer / [editor, Marianne Wait].
       p. cm.
  Includes index.
  1. Nutrition—Popular works. 2. Diet therapy—Popular works.
    3. Medicine, Popular. I. Wait, Marianne, 1967–
    RA784.F62   2007
    615.8'54—dc22

      ISBN 978-1-62145-421-2 (ppb)
      ISBN 978-1-62145-422-9 (e-pub)

Food Photography: Rita Mass
Food Stylist: Anne Disrude
Additional photography courtesy of: BrandXPictures, BananaStock,
 Corbis, Getty Images, Image Source, Jupiter Images, PhotoAlto,
 Reader's Digest, Shutterstock, and Stockfood.

We are committed to both the quality of our products and the service we provide
to our customers. We value your comments, so please feel free to contact us.

    Reader's Digest Adult Trade Publishing
    44 South Broadway
    White Plains, NY 10601

For more Reader's Digest products and information, visit our website:
    www.rd.com (in the United States)
    www.readersdigest.ca (in Canada)

Printed in China

1 3 5 7 9 10 8 6 4 2

NOTE TO OUR READERS

The information in this book should not be substituted for, or used to alter, medical therapy without your doctor's advice. For a specific health problem, consult your physician for guidance.

Chief Consultants

Susan Allen, RD, CCN
Private Practice
Past Chair, American Dietetic Association's
Nutrition in Complementary Care Practice
Group

Mary M. Austin, MA, RD, CDE
Private Practice
Past President, American Association of
Diabetes Educators

William G. Christen, ScD, OD
Associate Professor in Medicine
Harvard Medical School

Karen Collins, MS, RD
Nutrition Advisor
American Institute for Cancer Research

Randy J. Horwitz, MD, PhD
Medical Director, Program in Integrative
Medicine
University of Arizona, Tucson

David L. Katz, MD, MPH
Associate Clinical Professor
Public Health and Medicine
Yale University School of Medicine

Ben Kligler, MD, MPH
Associate Professor of Medicine (Family
Medicine)
Albert Einstein College of Medicine
Research Director
Continuum Center for Health and Healing

Ashley Koff, RD
Private Practice

Victoria Maizes, MD
Executive Director
Program in Integrative Medicine
University of Arizona

Daniel Muller, MD, PhD
Associate Professor of Medicine
(Rheumatology)
University of Wisconsin-Madison

Jeri W. Nieves, PhD
Associate Professor of Clinical Epidemiology
Columbia University

David Perlmutter, MD
Board-Certified Neurologist
Private Practice

Rebecca Reeves, DrPH, RD
Assistant Professor of Medicine
Baylor College of Medicine

Steve L. Taylor, PhD
Professor and Director
Food Allergy Research & Resource Program
Department of Food Science & Technology
University of Nebraska-Lincoln

SPECIAL THANKS TO Eugene Arnold, MD;
Neil Barnard, MD; Scott Berliner, RPh;
Amy Brown, PhD, RD; Laura Coleman,
PhD, RD; Tanya Edwards, MD; Evan
Fleischman, ND; Marc Greenstein, DO; Jon
D. Kaiser, MD; Penny Kris-Etherton, PhD;
Jessica Leonard, MD; Alan Magaziner, DO;
Alexander Mauskop, MD; Eva Obarzanek,
PhD; Alexandra J. Richardson, PhD; Michael
Rosenbaum, MD, MSc; Roseanne Schnoll,
PhD, RD, CDN; Suzanne Steinbaum, DO;
Bonnie Taub-Dix, MS, RD; Mark Toomey,
PhD; Jan Zimmerman, MS, RD.

contents

PART
three

Food Cures for Common Conditions 86

PART
four

Healing Recipes 284

Food, Wonderful Food

For those who follow news from the world of medical research, the past few years have been filled with intriguing announcements. All kinds of breakthrough healing medicines have been "discovered"—but many of them aren't pills. Instead, they're oatmeal for heart disease, salmon for asthma, peanuts for high cholesterol, and yogurt for eczema. Forget about wonder drugs; we're living in a time of wonder foods.

Of course, the concept of food as medicine is many thousands of years old. Hippocrates, considered the father of medicine, prescribed a veritable pharmacy of edibles, from bread soaked in wine to boiled fish. Yet somehow, over the past century, this message got lost. Until recently, few doctors ever recommended a food as a potential solution to a health problem. So what has changed?

Primarily, we have become far smarter about the underlying causes of common diseases. Researchers have discovered, for instance, that arthritis isn't a simple case of wear and tear but rather a destructive process spurred by molecules called free radicals. This knowledge opened the door to the next discovery: that getting more leafy greens and orange and yellow produce, rich in antioxidants that neutralize free radicals, helps stave off this crippling condition. We've also learned more about the healing powers of specific foods. We now know that pumpkin seeds improve symptoms of an enlarged prostate, that regularly eating yogurt effectively suppresses the bacteria that cause most ulcers, and that cabbage helps the stomach lining heal.

What else has changed? The medical community is finally taking the research to heart. Doctors are talking about nutrition and food solutions to everyday ailments more often than ever before. And what outstanding news this is! Who wouldn't rather eat a piece of dark chocolate than swallow a high-cost, potentially dangerous pill? Best of all, in contrast to most prescription drugs today, most healthy foods provide multiple benefits to your body. Our message: Food can be a source of both pleasure and healing. So take a few minutes now and turn to one of the health problems that concerns you, then follow our food and supplement prescriptions. Even better, try some of the healing recipes that we've included—they're as delicious as they are healthy! You'll see for yourself the very real power of food as medicine.

The New Food Medicines

An apple a day can keep the doctor away—and now researchers finally know why. Welcome to the new world of food as medicine, where nature's bounty has the power to ease, erase, and abolish many of the nagging health problems and major killers of our day.

food medicir

There's a new frontier in medicine. Researchers at the forefront say the key to a longer, healthier life is an idea that's radical—some old-school doctors still don't seem to get it—yet simple: Food can help heal what ails you. That is, adding the right foods to your diet, while leaving others off the menu, can bolster your body's defenses against disease, treat disease directly, and even slow the aging process.

The tools of this discipline aren't scalpels and scanners but rather serving spoons and spatulas. Nevertheless, it's strong medicine. The studies are piling up fast, and they're impossible to ignore: Choose wisely in your grocer's produce section, the data shows, and you may spend less time in line at the pharmacy. Get to know your local fishmonger, and you may never meet a cardiologist. Start thinking about food in a novel way—as a form of therapeutic and preventive medicine—and you may need a lot less of the kind of medicine that gets itemized on insurance bills.

Maybe you already make occasional forays into this new frontier. Have you skipped the porterhouse steak and potato in favor of salmon and a green salad lately? Made breakfast toast with dense, chewy slices of whole-grain bread instead of the nutrient-challenged white variety? Snacked on a tangerine instead of a candy bar or finally switched to fat-free milk?

Taking simple measures such as these can have profound effects on your health and well-being—and not just because they spare your body from a lot of *un*healthy stuff, such as saturated fat and refined sugar, though that certainly is a good start. Exciting new studies have confirmed what some healers have believed for thousands of years: Many foods are packed with beneficial chemicals that can promote health and protect your body from the ravages of disease.

The idea of nutrition therapy goes all the way back to the beginning. "Let food be thy medicine and medicine be thy food," said Hippocrates, the ancient Greek who is widely regarded as the father of modern medicine. True to his word, Hippocrates prescribed a grocery list of edible cures, everything from bread soaked in wine to boiled fish. If those remedies don't exactly pique your appetite, don't worry. In the pages that follow, you'll learn about a cornucopia of foods that please the palate *and* contain remarkable medicinal qualities. Almonds and avocados. Strawberries and sweet potatoes. Fruity extra-virgin olive oil and delicacies from the sea.

You probably already know that these foods are good sources of vitamins, minerals, and nutrients. But you may not realize that fruits, vegetables, and other plant foods also contain thousands of newly discovered compounds, known as phytochemicals or phytonutrients, that scientists are still busy cataloging.

These chemicals provide flavor and color, yet cutting-edge research suggests that many of them are also important—some scientists say essential—to your health. For instance, a cup of green tea contains 30 to 40 different catechins, which are chemicals that fight cancer, lower cholesterol, and may even help you drop a few pounds.

In short, the foods described in these pages are nutritional powerhouses bursting with compounds that have specific and well-defined health benefits. They have another advantage: You won't find many reports in the medical literature of broccoli overdoses, and the only way a banana can hurt you is if you slip on the peel—which isn't something you can say about those medicines you store in a cabinet over the bathroom sink.

Rare is the medication that doesn't have at least some potential for problems. Can you spell "Vioxx"? Maybe so, but you can no longer find it at your pharmacy; manufacturers were forced to pull the once-popular prescription

> Many foods are packed with beneficial chemicals that promote health and protect your body from the ravages of disease.

painkiller and several similar drugs off the market due to concerns that they damage the cardiovascular system. Some studies suggest that over-the-counter pain relievers, such as ibuprofen, slightly increase the risk of heart attacks, too. In fact, a report by the Institute of Medicine estimated that at least 1.5 million Americans become ill or die each year due to errors in prescribing, dispensing, and taking medications.

Changing your diet won't guarantee that you'll never need drugs or get sick, of course. But according to the Harvard School of Public Health, if all Americans ate the right foods—and exercised regularly and avoided tobacco—the number of heart attacks in the United States would drop by about 82 percent. Strokes would diminish by roughly 70 percent. Type 2 diabetes would practically disappear, and colon cancer rates would decrease by 70 percent. This book will teach you the steps that can put you on the right side of those numbers.

Fat Gets a Facelift

The less fat you eat, the better—right? Not necessarily. Although fat was once the very face of dietary evil, recently it's gotten a major facelift of sorts. It's no wonder we equate "fat" with "bad." A half century

ago, scientists made a discovery that made us think hard, almost for the first time, about our food and our health: People who live in countries where the diets are rich in saturated fat have far more heart attacks than people who eat less meat, dairy foods, and other sources of the stuff. Later research showed that eating saturated fat raises blood levels of cholesterol, causing this waxy substance to build up in the arteries and block blood flow to the heart.

Fat eventually became nutrition enemy number one. Remember the old USDA Food Guide Pyramid? Fats and oils (which are simply liquid fat) were lumped together with sweets in the tiny uppermost wedge of the pyramid, accompanied by the stern recommendation: USE SPARING-LY. Cookbooks loaded with fat-free recipes filled bookstore shelves. "Nonfat!" and "Fat-Free!" were stamped on food labels, often on products that never contained fat in the first place. Doc-tors-turned-authors, such as Dean Ornish, M.D., preached the virtues of very low fat diets.

These messages may have convinced you to make some very good, important changes, such as switching from whole milk to fat-free and stripping bacon from your diet. But they also led consumers to make some unfortunate choices, and we're not just talking about those tofu dogs you bought a few years back. One consequence of the anti-fat movement was that many people cut back on *all* fats—a trend that may have actually made us sicker, according to some prominent experts.

"There was no benefit, and there was likely some harm," says Walter Willett, M.D., of the Harvard School of Public Health.

"Vitamin F"

Your body can store about 80 percent of the fat you consume. Ideally, you burn off most of this reserved energy by staying physically active. If not, the fat you eat becomes the fat you fear, the kind that makes your clothes too snug and imperils your health.

However, about 20 percent of the fat in your diet is not stored. Instead, your body puts it right to work, since an astonishing variety of tissues and biological processes require a daily infusion of fat. Without fat, your hair and skin would be dull and dry. More important, fat in the diet allows your body to absorb the so-called fat-soluble vitamins, including A, D, E, and K. Every cell in your body needs fat to build a healthy protective membrane. Fat also provides the raw materials that your body uses to produce chemicals that control blood pressure, prevent blood clots, and regulate the body's response to injury and infection. In fact, the stuff that gives many foods that familiar luscious texture is so important to hu-man health that scientists in the 1920s briefly called certain forms of fat "vitamin F."

If you crave fudge or filet mignon with béar-naise sauce, blame evolution. Our ancestors developed a taste for fat as a way to be sure of packing on extra pounds to survive in times when food was scarce. A gram of fat has twice as many calories as an equal amount of carbo-hydrate or protein. No wonder survival food rations are often laden with fat.

Of course, few of us need extra calories today. And it's still as important as ever to cut back on saturated fat—think beef, butter, and cheese—an inflammatory culprit behind heart disease and insulin resistance, the problem at the core of diabetes. But cutting out all the fat in your diet might not pay off as you'd expect. That's because experts have discovered that far from being deadly, daily doses of certain fats actually fight disease. Many scientists and nutrition experts now believe that these unsaturated fats—a.k.a. the "good" fats—inhibit everything from diabetes, depression, and dementia to cancer, joint pain, and yes, even heart disease.

Replacing some of the calories in your diet that come from saturated fat with calories from unsaturated fat (trading a hamburger for a salmon burger, for instance) may be even better for you than replacing them with carbohydrate calories. Studies show that swapping saturated fat in your diet for carbohydrate-rich foods, such as rice or pasta, has only a modest effect on heart disease risk. On the other hand, Harvard researchers studied the diets of 80,000 nurses for 14 years and determined that replacing just 5 percent of calories from saturated fat with an equal amount of good fat can reduce the risk of heart disease by 42 percent.

It's not just your heart that benefits from these fats, though. They also fight an impressive range of other diseases, as you'll read shortly. But first let's explain which fats we're talking about.

Defining Good Fats

As anyone who has ever struggled to lose weight knows, the body is very good at making its own fat, which it stores most prominently on the hips, thighs, and midsection. That's because even if you eat nothing but rice cakes and carrot sticks, but you eat too many of them, your body converts the sugars in those foods that it doesn't burn as energy into triglycerides, the storage form of fat.

However, your body can't make some types of fatty acids—the building blocks of fat—that

> Far from being deadly, daily doses of certain fats actually fight disease.

are essential to health. That's why your diet must include the aptly named essential fatty acids, which come primarily from fish and plant oils and fall into the broader category of polyunsaturated fats. Meanwhile, you can live without eating monounsaturated fats, which form the other major category of unsaturated fat—but mounting research suggests that you may not live as long or as well as people who enjoy these good fats.

Monounsaturated fats: Olive oil and beyond

You may have been surprised to learn a few years back that a bit player in your cupboard was in fact a nutritional marvel. Scientific trials, such as the Lyon Diet Heart Study, found that eating a so-called Mediterranean diet appears to protect the cardiovascular system more effectively than a typical low-fat one. The cornerstone of a traditional Mediterranean diet? It's olive oil, one of nature's richest sources of monounsaturated fat.

In fairness, some of the wonders of the olive may have been overhyped by the cooking oil industry. After all, the traditional Mediterranean diet also includes frequent servings of fruits and vegetables as well as plenty of fish. But it's hard to ignore the fact that people in the Lyon Diet Heart Study who ate a Mediterranean-type diet consumed plenty of fat, much of it in the form of monounsaturated fatty acids in olive oil, yet they had four times *fewer* heart attacks than people asked to eat a standard low-fat diet.

Olive oil isn't the only good source of monounsaturated fat that may already be in your kitchen. Its shelf mate, canola oil, is another. Nuts are packed with monos, too, so add peanut butter and peanut oil to the list. Need an excuse to eat avocados? The green flesh of these nubby-skinned fruits contains nearly as many grams of fat as a cheeseburger, but the fat is mostly monounsaturated.

Polyunsaturated fats: Go fish, go nuts

Remember the cod-liver oil of your grandparents' day? It used to be fashionable to joke about this favorite all-purpose remedy. But

Don't Spoil Your Oil

Olive oil and canola oil are excellent sources of healthy fats and antioxidants. But cooking oil is a fragile food that turns rancid and loses antioxidants in a hurry if it's not stored properly. Protect yours from these four influences to keep it fresh and nutritious.

Light: Oils spoil faster when kept in clear containers. Ceramic or tinted-glass bottles are better choices. A dark, dry cupboard is ideal for storing most cooking oils.

Heat: Make sure that cupboard isn't next to the stove. Storing oil in the refrigerator is another option if you live in a warm climate or don't plan to use it promptly. (Nut oils turn rancid quickly, so they must be refrigerated.) Some oils become thick and cloudy when chilled but reliquefy when raised to room temperature.

Air: Oxygen and oil don't mix, so make sure whatever container you choose has an airtight lid or cover.

Age: Even under the best conditions, cooking oils have a limited shelf life. Most taste best and retain more nutrients when used within one year of opening the original container.

now? Fish oil is the best source of omega-3 fatty acids, one of the two main types of polyunsaturated fat and probably the best-for-you fat around. In recent years, scientists have linked a boatload of new health benefits to consuming this form of fat, such as lower rates of heart disease and depression. (You'll read more about the benefits of omega-3s in a bit.)

You don't have to swallow cod-liver oil to get omega-3s, though. Eating seafood, especially cold-water fish, is your best option. The fat that protects all marine creatures from cold water, from arctic char to Atlantic salmon, is packed with omega-3s. Unlike with beef or pork, you want to go for the fattiest fish possible, such as salmon, since more oil means more healthful omega-3s. Albacore tuna is another good choice, as are Atlantic mackerel, lake trout, herring, and sardines. (But think twice before gulping cod-liver oil, even if you can stand the taste; the recommended doses may contain toxic levels of vitamins A and D.)

Fish-phobes, fear not: There are other ways to put these fats to work in your body. Fish-oil capsules are one option, though you should talk to your doctor before taking them because they can thin the blood. Walnuts, walnut oil, flaxseed, and flaxseed oil won't give you omega-3s exactly, but they do supply a type of fat called alpha-linolenic acid (ALA), which your body can turn into omega-3s.

Less famous than the omega-3s are their cousins, the omega-6s, the primary type of fat in corn, sunflower, or safflower oils. Soybean oil, which is used in a wide range of products, is another major source of omega-6s. Some experts state that omega-6s are inflammatory types of fat and should be limited in our diets.

In 2009, however, a Science Advisory Committee of the American Heart Association took a hard look at the evidence on omega-6s and found that higher intakes (at levels that provide 5 to 10 percent of our daily energy) are not only safe but may be beneficial to decrease our risk for heart disease.

By the way, all fats and oils contain a blend of saturated, monounsaturated, and polyunsaturated fatty acids, along with smaller amounts of other elements. But any given fat or oil tends to have a higher concentration of one type. For example, 68 percent of the fat in butter is saturated, while 29 percent is monounsaturated and a trace is the polyunsaturated variety. By contrast, just 14 percent of the fat in olive oil is saturated, while 75 percent is monounsaturated and 11 percent is polyunsaturated.

Better Fats, Better Health

Are you getting enough fat in your diet? Just a few years ago, the question would have sounded crazy, but many scientists and nutrition experts now believe that mono- and polyunsaturated fats have a critical role in any healthy eating plan. These versatile fats seem to offer a variety of benefits for the cardiovascular system; likewise, they fight an impressive range of diseases.

Fish, Not Defibrillators

Each year, about a third of a million people in the United States with no prior history of cardiovascular disease die of sudden cardiac death, which occurs when the heart starts beating erratically. To battle this problem, health officials are encouraging people to learn how to use defibrillators, which shock the heart back to steady rhythm. But one study determined that even if every home and public place (such as airports and restaurants) in a community had defibrillators, only about 1 percent of sudden cardiac deaths would be prevented.

By contrast, raising blood levels of omega-3 fatty acids within a population would avert *eight times* as many deaths, according to an analysis in the *American Journal of Preventive Medicine*. To get the necessary level of protection, people would need to take fish-oil supplements, the authors of this study say. However, one study of 20,000 men found that simply eating fish once a week slashes the risk of sudden cardiac death in half. Another study found that dining on fish just once or twice per month provides similar protection against strokes. The American Heart Association recommends eating several servings of fish each week.

It's not just the polyunsaturated fats in fish that protect the cardiovascular system. The good fats in nuts, most of which contain a healthy dose of both kinds of unsaturated fat (mono and poly), also offer this benefit. Scientists who pooled the results of 61 intervention trials reported in the

Anatomy of "Good" Fats

Chemical structure distinguishes good fats—the unsaturated ones—from saturated fats. The details get pretty technical but boil down to this: All fat molecules are made of carbon, hydrogen, and oxygen atoms. Saturated fats are full of hydrogen atoms, and monounsaturated fats are missing a pair, while polyunsaturated fats lack two or more pairs. These differences, among other chemical attributes, affect the appearance of a fat—and influence how it behaves inside your body. They're why saturated fats tend to be solid at room temperature, while unsaturated fats are easily converted to oils once they're liberated from the fish, nuts, seeds, and other foods they come from.

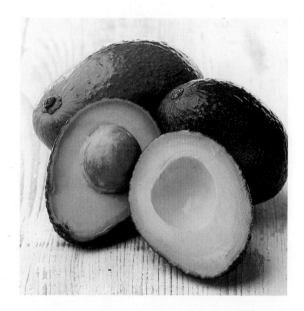

THE HEALING POWERS OF
nuts

Brazil nuts contain more selenium, an antioxidant trace mineral, than any other food.

Nuts are loaded with monounsaturated fats that benefit the heart, stabilize blood sugar, and help control your appetite.

Most nuts are significant sources of antioxidants.

An ounce of almonds has more fiber than a cup of strawberries.

Not a fish fan? Go nuts with walnuts, one of the best nonfish sources of omega-3 fatty acids.

Almonds are one of nature's best sources of vitamin E and are rich in calcium, too.

American Journal of Clinical Nutrition that each daily serving of tree nuts (walnuts, pistachios, macadamia nuts, pecans, cashews, almonds, hazelnuts, and Brazil nuts) significantly lowered total and LDL cholesterol levels as well as triglycerides in the blood. The fat in vegetable oil helps lower cholesterol, too. (The fat in fish has little effect on cholesterol, but it does lower levels of triglycerides, another blood fat linked to heart attacks, by up to 33 percent.)

Add Oil, Hold the Sugar

Eating more nuts, olive oil, and other foods rich in monounsaturated fats may also help safeguard you from the threat of type 2 diabetes. For starters, filling up on these good fats means you'll have less room for fatty meat, whole milk, and other sources of saturated fat, which contributes to insulin resistance—and high blood sugar. Left unchecked, chronically elevated blood sugar can cause type 2 diabetes—yet another reason why trimming the saturated fat from your meals is a no-brainer.

Exchanging saturated fat for monounsaturated and polyunsaturated fats appears to be a better approach to control blood sugars and keep cholesterol levels in check than exchanging it for carbs. That's according to the standards published in 2018 by the American Diabetes Association. To prevent and control diabetes, these experts recommend that saturated fats be decreased in the diet and replaced with unsaturated (polys and monos) fats, not with refined carbohydrates such as sugar and highly processed starches.

What's more, increasing your intake of monounsaturated fats appears to have other benefits you don't get from a high-carb diet, such as lowering levels of triglycerides. A study by Mexican researchers found that diabetes patients were able to lower their blood sugar while eating diets rich in olive oil and avocados. The study found that switching over to a high-carb diet worked, too. However, the patients' triglyceride levels dropped by 20 percent while eating the high-mono diet, compared to just 7 percent when they followed the high-carb meal plan.

Fighting Cancer, Mediterranean Style

The Lyon Diet Heart Study mentioned earlier showed the apparent cardiovascular benefits of

Inside Omega-3s: Alphabet Soup

The two major components of omega-3s are a mouthful to pronounce—docosahexaenoic acid and eicosapentaenoic acid—but you can call them DHA and EPA. You may have begun to notice these letters on products such as packages of eggs enriched with DHA. The FDA allows food manufacturers that add DHA or EPA to their products to state on labels that consuming these omega-3 fatty acids "may reduce the risk of coronary heart disease."

DHA, a fatty acid found in some eggs and in fish, may be one of the best nutrients for the brain.

the Mediterranean-style diet. But here's more good news: Those same study subjects, who ate plenty of fish and olive oil, cut their risk of cancer by 61 percent.

Although many questions remain about the link between diet and cancer, intriguing evidence suggests that healthy fats may protect against some forms of the disease. For example, studies in the 1990s showed that women who consume plenty of olive oil lower their risk of breast cancer by about 25 percent. More recently, a team of researchers at Northwestern University in Chicago discovered that oleic acid, the main form of monounsaturated fat in olive oil, reduces activity of a gene that causes an aggressive form of breast cancer by 46 percent. What's more, oleic acid appeared to increase the effectiveness of trastuzumab (Herceptin), a drug used to treat breast cancer. A second study found that fish oil may offer similar benefits.

Salmon, the Edible Antidepressant

If you ever travel to Iceland in the middle of January, don't count on seeing much of the sun: It rises at about 10 a.m. and disappears by 5 p.m. However, don't expect to find a bunch of gloomy natives, either. Icelanders have surprisingly low rates of seasonal affective disorder, the mood condition caused by low exposure to sunlight. Their secret to happiness? Some scientists think it's fish oil.

Consider this: The typical Icelander eats five times more seafood than do people in the United States or Canada. Several other studies have shown that rates of depression tend to be lower in countries where fish is frequently the main course. What's more, in 2011, the *Journal of Clinical Psychiatry* published a review and analysis of existing clinical trials and concluded that fish oils (EPA and DHA) were effective in the treatment of depression.

No one is certain why fish oil may help fight the blues, although DHA may affect the formation of chemicals linked to depression. While there's no guarantee that eating more salmon and tuna will make you happy-go-lucky, some scientists are studying whether having low levels of omega-3s contributes to depression. One scientific trial found that people with bipolar depression who added fish-oil supplements to their medication regimen had milder symptoms and fewer relapses than similar patients given placebo supplements.

> Diets high in monounsaturated fat control blood sugar just as effectively as the typical high-carb, low-fat diet many doctors recommend.

Feed Your Memories Well

Think of fish oil as brain food. The body uses its DHA to build and repair the membranes that protect brain cells. DHA also seems to be necessary for brain cells to communicate with one another. Eating plenty of fish may even lower your risk of dementia, the gradual loss of mental ability that sometimes accompanies aging. For example, researchers at Chicago's Rush-Presbyterian-St. Luke's Medical Center found that people who ate fish just once a week reduced their risk of Alzheimer's disease by 60 percent. The same research group also found that diets high in saturated fat and trans fats (the kind in hydrogenated cooking oil used by restaurants and food processors) seem to increase the risk of dementia. "What appears to be healthy for preventing cardiovascular disease also appears to be helpful for preventing Alzheimer's disease," says lead scientist Martha Clare Morris, Ph.D.

Scientists have also linked a deficiency of omega-3s to other cognitive problems, including attention deficit hyperactivity disorder, or ADHD. Blood tests show that children who struggle with the impulsivity, tantrums, and learning difficulties associated with this condition tend to have unusually low levels of DHA. Preliminary research hints that correcting that deficiency may help kids with ADHD settle down and focus. For example, one study by researchers at McLean Hospital near Boston showed that dietary supplements containing salmon oil and other fatty acids (as well as vitamins and plant nutrients) controlled ADHD symptoms as well as Ritalin, the widely prescribed stimulant drug.

Nature's Advil:
THE NEW SUPER-HEALERS

We've talked about the benefits of unsaturated fats, particularly the omega-3 fats in fish. But we haven't even touched on the biggest, most far-reaching benefits of omega-3s—and no doubt the most important

new breakthrough in our understanding of how our diets affect our health.

Here's a conundrum: About half of all heart attacks strike people who have normal cholesterol levels. Most cardiologists now agree that much of the "cholesterol gap" can be explained by a natural phenomenon gone awry: inflammation. In fact, inflammation has taken center stage as a major contributor to just about every chronic disease, from heart disease to diabetes to cancer. And fighting inflammation, as it turns out, is one of the jobs that omega-3s do best.

Inflammation plays a useful, even lifesaving role when it's acting as nature intended—to help an injury heal. Without it, a paper cut on your pinky finger could be fatal. That cut, or any other type of injury, from a scraped knee to a tongue burned by hot coffee, sets off a chain of events intended to limit the damage. First, the body increases blood flow to the injury site, delivering white blood cells that begin mopping up dead cells and bacteria, if any, to prevent infection. Other proteins arrive and seal off the area to stop germs and other harmful stuff from spreading to neighboring tissue. Inflamed skin feels warm to the touch because your body turns up the metabolic rate in the damaged tissue to speed the healing process. Even the pain and swelling that can accompany inflammation are beneficial, since the discomfort forces you to take it easy, which allows cells in the injured body part to repair and heal.

A scraped knee is one thing, but there's much more to inflammation than most of us—even

most experts—ever thought. Cardiologists now agree that inflammation triggers many heart attacks by causing artery-clogging plaques filled with cholesterol and other gunk to burst and form blood clots. In fact, studies show that having very high levels of inflammation-causing chemicals in the blood increases the risk of heart attack up to fourfold.

It's also increasingly clear that controlling inflammation with omega-3s can lower heart attack risk and also quiet the symptoms of some common conditions, such as rheumatoid arthritis. It may even offer protection against diseases as diverse and deadly as diabetes and cancer.

A Case of "Global Warming"

When inflammation is short-lived, it's not a problem. But thanks in part to our modern-day lifestyles, including the foods we favor and the extra weight that many of us carry, our bodies are living in a state of chronic inflammation—a sort of biological "global warming." To a growing number of scientists from many fields, this chronic inflammation is a silent scourge that causes premature aging and disease.

Intriguingly, scientific evidence is emerging to suggest that inflammation is the link between apparently unrelated diseases. For instance, a study at Weill Medical College at Cornell University found that people with rheumatoid arthritis have a threefold increase in their risk of developing early signs of heart disease. People with lupus and the inflammatory skin disease psoriasis have an unusually high risk for heart attacks, too.

Chronic inflammation is silent; you can't feel it the way you can feel a sore thumb. That doesn't mean it can hide, however. Inflammation leaves behind a trail in the form of a marker called C-reactive protein, or CRP, which can be measured with a simple blood test. Some doctors use the CRP test to decide how aggressively to treat patients who have other risk factors for heart attacks and strokes, such as high cholesterol and obesity.

Dousing the Flames with Fish Oil

If inflammation's so bad for you, you may wonder, why not control it by popping an ibuprofen tablet or two every day? Ibuprofen and other nonsteroidal anti-inflammatory drugs (NSAIDs), including aspirin, have a place in any medicine chest; nothing beats them for relieving an occasional headache or sore muscles after exercise. But using them too much can lead to gastrointestinal problems—and worse, in some cases. As you probably know, prescription drugs used to treat pain and inflammation, such as Vioxx, have been linked to heart trouble. However, according to recent studies, even over-the-counter NSAIDs such as ibuprofen may increase the risk of heart attacks, particularly in people who already have cardiovascular disease.

It's enough to make you padlock your pill box. Fortunately, you can help control inflammation and the destruction it can cause by eating more fish and other foods rich in omega-3 fatty acids, nature's own anti-inflammatories. Scientists first began to suspect there was something special about omega-3s when they noticed that heart disease is rare among people who eat a lot of seafood. And we do mean a lot—the original research involved Greenland Eskimos, who at the time survived largely on whale and seal meat.

> Inflammation has taken center stage as a major contributor to just about every chronic disease, from heart disease to diabetes to cancer.

However, scientists also discovered that these Eskimos rarely developed certain other diseases, including asthma, psoriasis, and rheumatoid arthritis. The common link? Out-of-control inflammation. Researchers eventually showed that omega-3 fatty acids appear to stifle inflammation in several ways. For one, they prevent the body from using other fatty acids needed to create prostaglandins and other hormone-like compounds that cause inflammation. They also block and reduce the number of hostile white blood cells the immune system dispatches to inflamed regions of the body. Consuming more omega-3s may be the key to quelling these and other common conditions.

Heart disease

An idea that seemed kooky not so long ago has gained wide acceptance. Doctors now believe that persistent low levels of inflammation create an unstable environment in the arteries, causing clumps of cholesterol and other gunk to burst open and form heart-stopping clots.

But cheer up: Help is as close as the fish counter or natural foods aisle at your supermarket. In one study, women who ate the most fish, flaxseed, and other foods rich in omega-3s had 29 percent less inflammation in their arteries (as indicated by levels of CRP) than women who consumed the least. Eating more fish appears not only to reduce inflammation but also to protect the heart in several other ways—by lowering levels of triglycerides and stabilizing heart rhythm, for example.

Cancer

Many oncologists now believe that excessive inflammation causes or speeds up the growth of many types of cancer. According to one theory, inflammation increases the rate at which cells "turn over," which raises the odds that defective cells will emerge in their place, leading to the out-of-control cell growth that produces malignant tumors. In some cases, persistent inflammation from common infections may increase cancer risk. For example, it's well known that some types of the human papillomavirus can cause cervical cancer, while stomach cancer primarily strikes people who have been infected with *Helicobacter pylori*, the bacteria that cause ulcers. Other sources of chronic inflammation have been linked to malignancies, too. People plagued by inflammatory bowel diseases, for example, have an unusually high risk of colon cancer.

Scientists are still studying whether dampening inflammation by consuming more omega-3 fatty acids prevents cancer, but some tantalizing clues have emerged. For instance, high doses of fish oil block colon tumors from forming in lab animals, apparently by cooling inflammation. What's more, eating fish three times a week halved the risk of prostate cancer in one study of nearly 48,000 males, while a Swedish study found that men who never ate seafood had double or triple the risk for the disease.

Asthma

Asthma rates are rising persistently, and some doctors believe our diets may be to blame. The wheezing and gasping brought on by an asthma attack occur because the bronchial tubes, which deliver air to the lungs, become inflamed. Inflammation causes the airways to narrow, which causes the asphyxiating symptoms. Recently, some scientists have speculated that a high intake of omega-6 fatty acids in many types of cooking oil along with a low intake of omega-3s may be the culprits. (Read more on these fats starting on page 27.) Many Americans consume large amounts of omega-6s and not enough omega-3s, which may allow the body to produce chemicals that cause inflammation.

Since omega-3 fatty acids reduce inflammation, consuming more fish oil may help prevent asthma attacks, at least in theory. Some evidence supports this idea. For example, an Australian study found that children who ate fish regularly cut their asthma risk by 75 percent. A study by Dutch researchers found a 50 percent reduction in asthma rates among children who had the highest intake of fish and whole grains.

Choosing Safe Seafood

In recent years, concerns about toxicity have threatened to sink fish's reputation as a healthy food. Seafood is one of nature's best sources of disease-fighting omega-3 fatty acids, but some varieties pack high levels of mercury and other toxins. Is eating fish really worth the risk?

Yes, say many leading health experts. In 2006, the *Journal of the American Medical Association (JAMA)* and the Institute of Medicine (which advises the federal government on health policy) published separate reports examining fish safety. The *JAMA* study determined that eating one or two servings of fish per week reduces the threat of a fatal heart attack by 36 percent and the overall risk of dying by 17 percent. The authors flatly state that "the benefits of fish intake exceed the potential risks."

In 2017, the US Food and Drug Administration and the Environmental Protection Agency endorsed the following levels of fish consumption for pregnant and breastfeeding women and young children:

- Eat two to three servings (approximately 8 to 12 ounces) a week of a variety of fish. Children younger than age 10 require smaller servings.
- Limit some fish to one serving a week. This includes albacore "white" tuna, halibut, snapper, bluefish, carp and mahi mahi/dolphinfish.
- Avoid fish known to be high in mercury such as shark, swordfish, tilefish from the Gulf of Mexico (tilefish from the Atlantic have low levels of mercury), marlin, orange roughy, and bigeye tuna.

For other adults and older children, the 2015-2020 Dietary Guidelines for Americans recommend at least 8 ounces of a variety of seafood each week.

Another guideline for selecting healthy seafood:

- Favor varieties with the highest concentration of omega-3 fatty acids. The top 10 are salmon, Atlantic herring, anchovies, mackerel, halibut, tuna, mussels, oysters, trout, and sardines.

Flax for Fish-Phobes?

If you want the benefits of omega-3 fatty acids and the convenience of a pill, fish-oil supplements may seem like the answer. But many people can't bear the side effects, which can include fishy-smelling breath, skin, and even urine. Freezing the capsules or switching brands may help, although another strategy might seem more appealing: taking flaxseed-oil supplements instead. After all, flax contains alpha-linolenic acid (ALA), which the body can convert to the two most important omega-3 fatty acids, EPA and DHA.

Unfortunately, this conversion isn't very efficient. It's thought that only a small percentage of the ALA you consume turns into EPA, and the amount that converts to DHA is even smaller.

While many studies suggest that fish-oil capsules can reduce the risk of heart attacks, the evidence to support using ALA supplements is far less convincing. However, flax oil is certainly better than nothing. One recent survey found that women who eat frequent servings of food that contains ALA cut their risk of sudden cardiac death by up to 40 percent. The American Heart Association recommends including plenty of ALA-rich foods, such as flaxseed and flaxseed oil, walnuts and walnut oil, canola oil, and tofu, in your diet.

Diabetes

Most people who develop type 2 diabetes are overweight. Fat cells produce chemicals that contribute to insulin resistance, the hallmark of the disease. They also churn out proteins that cause inflammation. Several large studies, which included more than 50,000 subjects combined, found that women with the highest levels of chronic inflammation had a fourfold increase in their risk of type 2 diabetes.

Scientists aren't sure why, but inflammatory chemicals may interfere with the work of insulin, causing blood sugar to rise. Perhaps it's no coincidence that population studies show that fish lovers have unusually low rates of type 2 diabetes.

Battling Autoimmune Diseases

Fish oil may also help relieve symptoms of some autoimmune disorders, such as rheumatoid arthritis. These are diseases in which the immune system mistakenly recognizes a perfectly healthy organ or other tissue, such as your thyroid or knee joints, as the enemy. In its confusion, it orders battalions of inflammatory chemicals to attack the healthy body part, leaving a wake of inflammation.

Autoimmune disorders include many common conditions, including type 1 diabetes (this occurs when the immune system mistakenly destroys insulin-producing beta cells in the pancreas) and thyroid disease. In lupus, the body attacks tendons, cartilage, and other connective tissue.

Consuming more omega-3 fatty acids won't necessarily prevent any of these diseases, but it may help relieve their symptoms in some cases. Think of eating fish for dinner or sprinkling flaxseed on your cereal as giving yourself a low dose of natural pain-relief medicine. Research into omega-3 fatty acids for treating autoimmune disorders has focused on fish-oil supplements, which appear to offer promise for treating two particular autoimmune conditions.

Rheumatoid arthritis

Since the 1990s, an impressive number of studies has shown that fish oil prevents and treats rheumatoid arthritis (RA). Unlike the more common osteoarthritis, RA occurs when the immune system attacks joints in the fingers, wrists, toes, and other parts of the body, causing them to swell, ache, and feel weak. Patients with RA often rely on medications such as aspirin, ibuprofen, and other NSAIDs to ease their pain and stiffness.

Just as eating fish cuts your odds of having a heart attack, it also makes you less likely to develop RA. In fact, a recent review in the journal *Arthritis Research and Therapy* looked at the evidence from seven studies to determine the association between fish consumption and the risk of RA. These experts determined that the risk for RA was 20 to 24 percent lower for people who ate one to three servings of fish per week.

> Think of eating fish for dinner or sprinkling flaxseed on your cereal as giving yourself a low dose of natural pain-relief medicine.

Several studies have also found that EPA and DHA (the omega-3s in fish) may help reduce morning stiffness, joint swelling and pain, even reducing the need for NSAID use in people with RA. The Arthritis Foundation recommends two 3-ounce servings of fish a week for general health. Therapeutic doses of fish-oil supplements may also be prescribed for arthritis-related conditions.

Inflammatory bowel disease

Persistent inflammation causes several common and maddening gastrointestinal conditions. These so-called inflammatory bowel diseases (IBDs) include Crohn's disease and ulcerative colitis. While Crohn's disease can produce inflammation anywhere in the GI tract, it usually strikes in the small intestine, resulting in abdominal pain, fever, diarrhea, and fatigue.

Ulcerative colitis affects the colon and rectum. It's painful, too, but also causes bloody diarrhea and urgent bowel movements; left untreated, long-term inflammation from colitis can increase the risk of colon cancer.

Some IBD patients require powerful anti-inflammatory medications called corticosteroids, which can prevent or treat flare-ups but may also cause unwanted side effects. While adding a few servings of fish to your weekly menu may not relieve these troublesome disorders, there is reason to believe that fish-oil supplements can help. In one study, Italian researchers asked a group of people with Crohn's disease who had gone into remission to take 2.7 grams of omega-3 fatty acids per day in the form of fish-oil capsules. A similar group of patients took placebo pills. After one year, the people taking high doses of omega-3s were twice as likely to still be in remission. A few other studies of fish oil and Crohn's disease offer hope, too, although overall, the results have been mixed.

The outlook is somewhat less clear for ulcerative colitis, but research hints that increasing your intake of omega-3 fatty acids may be worthwhile. In particular, studies suggest that people with moderate to severe colitis may be able to reduce their doses of corticosteroid medication if they supplement their diets with fish oil. A recent review from the *World Journal of Clinical Cases* concluded that almost all studies suggest a beneficial effect of omega-3s in the treatment of ulcerative colitis or Crohn's disease, although more studies are needed.

THE HEALING POWERS OF
fish

Fish oils have emerged again and again as effective treatments for health conditions involving inflammation.

Good fats are a main reason people who eat plenty of fish have unusually low rates of type 2 diabetes.

DHA, one type of omega-3 fatty acid, cuts the risk of Alzheimer's. EPA eases skin conditions.

Ounce for ounce, a salmon steak has one-fourth the saturated fat of beef steak.

Most fish contains about the same amount of protein as meat and provides iron and vitamin B_{12}, important for energy.

A Cool Diet:
MORE WAYS TO CHILL INFLAMMATION

You've started dreaming up new ways to cook salmon. When you toss a salad, you sprinkle on some chopped walnuts. You've even learned to love flaxseed. So far, so good, but adding omega-3 fatty acids to your

diet is just the first step you should take to turn down the heat in your body. To gain total control over the damaging effects of chronic inflammation, cutting back on or eliminating certain foods may be just as important.

Which foods spark flames? Relax—you don't have to give up *chiles rellenos* or any other tongue-searing dishes you may enjoy. The main inflammation inducers in most diets are less obvious—and more omnipresent. Some may be staples in your kitchen. Others you may not think much about unless you read the ingredient lists on labels. All coax your body's immune system into producing more inflammatory chemicals than it needs to defend itself, which could increase your risk of developing one of many debilitating chronic illnesses.

If the thought of avoiding certain foods leaves you feeling deprived, don't worry. In some cases, the inflammation-inducing culprits described below have healthful counterparts that will fit nicely into your diet. In other instances, food processors have begun to replace such ingredients with safer alternatives.

Time for an Oil Change?

Omega-3 fatty acids may be nutritional superstars, but some nutritionists take a dimmer view of their fellow polyunsaturated fats—the omega-6 fatty acids, prominent in corn oil, sunflower oil, and safflower oil. However, they're not all bad by any means. After all, omega-6s aren't considered "essential" for

nothing—your body needs them for normal development and a strong immune system, among other roles. However, few of us need to worry about getting enough omega-6s, since deficiency of these fats is practically unheard of. Instead, some scientists say, our bodies suffer from an oversupply.

Consider this: Our cave-dwelling ancestors consumed a diet that included roughly equal amounts of omega-3 and omega-6 fatty acids. Today, the typical American consumes at least 10 times more omega-6s than omega-3s. Some experts, including Artemis Simopoulos, M.D., author of *The Omega Diet*, believe the ratio is even higher. "Our genes haven't changed in 10,000 years," says Dr. Simopoulos. "If you're on the standard American diet, we know you're not getting enough omega-3s. And we also know that you're getting an enormous amount of omega-6 fatty acids."

In fairness, some nutrition experts don't believe that the ratio of essential fatty acids we consume is making us sick. Says Harvard's Dr. Walter Willett, "It's amazing how strong that myth seems to have become. There's really no human evidence to support it and quite a bit to suggest that it's not true. The ratio is really irrelevant." For instance, population studies indicate that people who replace saturated fat with either monounsaturated or polyunsaturated fat (which includes omega-6s) reduce their risk of heart disease, he notes.

However, other nutritionists feel that cutting back on our high intake of omega-6s may be as important as increasing our woefully low consumption of omega-3s. The imbalance creates problems, explains Dr. Simopoulos, because the human body processes both of these fats with the same enzymes. When omega-6s outnumber omega-3s, there are fewer enzymes around to process omega-3s, robbing the body of an inflammation fighter. Not all experts agree with this theory, however. As mentioned previously, a committee of experts were commissioned by the American Heart Association in 2009 to review the evidence on the relationship between omega-6 polyunsaturated fatty acids and the risk of heart disease. In an extensive Science Advisory paper published in *Circulation,* they outline a large body of evidence that including up to 10 percent of our daily calories from omega-6s *reduces* the risk of coronary heart disease.

The debate is still not over, however. Dr. Simopoulos published a paper in 2016 that suggests a higher risk for obesity when the diet is higher in omega-6s than omega-3s.

As conflicting as it seems, no one argues that omega-3s are potent anti-inflammatory agents. That means olive, canola, peanut, and flaxseed oils are excellent staples for your everyday cooking.

What we've learned in 50 years, says Dr. Willett, is the importance of replacing saturated fat with polyunsaturated fat.

Trans Fats: "Metabolic Poison"

If there's still debate over corn oil, there is no argument among scientists over the threat posed by another form of cooking oil: hydrogenated oil, which is simply vegetable oil with added hydrogen. This molecular tweaking gives cooking oil a longer shelf life and other properties that make it ideal for use in packaged goods and fast foods. Unfortunately, hydrogenation also produces sinister compounds called trans fatty acids, which raise levels of LDL cholesterol and also seem to lower levels of HDL cholesterol. Gram for gram, trans fats increase the risk of heart disease more than any other food ingredient, according to a review in the

New England Journal of Medicine. No wonder Dr. Willett calls them metabolic poison.

Scientists now know that along with wreaking havoc on cholesterol, these fats increase the risk of a number of other diseases, including Alzheimer's, type 2 diabetes, and gallstones. Eating trans fats may even cause greater weight gain than eating other fats, according to a review of several studies published in the *International Journal of Obesity.*

One reason trans fats have such far-reaching effects on the body appears to be that they ignite inflammation. It's not clear why, but studies consistently show that eating foods that contain trans fats causes levels of inflammatory chemicals to soar. In one study, women who consumed the most foods containing trans fats had 73 percent more inflammation, as indicated by levels of CRP, than women who ate the least. So convincing is the evidence against trans fats that in 2015, the US Food and Drug Administration determined that partially hydrogenated oils—the major source of trans fats in our food supply were no longer "Generally Recognized as Safe." It then published regulations requiring manufacturers to remove them from processed foods. This, says the FDA, could prevent thousands of heart attacks and deaths each year.

You won't find many products manufactured after June 2018 with partially hydrogenated oils. Some may still be making their way through the marketplace until 2020, however. Until then, always check the ingredient list and Nutrition Facts label, especially on products like cookies, chips, and other snack foods that we should be avoiding anyway, right? Your goal is no "partially hydrogenated oils" and zero trans fats (the label must tell you if these are present).

Fighting Inflammation

Along with reconsidering which cooking oil you use and steering clear of trans fats, you can snuff out inflammation even further by adhering to some familiar advice. People who keep their weight down, avoid saturated fat, and

> Gram for gram, trans fats increase the risk of heart disease more than any other food ingredient.

eat plenty of fruits and vegetables live longer for many reasons. Additionally, choosing your carbohydrates wisely seems to help, too.

Watch Your Weight

Scientists now know that fat cells do more than simply add flab to your hips and thighs. They constantly churn out proteins that affect your health, including several that promote inflammation. One study of 16,000 adults found that obese males were twice as likely to have elevated levels of inflammation compared to normal-size men. Obese women were six times more likely than slender women to have high CRP levels. Many scientists now believe that inflammation is a key reason people who struggle with weight suffer disproportionately from heart disease and diabetes.

Fortunately, shedding pounds appears to lower inflammation. In one 2006 study, for example, women who lost an average of 13 pounds lowered their CRP levels by an impressive 41 percent.

Go Easy on Hamburgers

A study involving 2,500 men and women found that a high consumption (more than about 10 ounces a week) of red meat was significantly associated with an unhealthy level of CRP, a marker for inflammation. Interestingly, this study also found that higher levels of whole-grain bread had the opposite effect— lower CRP levels at higher intakes.

No need to give up meat entirely, however. Changes in feeding practices over the past few decades have resulted in leaner, healthier choices compared to the fat-ridden cuts of the past. In fact, less than half the fat in today's beef is saturated and a third of that is stearic acid—a unique saturated fat shown to have a neutral effect on blood cholesterol levels.

To avoid the health-robbing effects of grease-laden meats (high amounts of saturated fat can pack on inflammation-producing fat around your midsection), choose small portions of lean cuts such as sirloin or eye of round. These skinnier cuts contain more anti-inflammatory monounsaturated fats than saturated fat, according to the USDA National Nutrient Database.

If you need to lose a few pounds, chalk up yet another reason to eat more fish and flax: Several

Where Are Trans Fats Now?

The main source of trans fats is partially hydrogenated oils used in a variety of processed foods. Because of the strong evidence that trans fats contribute to thousands of heart attacks and deaths a year, the US Food and Drug Administration ordered manufacturers to stop using partially hydrogenated oils after June 2018.

Until they work their way through the marketplace, however, some foods may still contain trans fats until 2020, says the FDA. If a product contains trans fat, food producers are required to declare it, so check the label, especially on these processed foods:

- Cake, pie, and cookie mixes
- Frosting
- Frozen and canned biscuits
- Stick margarine
- Packaged doughnuts and sweet rolls
- Crackers
- Breaded frozen fish and chicken
- Microwave popcorn
- Frozen pizza

THE HEALING POWERS OF
vegetables

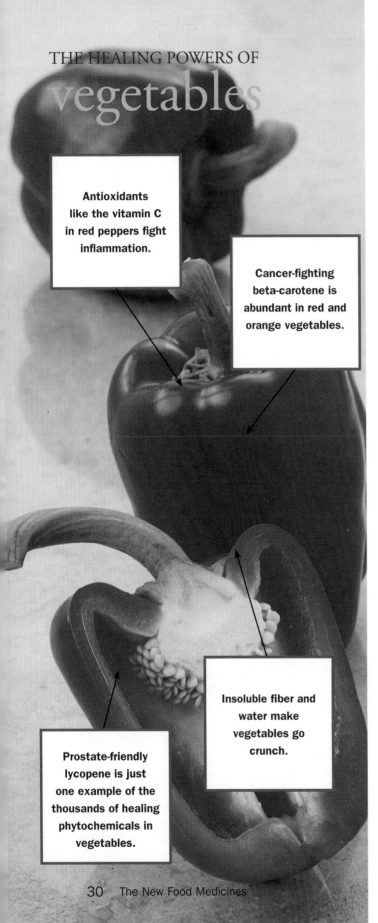

Antioxidants like the vitamin C in red peppers fight inflammation.

Cancer-fighting beta-carotene is abundant in red and orange vegetables.

Insoluble fiber and water make vegetables go crunch.

Prostate-friendly lycopene is just one example of the thousands of healing phytochemicals in vegetables.

studies show that circulating levels of chemicals that promote inflammation drop when over-weight people consume omega-3 fatty acids.

Listen to Mom

Your mother was right when she told you to eat your vegetables. Could adding carrots to a meal help dampen chronic inflammation? You bet.

Here's why: Produce is nature's most abundant source of antioxidants. As you'll learn later, these disease fighters neutralize the effects of naturally occurring molecules known as free radicals that attack and damage healthy cells. The body responds to this damage as it would to any injury: by producing inflammation. When fewer antioxidants are available to protect cells, that can mean more inflammation. A British study showed, for example, that men who consumed the least vitamin C had twice as much CRP in their blood as men who got plenty of this potent antioxidant.

The good news: In the first study of its kind, German researchers showed that men who increased their intake of fruit and vegetables from two servings a day to eight cut their CRP levels by one-third in just four weeks. Most of the inflammation-fighting punch came from fruit and vegetables rich in antioxidants called carotenoids, which include carrots, as well as tomatoes and red bell peppers.

By the way, Mom was also right when she told you to brush your teeth. No matter what or how much you eat, be sure to brush after meals and floss regularly. Gum disease increases inflammation throughout the body and seems to raise the risk of heart disease and diabetes.

Choose Your Carbs Carefully

In the pages to come, you'll learn what scientists have discovered in recent years about the complex—and controversial—role of carbohydrates in a healthy diet. For now, let's just say that in order to turn down the inflammation in your body, you may need to rethink your daily bread, among other carb choices.

Carbohydrates make up a vast and varied category of foods; some quell inflammation, while others make it worse. Learning to choose cooling carbs is easy once you get the hang of a few simple concepts that follow.

Smart Carbs:
FOODS FOR FIGHTING FLAB AND INSULIN RESISTANCE

Sometimes it seems like the carbohydrate story has taken more twists than a French braid. A generation ago, doctors concerned about rising rates of heart disease began advising patients to eat less fat—and more

carbohydrates. Waistlines bulged, and an epidemic of type 2 diabetes broke out.

Coincidence? Authors of the many low-carbohydrate diet books published in the 1990s didn't think so. These books blamed flabby thighs and bulging hips on carbohydrates, vilifying starches and sugars much the way many doctors demonized fat years earlier. Bad news about carbohydrates also began to turn up elsewhere in the library: namely in medical journals, as studies uncovered unusually high rates of diabetes, heart disease, and other conditions in people who eat carb-heavy diets.

The plot thickens, though, since carbohydrates are making a comeback—some carbs, that is. Thanks to important new research published in the past few years, it's now clear that carbohydrates share something in common with fats: Some are essential to a healthy diet, while others should be regarded as occasional treats.

Bashing *all* carbohydrates never made a lot of sense, given how many different varieties there are and how essential carbs are to human health. After all, soda pop and Skittles may be sources of carbohydrates, but so are snap peas and summer squash. What's more, carbohydrates provide ready fuel for your body, and they're the best source of energy for your brain cells.

Research shows that improving the quality of the carbs you eat can reap major benefits, and all it takes is making some simple exchanges on your daily menu. For instance, healthy vol-

unteers in one study who swapped white rice for brown rice experienced a 12 percent lower rise in blood sugars after eating the brown rice. In the same study, volunteers with diabetes who ate brown rice instead of white rice had a 35 percent lower rise in blood sugar! What's more, other research shows that you can dramatically slash your risk of heart disease and control your weight, too, if you learn to play your carbs right.

Quality Control: Choosing Better Carbs

Most doctors now agree that eating the wrong kinds of carbohydrates has helped to make Americans sicker and fatter. Extremely low-carb diets (a.k.a. high-protein diets) are the professed answer, at least according to the authors of some bestselling books. But these diets typically recommend a dramatic reduction in all carbohydrates—including healthful fruits, vegetables, and grains—especially in the early stages. And they can be loaded with saturated fat, which promotes inflammatory conditions like diabetes and cancer. In reality, kicking "good" carbs off your plate strips your diet of powerful disease fighters.

The Unrefined Truth about Whole Grains

When it comes to carb foods, white bread, sugary breakfast cereal, and other foods made from sugar and white flour remain the popular choices today. But overwhelming scientific evidence suggests that it's far healthier to go with the grain—the whole grain, that is.

Consider the irony: In the 17th century, milling techniques became sophisticated enough to turn coarse whole grains into the fine white flour needed to bake white bread, which became a coveted luxury. Dark bread became "peasant food." Little did the rich realize they were paying more for imperfection.

The milling and sifting needed to remove the bran (the outer layer) and germ (the portion that sprouts new plants) from whole grains also strip away nutrients, including B vitamins, trace minerals, and protein. Today food processors restore some lost vitamins and minerals, but not all. For instance, whole-grain bread (but not white bread) is a good source of magnesium, which your body needs to form enzymes that help burn glucose as energy. People with type 2 diabetes tend to have low levels of this important mineral.

Refining grains has another major downside: It removes a great deal of fiber. Whole grains are just one source of fiber, but most people don't eat anywhere close to the 20 to 35 grams of fiber per day that experts recommend. As you'll learn next, there have never been more reasons to fiber up.

Fiber: Nature's Secret Non-Nutrient

Technically, fiber is not a nutrient since it doesn't dissolve in the digestive tract and never enters the bloodstream. But it's still indispensable, and we're not just talking about its ability to promote "regularity." Insoluble fiber (the rough stuff in whole-wheat bread and broccoli) acts like a sponge by mopping up water in the intestines, which helps make stools bulky and soft. Soluble fiber turns into a sticky gel in your intestines. This gel pulls cholesterol along with it as it moves through the body, preventing cholesterol from entering the bloodstream and clogging arteries. The gel also removes bile acid, a digestive juice that's made from cholesterol. If you've ever wondered how humdrum oat bran

> Most doctors now agree that eating the wrong kinds of carbohydrates has helped to make Americans sicker and fatter.

became so fashionable, here's your answer: It's a soluble-fiber powerhouse. Other good sources include peas and dried beans, barley, apples, oranges, and carrots.

Fiber has another benefit that makes it a valuable disease fighter: It passes slowly from the stomach into the intestines. That makes fiber a must if you're trying to lose weight, since it makes you feel full longer. It also means that most high-fiber meals enter the bloodstream gradually. This is one instance where inefficiency is a good thing, since the sugars and starches that are part of your meal convert to glucose slowly, without overwhelming your body's capacity to store carbs as fuel and raising your blood sugar.

The Carbo-Rater: Using the Glycemic Index

One of the keys to choosing the best carbohydrates is knowing which ones raise blood sugar rapidly and which ones break down slowly. Avoiding the "fast-acting" carbs can help prevent diabetes and other devastating diseases. The reason: Chronically elevated blood sugar can damage organs and tissue throughout the body, leading to an alarming variety of health problems.

To identify how different carbohydrates affect blood sugar levels, researchers at the University of Toronto devised the glycemic index (GI) in the early 1980s. In 2008, the glycemic index for some foods was revised based on new data from current research studies. The GI is determined by measuring the effect of a food on an individual's blood sugar levels. Volunteers are fed whatever serving size of the food equals 50 grams of carbohydrate—to compare it against the effects of 50 grams of pure glucose—and then their blood sugar is measured two hours later. Glucose is assigned a GI value of 100. Jellybeans produce a rise in blood sugar that is 78 percent as high as the increase glucose produces. Jellybeans, then, have a GI value of 78. So does a boiled potato. The closer to 100 a food is ranked, the more it increases blood sugar. As a rule, a GI value of

bread

Coarsely ground breads with kernels and seeds digest the slowest.

The bran and germ are the most nutritious parts of the grain—and the parts that are stripped out in making white flour.

Magnesium relaxes arteries, and B vitamins such as folate lower homocysteine, which is linked with heart disease.

Cereal fibers like those in whole-grain bread actually lower the risk of diabetes and even the risk of breast cancer.

Buyer beware! Most "wheat breads" are simply white bread. Look for the word *whole* in the first ingredient.

55 or less is considered low, 56 to 69 is moderate, and 70 or more is high. That doesn't mean you can never eat another waffle (76) or bowl of white rice (72). But choosing lower-GI alternatives most of the time could help keep your blood sugar under control.

Critics have charged that the GI is too difficult for the average person to use, since most meals include not only carbohydrates but also fat and protein, which tend to blunt the rise of blood sugar. In other words, skeptics insist, you can look up the GI of a baked potato, but that number becomes irrelevant if you eat it with a steak or top the spud with butter and sour cream. However, in one recent study, researchers asked volunteers to eat 14 different typical meals (such as bagels and cream cheese with orange juice, for example), then measured the change in their blood sugar levels. They found that the GIs of the foods in each meal were about 90 percent accurate in predicting how much the volunteers' blood sugar levels changed, according to a study in the *American Journal of Clinical Nutrition*.

Some scientists and nutritionists prefer to use a fine-tuned version of the glycemic index known as the glycemic load (GL), which takes into account the amount of carbohydrate in a *typical* serving of the food instead of however much you'd need to eat to get to 50 grams. The GL turns some seemingly "unhealthy" foods (according to the GI) "healthy" again. Carrots, for example, have a high GI (71) but you'd have to eat about 1 1/2 pounds to get 50 grams of carbohydrate used to calculate the GI. A typical serving of carrots (about 1/2 cup) has a low glycemic load. So, say experts, unless you're going to eat a pound and a half of carrots at a time, you don't have to worry about them spiking your blood sugars.

Using either the GI or the GL may help prevent blood sugar spikes and reduce your risk of type 2 diabetes and other conditions, studies show. But if keeping track of all those numbers makes you dizzy, following a few simple rules can also keep your blood sugar in shape.

DON'T WORRY ABOUT FRUITS AND VEGETABLES (WITH A FEW EXCEPTIONS). Most produce contains only modest amounts of carbohydrate per serving. What's more, much of the sugar in fruit is fructose, a form that doesn't cause blood sugar to rise.

EAT SMALLER PORTIONS OF ROOT VEGETABLES. Here's the major exception to the first rule: Go easy on the potatoes, parsnips, and other starchy root vegetables. Starch is made from long chains of glucose, so it can cause a rapid rise in blood sugar levels if you eat large amounts. These exceptions have their own exceptions, however: Carrots, as mentioned previously, have minimal effects on blood sugars. And sweet potatoes are a good source of soluble fiber, which lowers their GI. (See "Eat more fiber" below).

CHOOSE YOUR OTHER STARCHES WISELY. Face it, you're not going to give up bread, but you can select better varieties. Most white bread, for instance, has a high GI (an exception is sourdough, which has a high acid content and slows digestion). Look for hearty-looking whole-grain breads, not whole-wheat breads that essentially look like white bread (see "Whole Grain Doesn't Always Mean Low GI" on the opposite page). If you're choosing between rice and pasta, take the latter; its starch breaks down more gradually.

EAT MORE FIBER. Especially look for soluble fiber, which causes blood sugar to rise gradually by slowing digestion. That's why oats, barley, apples and some berries, and legumes tend to have low GI values.

AVOID SUGARY FOODS. The truth is, many types of soft drinks and candy have only a moderately high GI value, not the sky-high one you'd expect, since sugar digests more slowly than pure glucose. But this is one form of moderation you can do without, since sugary foods provide empty calories and little else.

"Good" Carbs, Better Health

The science is unambiguous: Choosing better carbs not only crowds out empty-calorie, glucose-raising foods but also helps battle many of today's leading health threats. Here's what eating more high-fiber, low-GI foods will do for you.

Lower your risk of diabetes

The so-called diabetes epidemic has made headlines, and for good reason. The number of cases of type 2 diabetes (the most common type) is exploding, and many more people are in line for developing the disease. At the core is a condition called insulin resistance. Most people don't know they have it—or that the "wrong" kinds of carbs contribute to it.

Insulin resistance occurs when the body stops responding to this critical hormone. Think of insulin as a kind of doorman. Normally, it triggers a reaction that allows glucose to pass through cell walls, where it is burned to produce energy or stored for later use. In some people, however, cells start to ignore insulin, which means the pancreas must manufacture more of it. Insulin resistance is "silent" because often the pancreas can keep up with demand by working overtime. Eventually, however, it may fail to keep up, resulting in type 2 diabetes.

Your genes, excess body fat, and lack of exercise cause insulin resistance, but eating the wrong kinds of carbohydrates seems to worsen the problem. In one study, British researchers asked a group of nondiabetic women to eat a high-GI diet for three weeks, while a second group ate low-GI foods. An analysis of their fat cells detected more insulin resistance in the women who ate the high-GI diet. It's hardly surprising, then, that several large population studies have shown that people who eat diets filled with low-fiber, high-GI carbohydrates appear to double their risk of type 2 diabetes.

The good news: You can reverse the threat of diabetes by up to 42 percent simply by trading in your white bread, white rice, and sugary breakfast cereal for hearty dark loaves, brown rice, and oatmeal, according to a Harvard study of nearly 43,000 men.

Lower your risk of heart disease

Eating more whole grains could also lower your risk of heart attacks—by up to 29 percent, according to James W. Anderson, M.D., the University of Kentucky nutritionist whose research helped make oat bran a nutritional superstar in the 1980s. Dr. Anderson chalked up the benefits to oats' soluble fiber, which lowers cholesterol. But there's more going on than that.

Whole Grain Doesn't Always Mean Low GI

There's no doubt that whole grains are good for us. But just because a whole-grain food like whole-wheat bread has a lot of fiber doesn't necessarily mean it has a low GI. The grains used may have been ground into fine flour, which, like white flour, is digested quickly. Whole-wheat bread is still a good choice, but you can make it even better by choosing coarse breads that have intact grains. (These breads may be labeled with phrases such as "stone ground.") Or you can opt for oat bread and hot oatmeal over whole-wheat bread and breakfast cereal to eliminate this concern. Oats contain soluble fiber, which slows digestion, resulting in a modest increase in blood sugar. You can also simply consult the glycemic index (www.glycemicindex.com) and the 2008 revised list of GI foods to determine if a whole-grain food makes the grade.

Will More Protein Make You Lean?

As you rethink the kinds of carbohydrates you consume, you may also want to consider cutting back on sugars and starches altogether—and replacing them with protein. A growing body of research suggests that eating more protein, in the form of lean meat, poultry, seafood, eggs, and low-fat dairy foods, can safely promote weight loss and reduce your risk of heart disease.

For example, one 1999 study found that overweight men and women who followed a high-protein diet for six months lost about 8 pounds more, on average, than members of a similar group who ate a high-carbohydrate diet. One of protein's key benefits: It leaves you feeling full and satisfied longer than carbohydrates do, so you eat less. In fact, research shows that a high-protein meal helps curb appetite for up to a day. Most high-protein foods have low GIs, and they slow digestion, which reduces the overall effect a meal has on blood sugar and insulin.

Other studies suggest that you can shed pounds on any low-calorie diet, whether it's a high-carbohydrate or high-protein plan, and that most diets produce equal weight loss after a year or so. Yet high-protein diets may offer the fastest path to slimmer thighs and a taut belly, since they appear to burn flab more efficiently. Some trials comparing the two approaches show that high-protein diets produce up to 50 percent greater loss of stored fat. Increasing protein intake may also lower levels of dangerous blood fats called triglycerides.

Some doctors fear that consuming too much protein may damage kidneys and weaken bones. Recent diet studies don't support those concerns, though most have lasted only three to six months.

(In fact, one analysis published in the *American Journal of Clinical Nutrition* estimated that you'd have to eat three bowls of oatmeal a day to lower total cholesterol by only about 2 percent.)

Eating whole-grain carbs like oatmeal and whole-wheat pasta also keeps blood sugar levels in check, and there's little question that persistently high blood sugar increases the threat of heart attacks, perhaps by raising levels of destructive compounds called free radicals. These compounds "oxidize" cholesterol particles, making them more dangerous to your arteries. (You'll read more later about free radicals and how you can squelch them with the right foods.) People with prediabetes (high blood sugars that have not yet advanced to diabetes) are more likely to develop diabetes within 10 years and they are more likely to have a heart attack or stroke, according to the American Heart Association. And adults with diabetes are nearly twice as likely to die from heart disease or stroke as people without diabetes, says the National Institute of Diabetes and Digestive and Kidney Diseases (NIDDK).

Glucose begins to build up in the blood as insulin resistance worsens. No one is sure why, but people who have insulin resistance also tend to have high blood pressure, elevated triglycerides (a type of blood fat linked to cardiovascular disease), and low levels of heart-friendly HDL cholesterol—a recipe for disaster. This cluster of problems, along with obesity, comes together in insulin resistance syndrome, also known as metabolic syndrome.

Again, the right diet—and the right carbs—can help. A recent study on Japanese men found that those who were placed on a diet that included whole-grain bread lost visceral fat—the dangerous type of fat around the midsection that is part of the metabolic syndrome—while the men who ate white bread did not. Less visceral fat means less inflammation, another benefit of high quality carbs, as you'll see next.

Curb Inflammation

When cholesterol assaults artery walls, the immune system responds the way it does to any injury—with inflammation. Choosing carbs rich in soluble fiber may help put the chill on that process by clearing out some of that cholesterol.

You can cool inflammation by filling up your menu with both types of fiber—soluble and insoluble—according to a recent study at the University of Massachusetts Medical School. The researchers followed a group of more than 500 people for a little over a year, measuring their blood periodically for levels of CRP (the marker of inflammation we've mentioned before). They also asked the subjects to describe their diets. People who ate the most fiber—more than 20 grams per day, which is the minimum amount most experts recommend—had 63 percent less inflammation than others who ate low-fiber diets.

Help you lose weight

Can eating bran cereal and brown rice lead to slimmer hips and thighs? Population studies have shown that people who get most of their carbs from the low end of the GI tend to weigh less than others who gravitate toward more sugary or starchy foods. One reason appears to be that meals that include low-GI foods keep you full longer (probably by slowing digestion), which helps curb appetite later in the day.

A study that involved overweight adults from eight European countries found that those who ate a lower GI diet that was modestly high in protein lost weight and maintained it better than participants who followed a high-GI diet that was lower in protein. Interestingly, both diets contained the same amount of fat.

Additionally, the low-GI and higher-protein groups in this study were more likely to lose more than 5 percent of their body weight than were the high-GI groups. If a 5 percent weight loss doesn't sound like much, consider this: If you're overweight and have even a hint of insulin resistance, that modest amount of slimming can reduce your risk of diabetes by 58 percent.

For some reason, low-GI diets seem to be particularly effective in women. Compared with female subjects who ate a typical high-carb, low-fat diet, women who filled up on low-GI foods lost 80 percent more body fat. They retained more muscle, too. The high-carb, low-GI plan had a bonus: Not only did dieters who adopted this menu keep the pounds off, but their LDL cholesterol dropped, too.

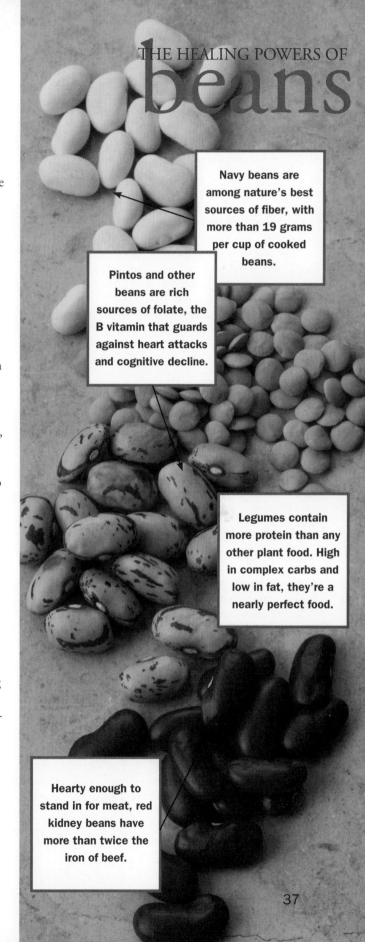

THE HEALING POWERS OF
beans

Navy beans are among nature's best sources of fiber, with more than 19 grams per cup of cooked beans.

Pintos and other beans are rich sources of folate, the B vitamin that guards against heart attacks and cognitive decline.

Legumes contain more protein than any other plant food. High in complex carbs and low in fat, they're a nearly perfect food.

Hearty enough to stand in for meat, red kidney beans have more than twice the iron of beef.

The *New* Antioxidant Revolution

A glass of orange juice. A side dish of steamed broccoli. Corn on the cob. All of these are simple pleasures that you may enjoy now and then without even realizing that these and other common foods and

beverages are brimming with antioxidants, which are critical disease fighters.

Remember antioxidants? Back in the 1990s, pills packed with these vitamins, minerals, and other natural compounds were touted as medical wonders. Many books, including bestsellers such as *Dr. Kenneth H. Cooper's Antioxidant Revolution* and *The Antioxidant Miracle*, insisted that antioxidant supplements could dramatically slash the risk of heart attacks and cancer and even slow the aging process.

Fast-forward to today: Mounting research suggests that the preventive and healing powers of antioxidants may extend beyond heart disease and cancer to include a wide range of chronic, painful, and potentially devastating conditions. For example, doctors once believed that daily wear and tear on the joints caused osteoarthritis, the most common type of this degenerative condition. However, recent studies show that damage by free radicals—the villainous molecules antioxidants were born to battle—may speed up the onset of osteoarthritis by attacking the cells that form cartilage. Studies also show that certain antioxidant compounds can slash the risk of cataracts and macular degeneration.

What has changed since the first "antioxidant revolution"—besides our knowledge that antioxidants are even more important than we thought—is that high-dose antioxidant supplements *aren't* the answer anymore. The answer is food.

In Sync: Antioxidants Work Better Together

There's no doubt about it: Many studies show that people who eat plenty of antioxidant-rich foods seem to lower their risk of heart attacks, cancer, and various chronic and debilitating diseases. This promising research led scientists to wonder whether high doses of these same antioxidants—extracted from food and packed into pills—would provide even greater disease protection.

Studies evaluating the benefit of antioxidant supplements have had mixed results. Take vitamin E, for example. Past research showed that people who consumed a lot of it from food had 30 to 40 percent fewer heart attacks than others whose diets included little. Yet several teams of scientists have compared large groups of people who took vitamin E supplements with others who took placebos. Most of these studies have found that people in both groups had the same risk of cardiovascular disease, raising doubts about whether vitamin E protects the heart.

There are several possible explanations for these disappointing results. For example, in some studies, people at risk for heart disease may have started taking the supplements too late for the pills to do much good. However, mounting research suggests that antioxidants simply work better as a team. That is, individual antioxidants such as vitamin E may be more potent when you toss them down the hatch with other antioxidants—the way they occur naturally in food.

"Antioxidants interact in a very dynamic interrelationship," says nutrition scientist Jeffrey Blumberg, Ph.D., chief antioxidant researcher at Tufts University in Boston. "It may be that for optimal health, we need to eat foods that have these complex mixtures of compounds." His research shows, for example, that vitamin E's antioxidant punch increases up to *300 percent* when the vitamin is combined in a test tube with certain flavonoids found in almonds.

That doesn't mean Dr. Blumberg and other scientists have given up on vitamin E pills or any other antioxidant supplements. In recent years, the National Institutes of Health has sponsored research on the use of antioxidant therapy to prevent or treat a long list of conditions. But the most powerful evidence on the books today suggests that eating foods rich in antioxidants is the best way to defend yourself against diseases that are caused or worsened by the daily assaults of free radicals.

> People who eat plenty of antioxidant-rich foods lower their risk of heart attacks, cancer, and various chronic diseases.

For instance, drinking a cool glass of orange juice at least three times a week may help reduce the risk of Alzheimer's disease by up to 76 percent, thanks to its high content of antioxidants called polyphenols, according to a study by Vanderbilt University researchers. Meanwhile, a study in the *Archives of Ophthalmology* found that women who eat plenty of corn, squash, and other yellow vegetables—which are full of antioxidants called carotenoids that protect the eyes from free radicals—halved their risk of macular degeneration, which can cause blindness. And an Italian study recently found that a small daily dose of antioxidants from a surprising source—dark chocolate—lowered blood pressure better than most standard medications. How sweet is that?

Free Radicals: Necessary Evils

Here's news that may leave you holding your breath: Oxygen is toxic. You can't live without it, of course, since every cell in your body requires oxygen to spark metabolism, or the production of energy. However, 1 to 3 percent of the oxygen you inhale never gets burned. Instead, it reacts with naturally occurring metal compounds in your body to produce renegade molecules called free radicals.

There are many different types of free radicals, but they all share one thing in common: Unlike normal molecules, they are missing a pair of electrons. This defect makes them dangerous, since they will attack anything in their path in order to replace their missing parts. Free radicals aren't entirely bad, though. In fact, your immune system produces them as part of your body's overall defense scheme, since free radicals kill bacteria and defuse viruses. However, in their quest for electrons, free radicals may also destroy healthy molecules, including proteins in cell membranes, fats, and even DNA.

In addition to the free radicals your body makes on purpose, exposure to certain triggers in the environment, including sunlight, air pollution, tobacco smoke, and radiation (from computers, for example), can produce these unstable molecules. It's also clear that the hormones that flood your body when you feel emotionally stressed produce free radicals.

Your body tries to keep these oxygen-borne baddies under control, but when levels rise too high, you experience a condition scientists call oxidative stress. Everyone undergoes at least a little oxidative stress now and then, but living in a chronic state of overwhelming oxidative stress seems to contribute to a long list of diseases.

Antioxidants to the Rescue

If free radicals are reckless marauders that disturb the peace in your body, antioxidants are the riot police. These various vitamins, minerals, and other natural compounds curb the chaos with generosity instead of brute force. An antioxidant neutralizes a free radical by first surrounding it, then giving it a pair of its own electrons, ending

Antioxidant Superstars

Could your diet use an infusion of antioxidants? The column on the left lists, in order, the food categories that offer the highest average antioxidant content. The column on the right lists the foods in each category with the highest concentration of antioxidants by weight.

Want to take a seasoned approach to better health? Cook with cloves, allspice, cinnamon, rosemary, and oregano, which are among the most concentrated antioxidant sources of all.

ANTIOXIDANT SOURCE	BEST CHOICES
Berries	Blueberries
Nuts and seeds	Walnuts, pecans
Chocolate	Dark chocolate
Fruits	Pomegranates
Vegetables	Kale, artichokes
Wine	Red varieties
Fruit juice	Grape
Coffee	Black, filtered
Tea	Green
Grains	Barley, buckwheat
Legumes	Kidney beans

the destructive behavior. This gesture turns the antioxidant itself into a free radical since it's now missing a pair of electrons, but the new molecule is toothless and does no harm.

As we mentioned earlier, your body produces its own lineup of antioxidants. Many have names that sound as if they came straight out of a science fiction novel, such as superoxide dismutase and coenzyme Q10. These homegrown antioxidants are a talented lot; one, called lipoic acid, is particularly versatile, capable of recycling used-up antioxidants and thus restoring their effectiveness. But your body makes only a portion of the antioxidant force needed to keep free radicals from taking over. What's more, your naturally occurring levels of antioxidants decline with age. That's why it's critical to get reinforcements from antioxidant-rich foods and, in some cases, dietary supplements. Many dietary antioxidants have been well studied and have familiar names, like vitamin C. Others belong to an emerging class of compounds that scientists are just beginning to identify and understand. All belong in your diet.

Vitamins and minerals

Your body can perform remarkable feats of chemistry, but it has limitations. While your inner chemist can build proteins from amino acids, for instance, it can't whip up many of the raw compounds needed to maintain daily functions and prevent disease. Instead, we rely on food for these critical compounds, known as vitamins and minerals. Not only is your body incapable of manufacturing its own vitamins and minerals, but it also has a limited capacity for storing them. That's why you must restock your inventory frequently by eating a well-balanced diet.

Most individual vitamins and minerals perform a lengthy list of chores. For instance, your body needs vitamin C to build a healthy immune system, brain cells, and bones, to name just a few of its roles. Vitamin E, meanwhile, is necessary for many tasks, such as forming red blood cells and muscle, lung, and nerve tissue. Both of these vitamins are powerful antioxidants, too. A healthy diet must also include a variety of minerals. One mineral, selenium, is needed to form certain enzymes that act as antioxidants.

Antioxidant Vitamins and Minerals

Here's a snapshot of the four most common and powerful antioxidant vitamins and minerals in the diet.

VITAMIN OR MINERAL	MAY HELP PREVENT OR TREAT	GOOD SOURCES
Beta-carotene	Some cancers, heart disease, cognitive decline	Carrots, squash, sweet potatoes, cantaloupe, peaches, apricots
Vitamin C	Some cancers, heart disease, arthritis	Citrus fruits; yellow, red, and green bell peppers; broccoli; strawberries
Vitamin E	Heart disease, some cancers, Alzheimer's disease, cataracts	Olive and canola oil, nuts, seeds, whole grains, avocado, spinach
Selenium	Some cancers, arthritis, HIV	Brazil nuts, beef, fish, pork, poultry, grains, vegetables (selenium content varies by region)

Source: Office of Dietary Supplements

Phytochemicals

You may be surprised to learn just how much you have in common with a tomato vine or blueberry bush. Just as your body makes antioxidants to fend off illness, plants produce chemicals that protect them against disease. Scientists have identified thousands of so-called phytochemicals (*phyto-* is Greek for "plant"). While they are not technically nutrients, many phytochemicals are now known to be critical for keeping your body up and running. "We may eventually discover that some of these phytochemicals are essential to human health," says antioxidant expert Dr. Blumberg.

Growing evidence shows that phytochemicals play a wide variety of roles in the body, such as preventing blood clots and slowing the spread of cancer cells. But perhaps the most attention has been focused on their potential as antioxidants. There are two main categories of phytochemicals that act as antioxidants.

CAROTENOIDS: Fruits and vegetables that are yellow, orange, or red tend to be good sources of these antioxidant plant chemicals. Think tomatoes, oranges, carrots, and pink grapefruit.

Some green vegetables, such as spinach and kale, are full of carotenoids, too. Everyone has heard of beta-carotene, which your body converts to vitamin A, but studies show that several carotenoids with less familiar names are critical to human health, too.

FLAVONOIDS: These blue, blue-red, and violet pigments are another important category of antioxidants (which technically belongs to a larger category called polyphenols) that may be particularly important in helping us fight diseases ranging from allergies to heart disease to cancer. One type of flavonoid, known as quercetin, appears to be particularly good for the cardiovascular system, since it prevents LDL cholesterol from being oxidized (making it less likely to stick to artery walls). Red and yellow onions, kale, broccoli, red grapes, and apples are all good sources of quercetin. Cocoa contains flavonoids called epicatechins, also thought to benefit the heart. These compounds, also found in tea, prevent blood clots, slow the oxidation of LDL cholesterol, improve blood vessel function, and even reduce inflammation.

Antioxidant Phytochemicals

Scientists have identified many thousands of phytochemicals; there are more than 6,000 flavonoids alone. Here are some of the most important antioxidant phytochemicals.

PHYTOCHEMICAL	MAY HELP PREVENT OR TREAT	GOOD SOURCES
Catechins	Heart disease, some cancers	Cocoa, tea, grapes, berries, beans and other legumes
Lutein	Cataracts, macular degeneration, heart disease, some cancers	Spinach, broccoli, and other leafy green vegetables; asparagus; brussels sprouts; artichokes
Lycopene	Prostate cancer; possibly osteoporosis and male infertility	Tomatoes (especially ketchup and other cooked tomato products), watermelon, pink grapefruit, red bell peppers
Proanthocyanidins	Heart disease, cancer	Tea, cocoa, berries, grapes, red wine, tea, apples
Quercetin	Heart disease, lung cancer, asthma, hay fever	Apples, onions, broccoli, kale, berries, grapes
Resveratrol	Heart disease, type 2 diabetes	Red wine, grapes, peanuts
Zeaxanthin	Cataracts, macular degeneration, some cancers	Leafy green vegetables, corn, egg yolk, tangerines, nectarines, orange peppers

Antioxidants in Action: The Benefits of Defusing Free Radicals

Free radicals don't sleep or take vacations. One expert quoted in *The Antioxidant Miracle* estimated that the DNA in every cell in the human body suffers about 10,000 "hits" from free radicals each day. It's not surprising then that the oxidative stress that can result when your antioxidant support isn't up to full strength can produce an array of debilitating conditions. However, if you choose your diet wisely and use supplements as necessary (always under your physician's guidance), antioxidants may do the following.

Protect your heart

Even though studies haven't shown conclusively that antioxidant supplements prevent heart disease, there's no doubt that your diet must include frequent doses of antioxidants to keep LDL cholesterol, the "bad" stuff, from turning even worse. Oxidized cholesterol—that is, cholesterol that's been attacked by free radicals—is more likely to burrow into artery walls. Once cholesterol makes its way there, it's even more likely to become oxidized. When this happens, your immune system senses trouble and responds by sending white blood cells to the scene. These defender cells devour cholesterol, turning into frothy blobs called foam cells. As these fat-filled cells accumulate, they form raised patches called plaques, which narrow arteries. Plaques can erupt, blocking the artery and causing a heart attack.

People who eat plenty of antioxidant-rich fruit and vegetables have a low risk of heart disease, many studies have shown. Other good sources of heart-healthy antioxidants include tea and wine; both beverages contain high concentrations of flavonoids. Studies suggest that eating a diet high in flavonoids may lower the risk of heart disease by up to 65 percent.

Want to lower the workload for your body's homegrown crew of antioxidants? Eat fewer sweets and starches, which seem to raise levels of free radicals. A study by University of California researchers found that people whose diets included the most high-GI foods had the highest levels of oxidized cholesterol, the kind most likely to cause heart attacks.

Protect your DNA

Free radicals can damage the DNA in healthy cells, which may alter their operating instructions and cause them to reproduce uncontrollably and form cancerous tumors. People who eat lots of fruits and vegetables have a low risk for some types of cancer. Lab studies show that phytochemicals stifle the growth of tumors in various ways, including by scavenging and demobilizing free radicals.

This news should have you seeing red—and orange and yellow—when you shop for vegetables, since carotenoids (the pigments that color these foods) may be one of the most potent types of antioxidants for fighting cancer. In particular, studies have revealed low rates of prostate cancer among men who consume a lot of tomatoes and cooked tomato products, which contain the carotenoid lycopene.

Control diabetes complications

High blood sugar seems to speed up production of some unusually nasty free radicals. These destructive molecules probably cause many of the complications that make diabetes so frightening, such as blindness, nerve damage, and kidney failure.

Some promising signs suggest that antioxidants could alleviate some diabetes symptoms. For instance, European studies have shown that dietary supplements containing alpha-lipoic acid (found in spinach, broccoli, and beef) may relieve the pain and discomfort of diabetic neuropathy. Scientists in India have shown that the antioxidant compound curcumin, which gives the spice turmeric its yellow color, slowed kidney damage in diabetic rats. The antioxidants resveratrol (found in

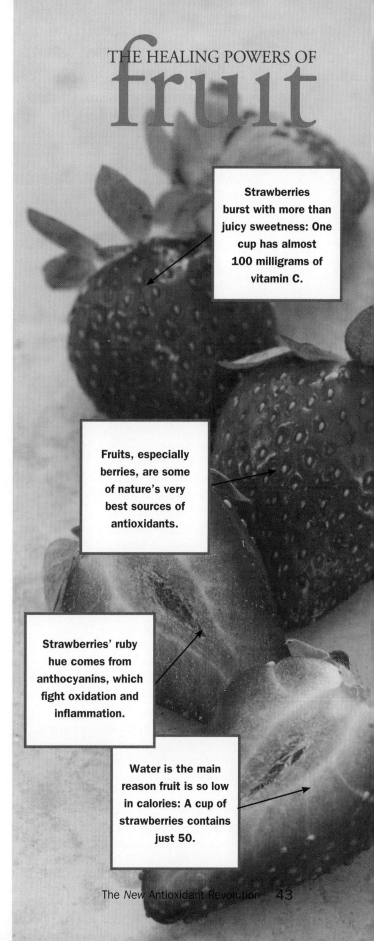

THE HEALING POWERS OF

fruit

Strawberries burst with more than juicy sweetness: One cup has almost 100 milligrams of vitamin C.

Fruits, especially berries, are some of nature's very best sources of antioxidants.

Strawberries' ruby hue comes from anthocyanins, which fight oxidation and inflammation.

Water is the main reason fruit is so low in calories: A cup of strawberries contains just 50.

red wine) and quercetin (apples and onions are good sources) had a similar effect.

Some phytochemicals may even offer protection against diabetes itself. In a Finnish study of more than 4,300 nondiabetic men and women whom researchers followed for 23 years, those who ate the most of a type of carotenoid found in citrus fruits, red bell peppers, papaya, cilantro, corn, and watermelon cut their risk of type 2 diabetes by 42 percent.

Defend against dementia

Brain cells of people diagnosed with devastating cognitive conditions show evidence of damage by free radicals. What's more, free radicals seem to be one cause of the clumps of proteins in the brain, called amyloids, that are characteristic of Alzheimer's disease.

No one is sure how to prevent Alzheimer's, but eating more oranges and whole-grain bread could be a good start. Human studies offer clues that vitamins C and E may be your brain's best defense. A 2015 study published in the *Journal of the Alzheimer's Association* found that people who adhered to a diet rich in green leafy vegetables, nuts, berries, beans, whole grains, and other antioxidant-rich foods lowered their risk of developing Alzheimer's disease by as much as 53 percent. No wonder they call this way of eating the MIND diet!

It's less clear whether taking high doses of antioxidants will do an even better job of safeguarding the brain. One study published in the *New England Journal of Medicine* found that taking daily supplements containing 2,000 IU of vitamin E—or about 66 times more than you'll find in a multivitamin—appeared to slow the onset of Alzheimer's. However, other studies have failed to show that vitamin E pills protect the brain. (The Alzheimer's Association doesn't recommend the use of antioxidant supplements.)

Save your sight

Tired jokes about rabbits not wearing eyeglasses aside, carrots are indeed good for your eye health (although they won't do anything to sharpen your eyesight). As anyone who tends a garden knows, rabbits eat many other plants besides carrots, and so should you. Here's why.

Carrots are loaded with beta-carotene, which the body converts to vitamin A—an essential nutrient for healthy eyes. But the latest research suggests that other antioxidant phytochemicals may also be critical for preserving vision. Take lutein, another carotenoid like beta-carotene, which is found in hefty amounts in spinach, kale, and collard greens. Retina cells at the back of the eyeball soak up lutein, apparently to ward off free radicals. When researchers analyzed the diets of more than 1,700 female volunteers in Iowa, Oregon, and Wisconsin, they found that women under 75 who ate plenty of foods rich in lutein and zeaxanthin, another carotenoid, appeared to halve their risk of macular degeneration, a leading cause of vision loss in older folks.

Consuming lots of foods filled with these antioxidants may help prevent cataracts, too. So eat your carrots, but don't skimp on the leafy greens, squash, corn, or peas, all of which are good sources of lutein and zeaxanthin, as are egg yolks, honeydew, and kiwifruit.

> Studies suggest that eating a diet high in flavonoids may lower the risk of heart disease by up to 65 percent.

Busting the Crockery:
FOOD MYTHS DEBUNKED

If you miss eggs, here's an invitation to get cracking again. And if you eat raw broccoli because you're afraid to steam away all the nutrients— and you *hate* raw broccoli—we've got some good news there, too.

Did you quit drinking coffee because you read somewhere that it causes cancer in lab rats? Too bad for lab rats; you should feel free to pick up a Starbucks card and savor some dark brew.

Over the years, myths and misconceptions have arisen about certain foods and scary diseases. To make matters worse, the allegedly evil dishes rarely turn out to be liver or lima beans. Instead, false and undeserved claims often end up tainting the reputations of favorite foods, some of which turn out to be good for you. One large study, for instance, found that women who drank up to 4 cups of coffee a day cut their risk of diabetes by 47 percent.

Here's the truth about some common—and stubborn—food falsehoods.

MYTH: Eggs are bad for you

This is a classic instance of good intentions but scrambled science. For years, nutrition experts cautioned that eggs were unhealthy. After all, those gifts from the henhouse are one of the richest sources of cholesterol in the human diet. Since cholesterol plugs up arteries, eggs must raise the risk of heart attacks and strokes, right?

Wrong. Large studies suggest that this theory is full of feathers. For example, the famous Framingham Heart Study, which first showed that high blood cholesterol causes heart attacks, found no connection between eating eggs and cardiovascular disease. Another study, involving more than 117,000 men and women, failed to show an increased risk of heart attacks in people who ate up to one egg per day.

How could that be? It turns out that only about 25 percent of the cholesterol in your blood comes from food. The other 75 percent is manufactured by the liver, which produces lots of cholesterol when you eat cheeseburgers, doughnuts, and other sources of saturated fat— something eggs are *low* in. Eggs are also filled with plenty of useful nutrients that may offset any damage done by their cholesterol content, including unsaturated fat, folate and other B vitamins, and minerals. And if you shop around, you can find eggs that are enriched with healthful omega-3 fatty acids.

Eggs can fit into a balanced diet. In fact, even two eggs a day won't budge most people's cholesterol. Just keep in mind that each little orb contains about 180 milligrams of cholesterol. The current Dietary Guidelines for Americans says that a healthy eating style includes up to 300 milligrams of cholesterol a day for most people . . . and is also limited in saturated fat. So enjoy your veggie omelet and stay clear of the bacon and sausage.

By the way, eggs aren't the only high-cholesterol food that has been exonerated by nutritionists. In the 1990s, research showed that eating another delicacy that's notoriously high in cholesterol—shrimp—had barely any effect on cholesterol levels.

MYTH: Coffee causes cancer

While we're on the topic of breakfast, coffee is another wrongly maligned staple of the morning meal. It's hard to say when doubts about this stimulating beverage first emerged, but it has been linked to cancer on several occasions over the past generation or so. In the late 1970s, for example, researchers reported that caffeine caused the growth of cysts in breast tissue. That finding raised concerns since women who frequently develop cysts often go on to have breast cancer. Then, in 1981, a Harvard study found an increase in pancreatic cancer among coffee drinkers.

However, other scientists later looked for links between coffee and these cancers, using superior research methods and studying larger groups of people. They found none. Likewise, major studies examining the risk of other cancers among coffee drinkers came up empty. In some cases, just the opposite appeared to be true. For instance, a recent review of 21 prospective studies found that coffee consumption was not associated with the risk for breast cancer. And in older women (past the age of menopause), 4 cups of coffee a day was associated with a 10 percent lower risk for breast cancer. In another review of scientific evidence, the American Institute for Cancer Research (AICR) concluded that drinking coffee "probably reduces the risk for endometrial and liver cancer."

Need another reason to raise your cup? Studies have also shown in recent years that drinking coffee appears to offer some protection against other conditions, including Parkinson's disease and type 2 diabetes A recent review in the *Journal of Agricultural and Food Chemistry* concluded that people who drank 4 cups of coffee per day had a 50 percent lower risk for type 2 diabetes. Some people also worry that consuming too much caffeine will raise their blood pressure. It now appears that caffeine's effect on blood pressure varies among individuals depending on how much they consume. Caution is always advised.

MYTH: To protect your heart, drink red wine

It's called the French paradox: French men and women have far fewer heart attacks than Americans do, despite their fondness for some notably unhealthy lifestyle habits. (They smoke more cigarettes, for example. And don't forget—these people invented french fries.) Some scientists have speculated that their love of wine, especially red wine, at least partly explains their superior cardiovascular health. It seems logical, since red wine contains high levels of a phytochemical called resveratrol, which acts as an antioxidant and reduces inflammation. (What's more, recent research offers intriguing clues that resveratrol may actually slow the aging process.)

As it turns out, though, it's the alcohol in red wine—and white wine and beer—that's responsible for most of its heart-related benefits. Large population studies suggest that most people enjoy at least some health benefits from sipping *any form* of alcohol in moderation. For example, the Harvard School of Public Health asked more than 38,000 men about their drinking habits, then checked up on them 12 years later. Men who had up to a drink or two per day were 37 percent less likely to have had heart attacks than men who rarely or never indulged.

Alcohol—no matter how you drink it—raises HDL ("good") cholesterol and seems to make blood less likely to clot. If you enjoy alcoholic beverages, most health authorities agree that having no more than a drink or two per day (one for women, two for men) may offer some benefits and probably can't hurt.

MYTH: Fat-free and low-fat foods are always healthier than full-fat varieties

When it comes to dairy products and some other foods, such as meat, you can reliably adopt a simple rule: The less fat, the better. But that's not always the case with other foods. Take salad dressing. If you're trying to lose weight, switching from an oil-based dressing to a low-fat or fat-free dressing may make sense. But sparing yourself 100 calories or so (per 2 tablespoons) comes at a cost.

For starters, salad dressings made with healthy monounsaturated fats, such as olive or canola oil, may help prevent heart disease and other conditions. What's more, a recent study shows that you may be missing out on important disease protection by going oil-free. That's because without some fat in the meal, your digestive tract won't absorb some of the nutrients in a salad.

Researchers at the University of Iowa demonstrated this phenomenon by asking volunteer diners to eat three different salads. Each included romaine lettuce, spinach leaves, grated carrots, and cherry tomatoes. But the first was topped with fat-free Italian dressing, the second with reduced-fat dressing, and the third with conventional full-fat dressing. The researchers took blood samples from the volunteers after they ate each salad and measured levels of carotenoids, the important antioxidants we've talked so much about. After eating the salad with fat-free dressing, the volunteers absorbed just a tiny amount of carotenoids, including beta-carotene and lycopene. The reduced-fat dressing improved matters only slightly, while the volunteers' bodies absorbed an adequate amount of carotenoids after eating the salad with the full-fat dressing. There's no need to drown your greens in oil, however; 1 or 2 tablespoons will get the job done.

MYTH: Raw fruits and vegetables are more nutritious than cooked ones

The idea sounds logical enough. Doesn't it make sense to eat fruits and vegetables in their natural state? Some "raw food" enthusiasts take this theory to the extreme, unwilling to eat so much as a pea pod if it's been boiled, steamed, or exposed to any form of heat.

However, the theory that cooking foods makes them less nutritious is a bit half-baked. Raw-food advocates note that heat destroys enzymes in foods that make them more easily digested. While that's true, cooking also breaks down fiber, making it easier for your body to process. (Just imagine trying to chew, much less digest, a spear of raw asparagus.) Subsisting primarily on raw fruit and vegetables could even backfire if your goal is to get healthier. German researchers studied 201 men and women who adopted raw-food diets and found that their total cholesterol and triglyceride levels dropped. However, the raw-food diet also lowered their HDL cholesterol. Meanwhile, their levels of homocysteine (an amino acid linked to heart attacks and strokes) rose.

Scientists have discovered in recent years that cooking actually *boosts* levels of important

Raw Sugar: A Raw Deal?

Should you pay more for so-called raw sugar? Sure, if you like its taste and texture. But don't buy the hype suggesting that it's more nutritious or wholesome than plain old table sugar.

Most "raw" sugar sold in the United States is turbinado sugar, so named because it is partially refined in turbines, or centrifuges. While common white sugar crystals are stripped of molasses during processing, turbinado sugar retains some of this syrup, so it has a yellow-gold or tan color. Similar sweeteners include demerara and muscovado sugars.

While these sugars have unique taste and cooking properties, they are scarcely more healthful than other sweeteners. Unlike table sugar, they contain minerals, but only a trace. Nor do turbinado and related sugars offer any edge for dieters; like table sugar, they provide 15 calories per teaspoon.

What's more, using the term *raw* to advertise any sugar sold to consumers in the United States is misleading. Strictly speaking, *raw sugar* is the term used for the tan or brown granules produced when mills process sugarcane stalks. Raw sugar is then refined to make table sugar and other forms of the sweetener. You can't buy true raw sugar, since the FDA declares it unfit for human consumption—and you wouldn't want to, since it contains yeast, mold, bacteria, dirt, bug parts, and other undesirable stuff.

THE HEALING POWERS OF
olive oil

Dieters were once advised to shun salad dressing, but eating some fat makes a healthy diet easier to stick with.

Olive oil, especially extra-virgin oil, is considered "liquid gold" because of its antioxidants and its ability to tame inflammation.

Rosemary is a highly potent source of antioxidants, as are other spices such as oregano.

Dressing a salad with a bit of oil makes the nutrients in the veggies much easier for your body to absorb.

Monounsaturated fats like those in olive oil can dramatically slash the risk of heart attacks.

Vinegar, thanks to its acids, can blunt postmeal spikes in blood sugar by 30 to 55 percent.

compounds in some fruits and vegetables. For instance, ketchup contains five to six times more of the antioxidant lycopene than raw tomatoes do, making it much more useful against diseases such as prostate cancer.

Heat does rob fresh produce of some nutrients, especially vitamins that dissolve in water. For example, cooking fruits and vegetables tends to reduce their levels of vitamin B_6, vitamin C, and folate in particular. But it increases the antioxidant levels of some vegetables, such as sweet corn and carrots. The bottom line: If you like raw produce, crunch away—but don't fear the vegetable steamer or stir-fry pan.

MYTH: Frozen and canned fruits and vegetables are less nutritious than fresh ones

Fresh fruits and vegetables *are* more nutritious than the frozen and canned variety—at the instant they are picked. However, the foods you find in the produce section have often had a long journey from the moment they were packed in crates, spending days or even weeks in transit from the farm or orchard. During shipping and storage, natural enzymes are released in fresh fruit and vegetables that cause them to lose nutrients.

By contrast, food processors quick-freeze fresh-picked produce, which preserves much of its vitamin and mineral content. "With some fruits and vegetables, you actually lock in a higher nutrient content by freezing," says Douglas Archer, Ph.D., a professor of food science at the University of Florida. A 1992 University of Illinois study found, for instance, that frozen beans retained twice as much vitamin C as fresh beans purchased in a grocery store. Contrary to common belief, canning does not deplete fruit and vegetables of significant amounts of nutrients either. While heat processing may reduce levels of some vitamins, certain canned foods—such as spinach

and pumpkin—actually have higher levels of vitamin A than fresh versions.

But what about taste? You'll never mistake a frozen strawberry for a fresh one, but freezing technology has made huge leaps in recent years. "Frozen vegetables used to have both texture and taste problems," says Dr. Archer. "Now they're quite good and are even used by professional chefs."

MYTH: Nuts are too fattening—eat them sparingly

And deprive yourself of a nutritious and satisfying food? To be sure, nuts contain a lot of fat, but it's mostly the good kind. Dry-roasted peanuts, for example, have three to four times more heart-healthy monounsaturated fat than saturated fat. Recent research suggests that eating nuts as part of a healthy diet may even help you lose weight.

Researchers believe that the fat in nuts helps people feel full, and the protein may use up calories as it digests. What's more, a study by British researchers shows that high-protein foods help trigger the release of a hormone known to reduce hunger.

Nuts' high concentration of healthy fats makes them a guilt-free way to satisfy hunger without raising cholesterol or other blood fats. What's more, nuts are an excellent fiber source and provide a long list of nutrients, including vitamin E, magnesium, folate, and copper. It's no wonder people who include nuts in their diet tend to be so healthy. For instance, women who eat just 1 ounce of nuts most days of the week are 35 percent less likely to have heart attacks than those who avoid nuts, according to a Harvard study of more than 80,000 nurses. Prefer peanut butter sandwiches? Eat one five days a week (preferably on whole-grain bread), and you may lower your risk of type 2 diabetes by 21 percent.

Your Food Cures
Arsenal

Food heals! That's the happy message we shouted in Part One. Now read on to learn which foods make our "top 22" list, plus our top 10 healing herbs and spices. Also discover which pantry staples are treasure troves of specific vitamins, minerals, and other key nutrients that show up again and again in our "food prescriptions" in Part Three.

Ancient Grains

What You're Eating

Ever wonder what's up with all these new grains, sometimes called Ancient Grains, popping up on restaurant menus and store shelves? While all grains have been around since the beginning of time, according to the Whole Grains Council, ancient grains are ones that are largely unchanged over the last several hundred years. These include amaranth, blue corn, einkorn, emmer/farro, kamut, millet, quinoa, sorghum, spelt, and teff. Bursting with complex carbohydrates and fiber, ancient grains provide protien, iron, copper and more, start adding ancient grains to your meals. They are usually prepared like brown rice but be sure to read the package as amounts of water and cooking times vary.

Healing Powers

The fiber and nutrients in these whole grains are important for staying slim and living a longer, healthier life. Studies have shown that people avoiding grains were more likely to be overweight or obese than those who ate grains. Additionally, those who eat more whole grains have less inflammation and lower risk of type-2 diabetes, stroke, and heart disease.

Healthful Hint

Ancient grains store well either in the refrigerator or freezer. When preparing, double or triple the amount needed so that you will have them on hand for last minute meal prep.

HOW MUCH IS ENOUGH

Three to five servings a day to increase fiber. A serving is a 1/2 cup cooked grain or an ounce of bread or cereal.

BUYING RIGHT

Look for the whole grain stamp when purchasing anceint grains. Any food bearing the Whole Grain Stamp contains at least 8 grams of whole grains, a half serving. Those with a 100 percent on the stamp provides 16 grams or one serving of whole grains.

Three Clever Ideas

1. Quinoa (pronounced keen-wah) contains a naturally occurring bitter coating to protect it from predators. Always rinse quinoa before cooking to remove the bitter flavor.

2. For variety in soups, salads, stir-fries, and stews, substitute one of these ancient grains for rice or pasta.

3. Following a gluten-free diet? Many ancient grains are naturally gluten-free. These include amaranth, buckwheat, corn, millet, quinoa, rice, sorghum, teff, and wild rice.

Avocados

What You're Eating

The reproductive part of the tree—and the fattiest fruit on Earth (even fattier than olives). Like olives, these odd-looking fruits, dubbed alligator pears for their shape and bumpy green skin, are an incredibly concentrated source of good-for-you monounsaturated fat. The dark-skinned, rough-textured California-grown variety (Hass) is fattier than the smooth-skinned, bright green Florida-grown variety. Avocados contain more soluble fiber and protein than any other fruit, and half a medium avocado provides more potassium than a banana.

Healing Powers

Despite their fat, or actually because of it, avocados can lower your cholesterol. Researchers find that replacing just 5 percent of your calories from saturated fat (think butter or cheese) with monounsaturated fat—the kind in avocados—could slash the risk of heart attack by more than a third. An added benefit: Avocados are also high in beta-sitosterol, a plant sterol (also found in cholesterol-lowering margarines such as Benecol) that blocks the absorption of cholesterol from food, and the anti-cancer compound glutathione, a powerful antioxidant.

Healthful Hint

Use avocados to replace other fat sources in your diet, not add to them.

KEY NUTRIENTS

> Monounsaturated fat
> Folate (a B vitamin)
> Vitamin A
> Potassium
> Sterols

HOW MUCH IS ENOUGH

At about 227 calories per Hass avocado, a little goes a long way. Cut an avocado into five pieces and enjoy one piece for just 45 calories—half the calories of a tablespoon of mayonnaise and much more healthful.

BUYING RIGHT

Hold a few fruits in the palm of your hand and choose one that seems heavy for its size. Store it on the kitchen counter until it's ripe or place it in a paper bag to hasten ripening. Hass avocados become very dark when ripe. To tell if the fruit is ready to eat, pull the stem off the end. If it comes off easily and the flesh of the fruit is green, the avocado is ripe.

Three Clever Ideas

1. To prevent a cut avocado from turning brown in the refrigerator, remove the seed and spray the flesh with cooking spray, then wrap in plastic. Use within three days.

2. Mashed avocado makes a healthy replacement for condiments. Spread on sandwiches in lieu of mayo or add to hot baked potatoes instead of sour cream.

3. If avocados are ripening faster than you can eat them, mash them with 1/2 table-spoon lemon or lime juice per avocado. Place in an airtight container, cover, and freeze. Use within four months.

Beans

What You're Eating

We don't normally think of beans as seeds, but that's what they are. Dry beans (legumes) grow inside pods, just as green beans do. After they're picked and cleaned, beans are often polished to command a better price. Because they're the plant's seeds, or embryos, beans are loaded with nutrients, including folate and iron. They're also stuffed with protein, with a cup of cooked lentils providing nearly 18 grams—about as much as a serving of T-bone steak.

Healing Powers

Beans are in fact good for your heart, thanks in large part to their soluble fiber, which soaks up cholesterol so the body can dispose of it before it can stick to artery walls. Studies find that diets high in soluble fiber can cut total cholesterol by 10 to 15 percent. The same soluble fiber, combined with beans' protein, makes beans beneficial to blood sugar. Their magnesium helps relax arteries, giving blood more room to flow and lowering blood pressure. Finally, beans are ranked among the top antioxidant foods.

Healthful Hint

Choose small red beans for truly astounding antioxidant power, followed by red kidney beans, then pinto beans. Beans contain more protein than any other plant food, but the protein is incomplete. Eating a grain such as rice or any other protein-containing food at any time during the day will "complete" the protein. Rinse canned beans before using to remove up to 40 percent of the salt.

KEY NUTRIENTS

> Folate (a B vitamin)
> Vitamins A and C
> Protein
> Iron

HOW MUCH IS ENOUGH
1/2 cup a day.

BUYING RIGHT
If you're buying your beans in a bag rather than a can, note that older beans take longer to cook than fresh ones—ideally, they should be less than a year old. For freshness, purchase from a busy, reputable store.

Three Clever Ideas

1. Store dry beans in a glass jar with a dried chile pepper, which will ward off pantry bugs. For a spicy dish, include the pepper; otherwise, discard it.

2. To prevent gas, change the soaking water several times when preparing beans. Never cook the beans in the soaking water. Or opt for canned beans, which contain less flatulence-causing substances, and rinse them first.

3. Snack on baked chickpeas! Toss about 2 cups drained and patted dry beans with one beaten egg white and a mix of spices such as cumin, chili powder, and cayenne pepper or cinnamon, ginger, and nutmeg. Bake, stirring occasionally, at 400°F (200°C) until golden.

Blueberries

What You're Eating

A lot of antioxidants. These berries have more antioxidants—those magical molecules that can help prevent cancer, heart disease, eye disease, memory loss, and a host of other maladies—than 40 other common fruits and vegetables tested. Blueberries are also one of only three fruits native to North America (Concord grapes and cranberries are the other two) and are the only truly blue food in nature, not counting some blue-purple potatoes from remote corners of the globe, a few fruits that can almost pass as blue, and blue corn. Blueberries may be small, but 1/2 cup contains almost 2 grams of fiber, the same as a slice of whole-wheat bread.

Healing Powers

The antioxidant plant pigments that make blueberries blue—flavonoids called anthocyanins—guard against heart disease, cancer, and age-related blindness and memory loss. Like their cranberry cousins, blueberries (and blueberry juice) are tops when it comes to preventing urinary tract infections, thanks to antioxidant epicatechins, which keep bacteria from sticking to bladder walls. Plus, the fiber in blueberries makes them powerful antidotes to constipation.

Healthful Hint

If you like blueberry pancakes, sprinkle on the blueberries at the last minute. Cooking the berries destroys valuable vitamin C. To get even more antioxidant power from berries, seek out elderberries, black currants, and chokeberries, all of which tested even higher than blueberries in antioxidant activity.

KEY NUTRIENTS

> Fiber
> Antioxidants
> Vitamin C
> Iron

HOW MUCH IS ENOUGH

1/2 cup blueberries equals one fruit serving.

BUYING RIGHT

Go for dry, plump berries full of fragrance and free of dents and bruises. They should have a silvery white coating called a bloom. If shriveled or lacking the bloom, they've been overhandled. Gently shake the container; fruit that doesn't move freely is overripe or damaged. Stains under the package also indicate overripe fruit. Wash just before serving.

Three Clever Ideas

1. Don't discard the little plastic container the blueberries come in; it makes a perfect mini-colander. Use it to rinse the berries, then save the container for rinsing small amounts of other foods.

2. To dry these delicate berries, place in a salad spinner lined with paper towels and give a quick spin.

3. Add blueberries to your lemonade. Place a few berries in each section of an ice cube tray, fill with lemonade, and freeze. Plop three cubes in each glass of lemonade.

Broccoli

What You're Eating

Broccoli is a member of the cabbage family, which helps explain its anticancer powers (all cabbages are anticancer foods). Almost 90 percent water, it's nevertheless loaded with nutrients. One stalk has as much fiber as a healthy breakfast cereal and as much vitamin C as two Florida oranges. By the way, the leaves are edible.

Healing Powers

Consider broccoli your number one cancer fighter, thanks to its sulfur compounds, such as sulforaphane, which you can smell as broccoli cooks. These compounds signal our genes to boost production of enzymes that detoxify potentially cancer-causing compounds. Eat more broccoli, and you could slash your risk of everything from breast and lung cancer to stomach and colon cancer by as much as half. Sulforaphane has also been found to kill the bacteria that cause ulcers. Broccoli's also a surprising nondairy source of calcium and potassium, making it good for your bones as well as your blood pressure. Its vitamin C and beta-carotene protect your eyes from cataracts and safeguard your brain cells from memory-robbing attacks by free radicals.

Healthful Hint

Steam broccoli for 3 to 4 minutes until it's crisp-tender to free up more of its sulforaphane. Don't cook it in a lot of water, or the nutrients will leach into the water. Eat the florets, where much of the beta-carotene is stored, but if you like the stalks, eat them, too—they also contain plenty of nutrients.

KEY NUTRIENTS

> Anticancer compounds (such as sulforaphane)
> Beta-carotene
> Calcium
> Fiber
> Folate (a B vitamin)
> Vitamin C

HOW MUCH IS ENOUGH

1/2 cup cooked broccoli is one vegetable serving.

BUYING RIGHT

Choose florets with a dark green, purple, or blue hue; they contain more beta-carotene and vitamin C than light green or yellow ones. Limp stalks or flowering buds are signs of poor quality.

Three Clever Ideas

1. Don't discard the leaves from broccoli stalks; they contain more vitamin A than the florets. Chop and add to the broccoli or toss in green salads. Eat the stalks, too. Peel away the tough outer skin before chopping or shredding.

2. If your broccoli has gotten limp, cut 1/2 inch off the bottom of each stalk. Place the stalks in a glass of cold water and chill. It will be crisp again in a few hours.

3. Although lemon juice keeps cut fruit from turning brown, it has the opposite effect on broccoli (or any other vegetable with chlorophyll), turning it a dull gray. Season with lemon or lime juice only after it has cooled.

Carrots

What You're Eating

Bugs Bunny's favorite food—and the vegetable that gave the all-important group of phytochemicals called carotenoids their name. Real rabbits, though, are more likely to eat the leafy green tops of the vegetable than its bright orange root, so they miss out on beta-carotene, which gives carrots their color and holds the key to their significant health benefits. One large raw carrot provides almost all the vitamin A you need in a day; a cooked carrot supplies even more. While most of us see orange carrots at the store, they come in many varieties and colors, including purple.

Healing Powers

Carrots won't prevent or correct nearsightedness, although they do help prevent night blindness, which is caused by a deficiency of vitamin A, as well as cataracts. Thanks to their soluble fiber, carrots also lower cholesterol. In one USDA study, eating 1 cup of carrots a day lowered cholesterol 11 percent after three weeks. Carotenoids like beta-carotene may also protect against certain types of cancer.

Healthful Hint

Cooked carrots contain more beta-carotene since cooking breaks down the cellular walls that encase this nutrient. To preserve carrots' natural sweet flavor and nutrients, cook them, covered, in as little liquid as possible, a technique known as sweating. To best absorb the beta-carotene, eat your carrots with a little fat (such as olive oil).

KEY NUTRIENTS

> Beta-carotene

> Vitamins B_6 and C

> Fiber

HOW MUCH IS ENOUGH

1/2 cup cooked carrots is one vegetable serving.

BUYING RIGHT

Go for the darkest orange carrots because they have the most beta-carotene. To ensure freshness, check that the roots are firm and bright in color and the carrots aren't wilted or cracked. If you purchase carrots with tops, remove them before refrigerating, or they'll rob the carrots of moisture and vitamins.

Three Clever Ideas

1. The fastest way to cut carrots into julienne strips is to start with packaged, peeled mini-carrots. They're the perfect size to simply slice length-wise into quarters and then cut into 1/8-inch strips.

2. For a change of pace, sauté sliced carrots in broth for 2 minutes. Cover and cook until crisp-tender. Finish by tossing with a few tablespoons of orange marmalade.

3. Add fiber and sweetness to hash browns, meat loaf, sauces, or casseroles by stirring in grated carrots—a great way to eat more vegetables.

Dark Chocolate

What You're Eating

Good-for-you candy loaded with antioxidants. It's made from the roasted beans of the cacao tree, native to South America. Columbus "discovered" these beans, and the returning crew of his fourth voyage took them to Europe. Originally cocoa was consumed as a beverage made by combining the ground beans with water. Chocolate was first introduced in bar form about 1910. It's made mainly from cocoa solids and cocoa fat (a.k.a. cocoa butter) plus sugar. Milk chocolate also contains milk or milk powder. White chocolate (mostly sugar and cocoa butter) lacks the cocoa solids that provide the health benefits of its darker cousins. Chocolate's melting point is just below human body temperature—the reason it melts so nicely in your mouth.

Healing Powers

Dark chocolate contains hefty amounts of disease-fighting flavonoids, antioxidants also found in red wine and many fruits and vegetables. In fact, it appears to have more flavonoids than most other foods. Studies find its antioxidants can significantly improve blood pressure, prevent blood clots, slow the oxidation of LDL cholesterol (making it less likely to stick to artery walls), and reduce inflammation. Some research suggests that eating 1.5 ounces a day can cut heart attack risk by 10 percent. Eating dark chocolate can also lower insulin resistance, the main problem behind diabetes.

Healthful Hint

For the most antioxidants, look for dark chocolate that contains at least 60 percent cocoa.

KEY NUTRIENTS

> Potassium
> Vitamins A, B$_1$ (thiamin), C, D, and E
> Iron
> Flavonoids

HOW MUCH IS ENOUGH

About 1.5 ounces is considered one serving.

BUYING RIGHT

Shop in a store with good turnover and look for bars with clean, neat packaging, a sign the chocolate is fresh. To store, wrap in foil, then in plastic wrap. Chocolate may develop a light coating or "bloom," but fear not; it won't affect flavor or texture.

Three Clever Ideas

1. Grate 1/2 ounce dark chocolate into your coffee cup. Fill with hot coffee and steamed milk for a delicious mocha cappuccino.

2. The easy way to melt chocolate: Put in a heatproof bowl, cover with a small plate, and place on your coffee-maker's heating plate. Turn it on, then stir the chocolate occasionally until melted.

3. Vanilla extract boosts the flavor of chocolate. Try doubling the amount called for in a recipe, adding as much as 1 tablespoon.

Flaxseed

What You're Eating

These seeds, also known as linseeds, come from the same plant that provides the fiber for linen. Flax is one of those plants in which every part is used: After the seeds are pressed to make the oil, the high-protein stuff left over is fed to horses to keep their coats shiny. It's just as healthy for humans, especially thanks to phytoestrogens called lignans. Flax is actually the richest source of these compounds ever discovered.

Healing Powers

A tablespoon of ground flaxseed sprinkled over cereal or yogurt provides an easy 2.3 grams of fiber, often more than what's in the cereal itself! But flaxseed is most revered for its lignans. These act like estrogen in the body, blocking estrogen receptors on cells and contributing to reduced rates of certain hormone-related cancers, such as breast cancer. Flaxseed is also a fantastic source of alpha-linolenic acid (ALA), an essential fatty acid the body uses to make omega-3 fatty acids. ALA thins the blood and makes it less sticky, reducing the risk of heart attack and stroke. The little seeds also can lower cholesterol, thanks to their big stores of soluble fiber. Their anti-inflammatory power may also help keep various conditions, from acne to asthma, at bay.

HOW MUCH IS ENOUGH

1 to 2 tablespoons ground flaxseed daily.

BUYING RIGHT

Purchase ground flaxseed, often called flax meal, or grind your own in a clean coffee grinder. Choose vacuum-packed packages to ensure freshness. If you buy flaxseed oil, which turns rancid quickly, look for it in refrigerated dark bottles and buy only as much as you can use in a month.

Healthful Hint

Make sure your flax is ground; otherwise, the seeds will come out the same way they went in (whole), and you won't reap any health benefits. Eat too much flaxseed, and you'll quickly discover its laxative effect.

Three Clever Ideas

1. Use flaxseed oil in salad dressings, replacing at least half of olive oil with flaxseed oil. Don't cook flaxseed oil, or "good" fat will turn to "bad."

2. If you don't have a spare coffee grinder for flaxseed, here's a simple way to "grind" it. Place the seeds on a cutting board and surround them with a few drops of water (just enough to moisten and hold them in place), then chop with a chef's knife.

3. Out of eggs? In a blender, combine 1 tablespoon ground flaxseed with 3 tablespoons water and process for 1 minute, then let stand until viscous. Use for adhering crumbs to chicken or fish; as filler in meatballs; or in muffin or pancake batter.

Garlic

What You're Eating

An edible antibiotic. The French chemist Louis Pasteur was the first to demonstrate garlic's antiseptic properties, which were put to good use in World War I. Long before that, the Egyptians fed it to slaves while they built the pyramids. Garlic has been used in folk medicine for everything from constipation to leprosy. And garlic breath? Blame garlic's sulfur compounds, which are also responsible for most of its healing powers.

Healing Powers

More health benefits have been ascribed to garlic than to just about any other food—and some of them even hold true. Garlic has antibacterial, antifungal, and antiviral properties; it even appears to banish some antibiotic-resistant bacteria, at least in test tubes. Most of its disease-fighting potential comes from its sulfur compounds, which act as antioxidants, providing many of its cardiovascular benefits. Garlic lowers cholesterol only modestly, but it also acts as a blood thinner, reducing the formation of blood clots and your risk of heart attack and stroke. Just six or more cloves a week can slash your risk of colorectal, stomach, and prostate cancer in half, compared to eating one clove a week or less. The sulfur compounds flush out carcinogens before they can damage cell DNA, and they force cancer cells that do develop to self-destruct.

Healthful Hint

Garlic makes its healing chemical compounds only when the cloves are chopped, crushed, chewed, or otherwise assaulted, which triggers the breakdown of sulfur-containing compounds in the cells. Chop or crush your garlic, then let it stand for 10 minutes to fully release its healing potential.

KEY NUTRIENTS

- > Copper
- > Iron
- > Zinc
- > Magnesium
- > Germanium
- > Selenium

HOW MUCH IS ENOUGH

At least a clove a day.

BUYING RIGHT

Garlic bulbs should be plump, with smooth, firm cloves. Store in an open container in a cool, well-ventilated place for up to two months; don't refrigerate. Cloves that have sprouted are fine to use, though they're less pungent. Mince the sprout and cook along with the garlic.

Three Clever Ideas

1. For perfectly minced garlic, rub a clove over a fine grater or zester. Before using the grater again, run it through the dishwasher to remove all flavor.

2. For a small amount of garlic paste, place one clove on a cutting board and mash with a fork, occasionally changing the direction of the tines.

3. To reduce the pungency of garlic when adding it raw to vinaigrettes or dips, simmer peeled cloves in a little water for 2 minutes, then drain.

Kale

What You're Eating

Kale is everywhere these days and with good reason. This nutrient powerhouse may be one of the world's healthiest foods and delivers rich sources of vitamins C and A along with 5 grams of fiber per cooked cup. Kale also boasts cancer-fighting carotenoids such as lutein and zeaxanthin, which are linked to the prevention of macular degeneration. A member of the cruciferous family, kale comes in varieties that include common curly kale with a peppery, bitter flavor and dense leaves; red, scarlet, or red Russian kale with flavors similar to curly but a distinct purplish, red color; and Tuscan or Lacinato kale (also know as dinosaur kale), featuring a more mild, somewhat sweeter flavor with tender leaves.

Healing Powers

Greens, including kale, are rich sources of beta-carotene, which may help strengthen the body's immune system against harmful free-radical compounds. Kale has the most, with 5.8 milligrams per cup of cooked, providing 72 percent of the daily recommended intake. Cook kale in a small amount of olive oil to enhance the bioavailability of the beta-carotene in the greens.

Healthful Hint

Kale is a packed with vitamin K, a bone-builiding nutrient that is being shown to reduce inflammation and help reduce the risk of heart disease and diabetes. However, it's anticlotting properties may interfere with blood-thinning medications. Speak to your doctor before adding kale to your meals if you are on any of these medications.

KEY NUTRIENTS

> Beta-carotene
> Calcium
> Folate
> Magnesium
> Vitamin C
> Vitamin A

HOW MUCH IS ENOUGH

1 cup raw or 1/2 cup cooked kale leaves is one vegetable serving.

BUYING RIGHT

Choose crisp, bright green leaves and stems with no sign of yellowing, wilting, or bruising. Choose baby kale for mild flavor and delicate texture; it's delicious in smoothies or salads. Opt for bunches with smaller leaves that are more tender and mild. For last-minute meals, grab a bag of chopped kale, but be sure to wash it.

Three Clever Ideas

1. Power boost your pesto by switching out the basil for a mixture of half kale and half parsley. You can increase the nutrients by using walnuts or almonds instead of the pine nuts.

2. To increase your consumption of kale, add it, chopped and cooked, into meat mixtures like meat loaf and meatballs, or cheese mixtures such as the filling for pasta dishes.

3. For quick Tuscan soup, cook a variety of chopped greens in vegetable broth. Add rinsed and drained canned white beans and red pepper flakes. Divide into bowls and drizzle with olive oil. Serve with crusty whole-grain bread.

Low-Fat Milk

What You're Drinking

The same thing mama cows feed their young—almost. In the United States, it's usually pasteurized and homogenized. Homogenization breaks up and disperses milk fat globules, making the liquid smoother; otherwise, the fat would rise to the top of the milk like oil lying on top of water. (Although milk is an excellent source of protein, it's 87 percent water.) Pasteurization destroys bacteria and disables certain natural enzymes. Until the 1950s, you could get your milk only one way—full fat, with 3.25 percent milk fat in 8 ounces. Today you can get milk with less than 0.5 percent fat (fat-free). Removing the fat also removes vitamins A and D, which are later added back.

Healing Powers

If you left milk behind with your childhood, you're missing out on one of the best sources of calcium. Fat-free milk actually has more calcium than whole milk because calcium is found in milk solids, not milk fat. Milk is also fortified with vitamin D, making it one of the only dietary sources of this nutrient, which is emerging as an anticancer vitamin. Dairy products are excellent sources of potassium and magnesium, which naturally reduce blood pressure. A daily glass of milk can also reduce the risk of colorectal cancer by 15 percent.

Healthful Hint

Skin forms on heated milk when water evaporates and calcium and protein combine. If you skim it off, you lose valuable nutrients. Heat milk in a covered pan to reduce evaporation.

KEY NUTRIENTS

> Calcium
> Vitamins A, B$_2$ (riboflavin), B$_{12}$, and D (vitamins A and D are added)
> Phosphorus
> Zinc
> Magnesium

HOW MUCH IS ENOUGH
At least 8 ounces a day.

BUYING RIGHT
Always check the sell-by date and don't buy more than you'll use by then. And of course, choose fat-free or 1 percent milk to keep your fat intake down. Also keep a can of low-fat evaporated milk in your cupboard. It makes a great substitute for cream in recipes, and it's an even better source of calcium than regular milk.

Three Clever Ideas

1. Dairy cuts the heat from spicy ingredients like chile peppers. If a dish comes out too spicy, remove it from the heat and stir in some milk. It will cut the spice and the acid as well.

2. For rich, creamy grains, such as oatmeal, rice, or barley, substitute milk for some or all of the cooking water.

3. Remember Creamsicles? Here's a way to get your milk and enjoy that flavor. In a blender, combine 3/4 cup milk, 3 tablespoons frozen orange juice concentrate, 1/4 teaspoon vanilla extract, and six ice cubes. Blend and enjoy.

Nuts

What You're Eating

Many of our top 22 foods, including avocados, beans, and flaxseed, have something in common, and it's no coincidence: They are the seeds or embryos of plants. Nuts are the embryos of various trees (peanuts, which don't grow on trees, aren't technically nuts but legumes). As such, they contain all the nutrients needed to grow a new plant. Americans eat about 600 million pounds of peanuts a year in addition to the more than 700 million pounds of peanut butter we spread, enough to cover the floor of the Grand Canyon.

Healing Powers

Nuts are high in calories, but most of them come from healthy mono- and polyunsaturated fats, which are behind nuts' ability to slash cholesterol and heart attack risk (by as much as 39 percent) when eaten in place of animal fats. Walnuts in particular are rich in omega-3 fatty acids, the reason they're considered heart-smart snacks. Some nuts, including peanuts, walnuts, and almonds, also contain plant sterols, which lower cholesterol. Nuts are a "slow-burning" food; studies show they can even help people lose weight. Their nutritional benefits vary. One Brazil nut delivers a day's supply of selenium, pecans are especially rich in antioxidants, and 1 ounce of almonds provides nearly half your recommended daily quota of vitamin E. Just don't overdo: A cup of walnuts has more calories than a Big Mac.

Healthful Hint

Eat your peanuts roasted, not raw or steamed. Roasting boosts levels of the antioxidant p-coumaric acid, believed to help prevent stomach cancer by 22 percent.

KEY NUTRIENTS

> Protein
> Omega-3 fatty acids
> Selenium
> Vitamin E
> Potassium
> Calcium
> Iron
> Magnesium
> Zinc

HOW MUCH IS ENOUGH

1 ounce at least five times a week.

BUYING RIGHT

When buying nuts in the shell, look for whole, clean shells without cracks or holes. Shelled nuts should be plump and firm. Since nuts contain fat, they will go rancid. Store them in the fridge for up to a month or freeze in a sealed container for a few months.

Three Clever Ideas

1. Walnuts are, well, a tough nut to crack. Forgo struggling with a nutcracker to break the shells. Reach instead into your toolbox for a vise grip (or curved-jaw locking pliers) for perfectly shelled nuts every time.

2. Avoid the mess from chopping nuts by placing them in a zipper-seal plastic bag and crushing with a rolling pin. Why not do more than you need and freeze the rest in the bag?

3. Toast nuts to bring out their flavor. Preheat the oven to 300°F (150°C). Place 1/2 cup shelled nuts in a single layer on a baking sheet and roast for 7 to 10 minutes. Don't let them burn.

Oats

What You're Eating

Oats are the seeds of the plant—packing all the future potential of the cereal grain into their tiny forms. Historically, oats were viewed in some countries as inferior, to be used only as horse feed because they couldn't be made into bread. But they're one of the best sources of plant-based protein. In 1997, Quaker Foods hit pay dirt when the FDA allowed the company to make the first-ever food-specific health claim on its oatmeal products. That claim—that oats, as part of a healthy diet, could reduce the risk of heart disease—has stood the test of time.

Healing Powers

Oats' cholesterol-lowering powers (and its blood pressure–lowering powers) come from beta-glucan, a type of soluble fiber. One cup a day of cooked oat bran, 1 1/2 cups of cooked oatmeal, or three packets of instant oatmeal provide enough beta-glucan to lower blood cholesterol by about 5 percent and heart attack risk by about 10 percent. Oats may reduce heart attack risk in other ways, too. They contain antioxidants, which help prevent "bad" cholesterol from being oxidized, making it less likely to stick to artery walls. The soluble fiber has another benefit: It forms a gel in the stomach that slows digestion (critical for heading off blood sugar spikes) and helps keep hunger under control.

Healthful Hint

Buy the type of oatmeal you'll eat. It doesn't matter much if it's steel-cut or instant. Just watch out for added sugar in most "instant" brands.

KEY NUTRIENTS

> Calcium
> Iron
> Manganese
> Zinc
> Vitamin E
> B vitamins

HOW MUCH IS ENOUGH

Aim for 10 grams of soluble fiber each day. Cooked oats contain 2 to 3 grams per serving.

BUYING RIGHT

The most commonly used oats are rolled oats. Old-fashioned rolled oats are grains that have been steamed, rolled into flakes, and dried. Quick-cooking oats are cut into small pieces before rolling. Store oats in a tightly sealed container for up to six months.

Three Clever Ideas

1. Add fiber to baked goods by replacing 1/2 cup of the regular flour called for with 1/2 cup oat flour. To make your own, finely grind quick-cooking or old-fashioned oats in a food processor or blender.

2. Toasting rolled oats boosts their flavor. Spread them in a single layer on a baking sheet and bake, stirring, at 350°F (180°C) for 3 to 5 minutes or until fragrant.

3. Make your own flavored oatmeal "packets." In snack-size zipper-seal bags, combine 1/2 cup quick-cooking oatmeal, 2 tablespoons raisins, 1 tablespoon wheat germ, 1 teaspoon brown sugar, 1/4 teaspoon cinnamon, and a pinch of salt.

Olive Oil

What You're Eating

Press an olive, and you get one of the healthiest fats in the world. Yet olive oil accounts for just 9 percent of world oil consumption and for about 2 percent in the United States, or about one quart per person per year. Compare that to Mediterranean countries like Italy (3 gallons per person per year), Spain (3.75 gallons), and Greece (5.3 gallons). Given the amount of olive oil Greeks consume, it's not surprising that Greece devotes some 60 percent of its cultivated land to olive growing. Don't just pluck one off a tree, though. Raw olives are incredibly bitter until processed (which often involves soaking them in a lye solution). Extra virgin is considered the Rolls Royce of olive oils for its low acidity.

Healing Powers

The main benefit of olive oil, and there are many, is that it lowers "bad" LDL cholesterol and raises "good" HDL cholesterol, thanks to its monounsaturated fats. Olive oil is also packed with antioxidants called phenols, which may protect artery walls from cholesterol buildup. Researchers even discovered recently that olive oil acts as an anti-inflammatory, which further protects your heart, and the rest of your body, too. Inflammation is strongly linked not only to heart disease but also to type 2 diabetes, Alzheimer's disease, and cancer.

Healthful Hint

Look for "virgin," "extra-virgin," or "cold-pressed" oils. They are extracted by pressing alone. The solvents and heat used to produce "light" or "extra-light" oils destroy antioxidants. All olive oils have 120 calories per tablespoon.

KEY NUTRIENTS

> Vitamins E and K
> Monounsaturated fats
> Antioxidants

HOW MUCH IS ENOUGH
Up to 1 tablespoon a day.

BUYING RIGHT
Delicate extra-virgin olive oil is best used uncooked for salad dressings or dipping. Virgin olive oil is perfect for sautéing, so you'll want to keep both on hand.

Three Clever Ideas

1. Best stored in the refrigerator, olive oil does solidify when chilled. A solution: Keep the bottle in the fridge, but fill a clean, pretty, dark wine bottle with 1 cup of oil in a cabinet for when you need it.

2. Using flavored oils saves you from having to add seasoning to dishes. Make your own by adding dried herbs and seasonings to a bottle of oil. Start with different combinations in small bottles until you find a favorite.

3. To prevent over-pouring, don't remove the safety seal from a new bottle. Instead, poke through the seal with the tip of a paring knife. To pour, squeeze or shake the oil into the pan or measuring spoon.

Red Wine & Grape Juice

What You're Drinking

The juice or, in the case of wine, the fermented juice, of grapes. Most wines are made from purple grapes. In making white wine, the grape skins are removed before their pigments add color. The skins contain most of the antioxidants that contribute to wine's health benefits. Grape juice also contains many of the antioxidant compounds found in grape skins. Alcohol, a byproduct of fermentation, is toxic to all living things at various doses; the yeasts that excrete it cannot tolerate an environment that's more than 15 percent alcohol, which is why fermentation stops at about this concentration. In small doses, though, alcohol can be good for the body.

Healing Powers

Most of the health benefits of wine come from the alcohol itself, which raises "good" HDL cholesterol A moderate intake (no more than one or two servings a day) of alcohol has been associated with a decreased risk for heart disease and diabetes. However, a 2018 systematic review of alcohol use in 195 countries caused some to question the healthfulness of alcohol at any level. If you choose to drink alcohol, red wine may offer some added benefits from the plant compounds found in grape skins, such as flavonoids, which help prevent blood clots, and resveratrol, which may lower the risk for heart disease. That said, alcohol promotes certain cancers, including breast cancer and colon cancer. If you have a family history of cancer, favor grape juice.

Healthful Hint

Drink alcohol with meals instead of by itself for the greatest protection from heart attacks.

HOW MUCH IS ENOUGH
One to two 4-ounce (118-ml) glasses of wine (one for women, two for men) or grape juice a day.

BUYING RIGHT
Whether for drinking or cooking, select wine you'll enjoy. Avoid cheap cooking wines loaded with sodium. One rule of thumb: If you wouldn't drink it, don't cook with it.

Three Clever Ideas

1. Red wine can be served with many dishes. Fish, chicken, and eggs need lighter wines like Beaujolais or Pinot Noir. Denser foods with more fat—beef, lamb, and stews—can handle Shiraz, Cabernet, or Zinfandel.

2. When you have just a touch of wine left over, instead of discarding it, place it by tablespoons in an ice cube tray. When frozen, transfer to a zipper-seal plastic bag. Add to sauces as needed.

3. To remove a broken cork from a bottle, place a coffee filter over a carafe or measuring cup and pour the wine through the filter. The cork will come out, too. Serve from the carafe or pour back into the bottle.

Salmon

What You're Eating

A healthier alternative to steak and one of the best sources of omega-3 fatty acids, particularly EPA and DHA—nature's heart medicines. About 70 percent of the salmon you see in supermarkets is farmed, also referred to as aquaculture. If you want wild salmon, choose Alaska salmon, which is wild caught. Most canned salmon in the United States is also wild caught. Because overfishing has caused a decline in the wild salmon population, experts estimate that the majority of fish we will eat in the next decade will be farm-raised. But that is not necessarily bad. Changes in seafood farming practices now produce salmon populations that are both healthful and sustainable. Find the most current recommendations for salmon and other fish at the Monterey Bay Aquarium Seafood Watch program (www.seafoodwatch.org).

Healing Powers

The fat in salmon is like liquid gold when it comes to your blood vessels. Just two servings of salmon a week can reduce your risk of dying from cardiovascular disease by 37 percent. And the benefits appear to go beyond the heart. Recent studies have found that high intakes of omega-3s from fatty fish like salmon may help protect against cancers of the prostate and breast. And although not conclusive, some research has shown that omega-3s may be helpful in the treatment of depression.

Healthful Hint

When food farming practices are used, farmed salmon is just as healthful as wild, say experts. Some farm-raised salmon actually has more omega-3s than its wild counterpart. (For more details, see page 23.)

KEY NUTRIENTS

> Omega-3 fatty acids
> Protein
> Vitamins A, B_3 (niacin), B_{12}, and D
> Zinc
> Magnesium

HOW MUCH IS ENOUGH

Two 4- to 6-ounce servings a week.

BUYING RIGHT

Fresh wild salmon, available from early summer to fall, should look moist and firm. It should smell sea-fresh, not overwhelmingly fishy. When fresh is out of season, go for frozen salmon fillets. Traditionally packed canned salmon offers many benefits, including increased calcium due to its tender edible bones. But since it's messy and time consuming to remove the skin and large bones, opt for ready-to-use boneless, skinless pink salmon sold in cans or pouches.

Three Clever Ideas

1. For a fun appetizer, cut salmon fillets into 1-inch-thick strips and thread onto wooden skewers that have been soaked in water for 30 minutes. Brush with teriyaki sauce and grill just until opaque.

2. To easily remove pin bones from a salmon fillet, place the fish skin side down over a bowl. The bones will stick up, ready for removal with tweezers or pliers.

3. Transferring a large fillet from a baking sheet to a serving plate can be tricky. Slide a flexible cutting board under the cooked fish and gently move to the plate.

Soy

What You're Eating

One of the most nutritious plant foods and the only legume that provides complete protein. All soy foods—from miso to tofu to edamame (green soybeans)—come from soybeans. Tofu is made from pureed soybeans processed into a "cake"; miso, used in soup broths, is fermented soybean paste; soy sauce is a byproduct of miso production; and tempeh is fermented cooked soybeans. While soybeans are native to Southeast Asia, today 55 percent of soybean production occurs in the United States, most of it for oil.

Healing Powers

Just a cup of boiled soybeans provides more than 7 grams of fiber—more than in a baked sweet potato. One cup of cooked soybeans contains more protein and iron than 3 ounces of beef and almost as much calcium as 1 cup of milk. But it's soy's phytoestrogens called isoflavones that take center stage. They may help cool off hot flashes, and there's some evidence they may block certain hormone-related cancers, including breast and prostate cancer. They're thought to help lower blood pressure and stave off bone loss. Soy foods may reduce your risk of heart disease, especially if you eat them in place of meat and full-fat dairy foods, which is easy to do since soy can mimic nearly any food product, from meat (think soy crumbles) to milk (soy milk) to nuts (soy nuts, which are roasted soybeans).

Healthful Hint

Minimally processed soy foods like tofu, soy nuts, and soy milk retain more isoflavones than processed soy products like soy-based deli "meat" or soy "bacon."

KEY NUTRIENTS

> B vitamins
> Protein
> Potassium
> Zinc
> Iron

HOW MUCH IS ENOUGH

There's no official overall recommendation. Some experts recommend 25 grams of soy protein a day. Others just recommend replacing meat with soy whenever you can.

BUYING RIGHT

Look for calcium-enriched soy milk in the refrigerated section of your supermarket and buy a low-fat brand. It keeps for about a week after opening. Choose soy sauce that's labeled "naturally brewed" to avoid artificial flavoring and coloring. Edamame is most readily available frozen, both in and out of the shell. Look for fresh edamame in summer.

Three Clever Ideas

1. Add soy flour to your baked goods by substituting it for one-third of the flour called for. It's best cooked at lower temperatures, so decrease the oven temperature by 25°F (4°C) and check for doneness 5 to 10 minutes early.

2. Soy nuts make great snacks, especially if you buy them un-salted. Also toss them into salads instead of croutons.

3. Snack on edamame in the pods by slipping the beans out of the pod and into your mouth. To add flavor, partially steam the pods, then add to a hot skillet with a bit of oil and stir-fry until lightly browned. Sprinkle with salt.

Spinach

What You're Eating

One of the best sources of the B vitamin folate—a cancer fighter—and carotenoids such as lutein, which helps prevent macular degeneration, the leading cause of blindness in older adults. One thing you're not eating: a lot of iron. The myth that spinach is rich in iron (which made Popeye strong) surfaced back in 1870 when a researcher's misplaced decimal point in a publication gave spinach an iron content 10 times higher than reality. Reality is that a serving (1/2 cup) of raw spinach contains less than 1 milligram of iron. Iron and calcium in spinach are not well absorbed by your body, thanks to high concentrations of oxalic acid.

Healing Powers

In addition to protecting your eyes from age-related macular degeneration, thanks to its carotenoids, spinach has high concentrations of vitamin K, which can help maintain bone density and prevent fractures. The green stuff is also a powerful source of potassium and magnesium as well as folate, all of which can keep blood pressure low, reducing the risk of stroke. Folate also appears to slash the risk of lung cancer in former smokers.

Healthful Hint

To absorb more of the iron from spinach, eat it with foods rich in vitamin C, such as red bell peppers or orange slices.

KEY NUTRIENTS

> Beta-carotene
> Vitamins B_2 (riboflavin), B_6, C, and K
> Folate (a B vitamin)
> Potassium

HOW MUCH IS ENOUGH

1 cup raw or 1/2 cup cooked spinach leaves is one vegetable serving.

BUYING RIGHT

Choose crisp, bright green leaves and stems with no sign of yellowing, wilting, or bruising. For mild flavor and delicate texture, buy baby spinach. The best way to remove sand is to swish the spinach in a sink or bowl of water; as the leaves float, the sand sinks. Opting for prepackaged, prerinsed spinach eliminates this step. Products that are triple-washed are safe to eat out of the bag.

Three Clever Ideas

1. A quick way to squeeze spinach dry is to place it in a single layer on a plate and top with an identical plate, then hold the plates together vertically over the sink and press them together.

2. Your teakettle will make preparing blanched spinach a breeze. Place clean, stemmed spinach in a metal colander in the sink and pour boiling water over it. Follow with cold water to stop the cooking.

3. Sneak some spinach into soups and stews by cutting it as you would an herb. To chiffonade, stack about 10 leaves on top of each other, roll them like a cigar, and slice crosswise into thin strips.

Sweet Potatoes

What You're Eating

A New World plant introduced to Europeans by Columbus and other explorers; not to be confused with white potatoes, to which they are unrelated. They are also unrelated to yams (starchy edible roots native to Africa and low in vitamins), although they are sometimes marketed as yams in North America. They derive their flavor from an enzyme that converts starches to sugars. Like other orange-yellow vegetables, they're an excellent source of beta-carotene, a precursor of vitamin A. Just one provides more than 100 percent of the RDA of vitamin A and more than a third of the RDA of vitamin C.

Healing Powers

Sweet potatoes are a great source of the soluble fiber pectin, which soaks up cholesterol, and of insoluble fiber (mostly in the skin), which helps prevent constipation and hemorrhoids and may reduce the risk of stomach and colon cancer. Their high levels of beta-carotene protect against heart disease and many cancers, help keep skin healthy, and fuel a healthy immune system.

Healthful Hint

Eat the skin of the sweet potato since that's where much of the fiber lies.

KEY NUTRIENTS

> Beta-carotene

> Vitamins B_6, C, and E

> Potassium

> Folate (a B vitamin)

> Iron

HOW MUCH IS ENOUGH

One medium (5-ounce) sweet potato is one vegetable serving.

BUYING RIGHT

Choose smooth, plump, dry sweet potatoes free of wrinkles, sprouts, or decay. Grab the ones with the darkest skin, as these also have bright orange flesh that offers the most nutrients. Store in a cool, dark place other than the refrigerator. Toss any that show the least sign of mold; once mold strikes, the entire potato will taste "off."

Three Clever Ideas

1. Cooking sweet potatoes in lots of water, as for traditional mashed potatoes, will leach nutrients and flavor. Instead, simmer over low heat in a bit of broth and mash without draining.

2. Not just for the holidays, sweet potatoes are great in the summer. Grill skewers of sweet potato chunks brushed with a touch of olive oil and sprinkled with cinnamon or ginger. They cook fastest on metal skewers that get hot and cook the potato from the inside while the flame sears the outside.

3. A simple way to prepare sweet potatoes is to cut them into cubes and toss in a bit of olive oil. Roast in the oven until tender and lightly browned. Sprinkle with spices such as cinnamon, ginger, or chili powder.

Tea

What You're Drinking

The world's most popular nonalcoholic beverage and one of the most potent sources of antioxidants in nature (more potent than any fruit or vegetable). Whether you're drinking black tea, green tea, or something in between, you're drinking a beverage made from the leaves of the *Camellia sinensis* plant. In black tea, the leaves are crushed and allowed to "ferment" in the tea's own enzymes; green tea is not fermented. The finest leaves are plucked from the youngest shoots and unopened leaf buds. Tea contains antioxidants that belong to a group called flavonoids and is especially rich in catechins, which give it most of its health benefits.

Healing Powers

Tea's antioxidants offer protection from heart disease, stroke, and cancer. They appear to protect against heart disease by slowing the breakdown of "bad" LDL cholesterol, preventing blood clots, and improving blood vessel function. People who drink a cup or two of tea a day have a 46 percent lower risk of developing narrowed arteries. The antioxidants also protect against the DNA damage that causes cells to turn cancerous. In cell studies, one of the most important catechins, called epigallocatechin gallate (EGCG), blocked an enzyme that cancer cells need to grow. While black tea may stain your teeth, tannins and fluoride protect against tooth decay.

Healthful Hint

Brew black tea for at least 5 minutes to draw out the maximum amount of catechins. Drink most of your tea between meals since the tannins interfere with the absorption of iron from food.

KEY NUTRIENTS

> Flavonoids (antioxidants), especially catechins
> Tannins
> Vitamin K (green tea only)

HOW MUCH IS ENOUGH

2 to 5 cups daily.

BUYING RIGHT

For the freshest tea, shop at a store that has a good turnover rate and buy only as much as you can use in a month. Tea is best stored in airtight dark glass containers in a cool, dry place since refrigerating or freezing can ruin its flavor. Caffeine content of teas varies, but generally has about half the caffeine of coffee.

Three Clever Ideas

1. The easiest way to remove tea bags from iced tea is to first tie the bags onto a skewer. Place the skewer over a pitcher with the tea bags hanging down, then add water. After the tea brews, simply lift out the skewer.

2. When boiling water to cook whole grains, add a green tea bag. Boil for 3 minutes, then remove the bag before adding the grains.

3. Sprinkle green or white tea leaves on salads or stir-fries or add to chicken- or fish-based soups or stews.

Whole Wheat

What You're Eating

Wheat in its "whole" form. That includes the bran, or outer husk of the plant, which is strong enough to protect the other two major parts of the plant—the germ and endosperm—from too much sunlight, water, and attacks from pests and diseases. The germ is the plant's embryo, which eventually becomes a new stalk of wheat. Many of the nutrients and much of the fiber in wheat are contained in the bran and germ—the parts that are removed when whole wheat is refined into white flour. That leaves the endosperm, which is mostly starch and protein.

Healing Powers

Whole grains are a surprising source of antioxidants. The high fiber and B vitamin content of whole wheat plays a major role in the grain's ability to reduce the risk of death from cardiovascular disease—and in fact from any cause. The fiber may also lower your risk of colon cancer. Whole grains such as whole wheat contain plant estrogens called lignans, which help lower estrogen levels and encourage cancer cells to self-destruct. On the whole (no pun intended), whole grains digest more slowly than refined grains do, so they don't raise blood sugar as quickly or dramatically. This keeps insulin levels low—a boon to both diabetes and cancer prevention.

Healthful Hint

Make sure the word *whole*, as in "whole-wheat flour," is part of the first ingredient listed in any grain product to make sure you're getting the real thing. If you see "wheat flour," that's white flour.

KEY NUTRIENTS

> Fiber
> Vitamins B_2 (riboflavin), B_3 (niacin), and other B vitamins

HOW MUCH IS ENOUGH

At least three servings of a whole-wheat or whole-grain food a day to help boost your daily fiber intake. A serving is a slice of bread or an ounce of breakfast cereal.

BUYING RIGHT

Since whole-wheat flour doesn't move as fast as white flour, be sure to purchase it from a store with good turnover. Whole-wheat flour contains some fat from the bran, so store it in a sealed container in the fridge for up to six months.

Three Clever Ideas

1. For baking, use white whole-wheat or whole-grain (wheat) pastry flour. These types are more finely ground than whole-wheat flour and work better in baking.

2. Although whole-wheat bread is readily available, whole-wheat crumbs are not. Make your own by saving bread ends and any stale slices in the freezer in a zipper-seal plastic bag. Pulse in a food processor to form crumbs.

3. Create a delicious, healthy topping for baked casseroles or gratins by sprinkling with toasted wheat germ before baking.

Yogurt

What You're Eating

Pasteurized milk to which live bacteria cultures have been added for fermentation. Once the desired acidity is reached, the fermentation is stopped by cooling the yogurt. The bacteria cultures consume much of the lactose, or milk sugar, found in milk—which is why even people who are lactose intolerant can often eat yogurt with no problem—and release lactic acid, the stuff that makes yogurt tangy. Yogurt contains the same amount of fat as the milk it's made with. Some brands contain pectin or gelatin for added body.

Healing Powers

Yogurt is a great source of bone-building calcium, but its real strength lies in live beneficial bacteria, known as probiotics, that keep down the growth of harmful bacteria in your gut. Too many "bad" bacteria can lead to gastrointestinal and other health problems. Eating more yogurt could help with inflammatory bowel disease, ulcers, urinary tract infections, and vaginal yeast infections, to name a few conditions. Getting plenty of "good" bacteria from yogurt is particularly important when you take antibiotics, which wipe out all bacteria, good and bad, in your gut. Probiotics also produce immunity-enhancing compounds and natural antibiotics that help reduce levels of nasty bacteria in the gut.

Healthful Hint

Look on the label for *Lactobacillus acidophilus, Bifidobacterium bifidum,* and *Streptococcus thermophilus,* among other active cultures.

KEY NUTRIENTS

> Protein
> Calcium
> Vitamin A
> B vitamins
> Zinc
> Phosphorus

HOW MUCH IS ENOUGH

1 cup a day of low-fat or fat-free yogurt with live cultures.

BUYING RIGHT

Choose low-fat yogurt that's not overly sweetened and look for "live bacteria" on the container. Also get the freshest yogurt you can find; the longer a product has been refrigerated and the more pasteurized it is, the fewer active bacteria it contains.

Three Clever Ideas

1. Yogurt can break down during cooking, so if you're adding it to a hot dish, stir 1 tablespoon flour or cornstarch into 1 cup yogurt. Remove the pan from the heat and stir in the yogurt until creamy.

2. Most store-bought chocolate yogurt doesn't contain as many live, active cultures as plain yogurt. Make your own by stirring cocoa powder and a bit of sugar into fat-free or low-fat plain yogurt.

3. When coating pork, chicken, or fish with bread crumbs, replace the eggs used to moisten the meat with plain yogurt. Plan on using about 8 ounces of yogurt per pound of protein.

10 Healing Herbs AND Spices

Imagine garlic bread without the garlic, apple pie without the cinnamon, and lamb curry without the turmeric (the stuff that makes curry powder yellow).

There's no doubt that herbs and spices add distinctive flavors to our cooking. But little do most people know that the red, yellow, and brown powders they sprinkle on their food—not to mention the fresh herbs they cook with—also add significant health benefits. After all, herbs and spices come from plants, and many plants, as scientists are learning, contain a variety of healing substances—often found in high concentrations in the seeds, oils, and other plant parts that make up herbs and spices.

You may think of blueberries when you think of antioxidants, but you should also think of cloves. You know by now that fatty fish combats inflammation, but so does ginger. Certain herbs and spices—garlic and turmeric in particular—may even help us stave off cancer. And many are potent killers of bacteria and viruses.

Dozens of herbs and spices contain useful plant compounds, but the following 10 are healing standouts.

Cayenne

That burning sensation in your mouth when you eat foods spiced with cayenne (red) pepper comes from capsaicin, the oily compound behind most of the health benefits of cayenne and its peppery cousins. Capsaicin is the active ingredient in many prescription and over-the-counter creams, ointments, and patches for arthritis and muscle pain. Over time, it short-circuits pain by depleting nerve cells of a chemical called substance P, which helps transfer pain signals along nerve endings to the brain. It's also used for treating shingles pain and diabetes-related nerve pain.

Cayenne's benefits don't end there, however. Sprinkle some onto your chicken soup to turbocharge that traditional cold remedy, since cayenne shrinks blood vessels in your nose and throat, relieving congestion. It's also a metabolism booster, speeding up your calorie-burning furnace for a couple of hours after eating. Cayenne is thought to act as an anti-inflammatory and antioxidant. Studies find that it also has some anticancer properties, and researchers are exploring its potential as a cancer treatment. Finally, in at least one study, published in the *American Journal of Clinical Nutrition,* researchers found that people with diabetes who ate a meal containing liberal amounts of chile pepper required less postmeal insulin to reduce their blood sugar, suggesting the spice may have antidiabetes benefits.

Cinnamon

Cinnamon on toast or oatmeal is so tasty it's hard to believe the brown powder has any health benefits at all, but it's actually one of the most powerful healing spices. It's become most famous for its ability to improve blood sugar control in people with diabetes, although recent clinical trials show inconsistent results. Still, some of its natural compounds may improve insulin function, which may help lower blood sugar with as little as 1/4 to 1/2 teaspoon a day. The same amount could cut triglycerides and total cholesterol levels by 12 to 30 percent. The apple pie spice can even help prevent blood clots, making it especially heart smart.

Like many other spices, cinnamon has antibacterial and anti-inflammatory properties. It's been shown to conquer *E. coli,* among other types of bacteria. Researchers have even discovered recently that it's rich in antioxidants called polyphenols—another reason it's good for your heart. It's also a source of fiber (after all, it comes from the bark of a tree) and can reduce heartburn in some people.

Cloves

Cloves, an aromatic spice common in Indian cooking, contain an anti-inflammatory chemical called eugenol. In recent animal studies, this chemical inhibited COX-2, a protein that spurs inflammation (the same protein that so-called COX-2 inhibitor drugs such as Celebrex quash). Cloves also ranked very high in antioxidant properties in one study. The combination of anti-inflammatory and antioxidant properties spells heaps of health benefits, from boosting protection from heart disease to helping stave off cancer, as well as slowing the cartilage and bone damage caused by arthritis. Compounds in cloves, like those found in cinnamon, also appear to improve insulin function.

Have a toothache? Put a couple of whole cloves in your mouth. Let them soften a bit, then bite on them gently with good molars to release their oil. Then move them next to the painful tooth and keep them there for up to half an hour. Clove oil has a numbing effect in addition to bacteria-fighting powers. In test tubes, cloves also killed certain bacteria that were resistant to antibiotics.

Coriander

Coriander seeds yield cilantro, also known as Chinese parsley, a staple herb in Mexican, Thai, Vietnamese, and Indian cooking. The seeds have been used for thousands of years as a digestive aid. Try making a strong tea from crushed seeds (strain before drinking). The herb can be helpful for some people with irritable bowel syndrome, as it calms intestinal spasms that can lead to diarrhea. Preliminary studies in animals support another traditional use for coriander— as an antianxiety herb. Its essential oil appears to fight bacteria, including *E. coli* and salmonella. It's also being studied for its potential cholesterol-reducing benefits and has been shown to lower cholesterol in animals.

Like many other herbs, this one acts as an antioxidant. According to one study, cilantro leaves provide the most antioxidant punch.

Garlic

Smash a clove of garlic and take in the pungent fragrance. That famous odor comes from byproducts of allicin, the sulfur compound believed to be responsible for most of the herb's medicinal benefits. It's what gives garlic its "bite."

When eaten daily, garlic may help lower heart disease risk by moderately reducing cholesterol levels (by between 5 and 10 percent in some studies), by thinning the blood and thereby staving off dangerous clots, and by acting as an antioxidant. Garlic's sulfur compounds also appear to ward off cancer, especially stomach and colorectal cancer. The compounds flush out carcinogens before they can damage cell DNA, and they force cancer cells that do develop to self-destruct.

Strongly antibacterial and antifungal, garlic can help with yeast infections, some sinus infections, and the common cold. It can even repel ticks (as well as friends and family, if you eat enough).

Ginger

This gnarled root has been a major player in Asian and Indian medicine for centuries, primarily as a digestive aid. Today researchers are most excited by ginger's ability to combat inflammation. Several studies have found that ginger (and turmeric) reduces pain and swelling in people with arthritis. It may work against migraines by blocking inflammatory substances called prostaglandins. And because it reduces inflammation, it may also play a role in preventing and slowing the growth of cancer.

Ginger's still good for the tummy, too. It works in the digestive tract, boosting digestive juices and neutralizing acids as well as reducing intestinal contractions. It's proven quite effective against nausea. In fact, at least one study found ginger to work just as well as Dramamine (dimenhydrinate) and other nausea-stopping drugs, with the added benefit that it doesn't make you sleepy. The trick is to take ginger (in tablet, powder, or natural form) *before* you think you may become nauseated, when it works best. It's also an effective, short-term treatment for morning sickness.

Mustard

Mustard is made from the seeds of a plant in the cabbage family—a strongly anticancer group of plants. Indeed, mustard seeds contain compounds that studies suggest may inhibit the growth of cancer cells.

Mustard also packs enough heat to break up congestion, the reason it was traditionally used in chest plasters. Like cayenne pepper, it has the ability to deplete nerve cells of substance P, a chemical that transmits pain signals to the brain, when used externally. A mustard compress also brings more blood to the fingers of people with Raynaud's phenomenon, a circulatory problem that causes frigid fingers.

Mustard is also said to stimulate appetite by increasing the flow of saliva and digestive juices. A bit of mustard powder added to a footbath helps kill athlete's foot fungus. Don't eat too many mustard seeds or more than a teaspoon of mustard powder; the former has a strong laxative effect, while the latter can induce vomiting.

Nutmeg

Like cloves, nutmeg contains eugenol, a compound that may benefit the heart. It was one of the key spices that give the Spice Islands their name, and some historians link its popularity in the spice trade to the hallucinatory effects that result from ingesting large amounts. The euphoria, which is due to nutmeg's active ingredient, myristicin, is described as similar to that caused by the drug ecstasy. Don't worry about your teens raiding your spice drawer for a quick high, however; it also packs some nasty side effects, and nutmeg poisoning is a very real risk.

Medically, nutmeg (the seed of an evergreen tree) and mace (the covering of the seed) have strong antibacterial properties. It's been found to kill a number of bacteria in the mouth that contribute to cavities. Myristicin has also been shown to inhibit an enzyme in the brain that contributes to Alzheimer's disease and to improve memory in mice, and researchers are currently studying its potential as an antidepressant.

Sage

Perhaps it's no coincidence that "sage" describes a wise person; the herb is a known memory enhancer and has been shown in some lab studies to protect the brain against certain processes that lead to Alzheimer's disease. In at least one human study, a sage-oil concoction improved the mood of participants, increasing their alertness, calmness, and contentedness. In a British study, healthy young adults performed better on word recall tests after taking sage-oil capsules.

Like so many other herbs and spices, sage has anti-inflammatory and antioxidant properties as well as anticancer actions. One of its phytochemicals is thujone, best known as a chemical in the liquor absinthe that is said (falsely) to have hallucinatory effects. Today sage shows potential as a diabetes treatment. It appears to boost the action of insulin and reduce blood sugar. As a result, sage is sometimes called nature's metformin since it performs like the common antidiabetes drug. Some researchers have already suggested that sage supplements may be beneficial for people with type 2 diabetes.

Turmeric

Turmeric, the spice that gives curry powder its yellow hue, is used in Indian medicine to stimulate the appetite and as a digestive aid. But lately it's grabbing some serious attention as a potentially powerful cancer fighter. The chemical responsible for turmeric's golden color, called curcumin, is considered a top anticancer agent, helping to quell the inflammation that contributes to tumor growth and working in much the same way as broccoli and cauliflower to clear carcinogens away before they can damage cellular DNA and to repair already damaged DNA. Preliminary studies found that substances in turmeric may reduce the number of heart attacks bypass patients had after surgery, control knee pain from osteoarthritis as well as ibuprofen did, and reduce the skin irritation that often occurs after radiation treatments for breast cancer.

Studies have also linked turmeric to reduced inflammation in a number of conditions, including psoriasis. In animal studies, curcumin decreased the formation of amyloid, the stuff that makes up the brain deposits characteristic in people with Alzheimer's disease.

WHERE THE Nutrients Are

Coming up in Part Three, you'll discover food prescriptions for 56 common ailments, which highlight foods rich in key nutrients and phytochemicals that science tells us can help treat what ails us or prevent new health problems. Look to the tables here to find more good food sources of these substances, such as macronutrients (like monounsaturated fats and omega-3 fatty acids), micronutrients (like vitamins and minerals), and phytochemicals (like beta-carotene and isoflavones). These are the compounds that put the healing power in nature's edible medicines. We've also included fiber here even though it's not technically a nutrient because it isn't absorbed by the body, but is important nonetheless.

One of the units of measurements you'll see in these tables is "µg," which stands for micrograms (a microgram is 1/1,000 of a milligram). Another unit is IU, which stands for international units. Used for some vitamins—especially those that come in different forms—it indicates the amount of a vitamin needed to achieve a certain biological effect. To convert milligrams of vitamin E to IUs of alpha-tocopherol (the natural form of E), multiply the number of milligrams by 1.5 (or by 2.2 to convert to IUs of synthetic vitamin E). To convert IUs of vitamin E to milligrams of natural vitamin E, multiply the number of IUs by 0.67 (or by 0.45 for synthetic E).

Researchers haven't yet discovered all of food's healing compounds. A good rule of thumb, then: Eat more fruits and vegetables, add fish to your weekly menu, and choose whole grains over refined grains.

NUTRIENT/PHYTOCHEMICAL	FOOD	AMOUNT
Antioxidants (measured by total antioxidant capacity)	Cloves, ground (3 tablespoons)	125.55
	Cinnamon (3 tablespoons)	77.0
	Oregano (3 tablespoons)	40.3
	Walnuts (2/3 cup)	21.9
	Turmeric (3 tablespoons)	15.68
	Dark chocolate (3 1/2 ounces)	14.98
	Artichokes (1/2 cup)	4.54
	Pecans (2/3 cup)	8.5
	Raspberries (3/4 cup)	2.3
	Strawberries (3/4 cup)	2.1
	Blackberries (3/4 cup)	2.0
	Blueberries, cultivated (3/4 cup)	1.85
	Yellow bell pepper (1 medium)	1.79
	Cranberries (3/4 cup)	1.64
	Pinto beans, cooked (1/2 cup)	1.15
	Hazelnuts (2/3 cup)	0.94
	Raisins (1/2 cup)	0.91
	Sweet potato, baked (1 medium)	0.79
	Almonds (2/3 cup)	0.53

NUTRIENT/PHYTOCHEMICAL	FOOD	AMOUNT
	Black-eyed peas, cooked (1/2 cup)	0.50
	Russet potato, cooked (1 medium)	0.42
	Avocado, Hass (1 medium)	0.41
	Small red beans, cooked (1/2 cup)	0.33
	Pear, green (1 medium)	0.23
	Apple, Red Delicious with peel (1 medium)	0.4
Beta-carotene	Sweet potato, baked, with skin (1 cup)	23,018 µg
	Carrot juice, canned (1 cup)	21,955 µg
	Pumpkin, canned (1 cup)	17,003 µg
	Spinach, frozen, cooked (1 cup)	13,750 µg
	Carrots, boiled (1 cup)	11,971 µg
	Collards, frozen, cooked (1 cup)	11,591 µg
	Carrots, raw (1 cup)	10,605 µg
	Turnip greens, frozen, cooked (1 cup)	10,593 µg
	Butternut squash, baked (1 cup)	9,368 µg
	Beet greens, cooked (1 cup)	6,610 µg
	Winter squash, all varieties (1 cup)	5,726 µg
	Cantaloupe (1 cup)	3,575 µg
	Dried apricots (1 cup)	2,812 µg
	Kale, frozen, cooked (1 cup)	2,043 µg
Calcium	Tofu prepared with calcium sulfate (1/2 cup)	434 mg
	Nonfat dry milk powder (1/4 cup)	377 mg
	Collards, frozen, cooked (1 cup)	357 mg
	Yogurt, fruit, low-fat (8 ounces)	345 mg
	Soy milk with calcium (1 cup)	340 mg
	Ricotta cheese, part skim (1/2 cup)	337 mg
	Milk, fat-free (1 cup)	306 mg
	Milk, 1% (1 cup)	300 mg
	Spinach, frozen, cooked (1 cup)	291 mg
	Cheddar cheese (1 ounce)	204 mg
	White beans, canned (1 cup)	191 mg
	Salmon, canned, with bones and liquid (3 ounces)	181 mg
	Soybeans, mature, cooked (1 cup)	175 mg
Fiber	Soybeans, roasted (1 cup)	30.0 g
	Navy beans, cooked (1 cup)	19.1 g
	Kidney beans, canned (1 cup)	16.5 g
	Split peas, cooked (1 cup)	16.3 g
	Lentils, cooked, (1 cup)	15.6 g
	Pinto beans, cooked (1 cup)	15.4 g
	Black beans, cooked (1 cup)	15.0 g
	Figs, dried (1 cup)	14.6 g

NUTRIENT/PHYTOCHEMICAL	FOOD	AMOUNT
	Oat bran, raw (1 cup)	14.5 g
	Lima beans, cooked (1 cup)	13.2 g
	Chickpeas, cooked (1 cup)	12.5 g
	Raspberries, frozen, sweetened (1 cup)	11.0 g
	Soybeans, mature, cooked (1 cup)	10.3 g
	Cornmeal, whole grain, yellow (1 cup)	8.9 g
	Green peas, frozen, cooked (1 cup)	8.8 g
	Cereal, Kellogg's All-Bran (1/2 cup)	8.8 g
	Bulgur, cooked (1 cup)	8.2 g
	Mixed vegetables, frozen, cooked (1 cup)	8.0 g
	Raspberries (1 cup)	8.0 g
	Soybeans, green, cooked (1 cup)	7.6 g
	Spinach, frozen, chopped, cooked (1 cup)	7.0 g
	Brussels sprouts, frozen, cooked (1 cup)	6.4 g
	Spaghetti, whole wheat, cooked (1 cup)	6.3 g
	Pearled barley, cooked (1 cup)	6.0 g
	Oat bran, cooked (1 cup)	5.7 g
	Winter squash, cooked (1 cup)	5.7 g
	Raisins (1 cup)	5.4 g
	Pear	5.1 g
	Sweet potato, cooked, with skin	4.8 g
	Carrots, cooked (1 cup)	4.7 g
	Potato, baked, with skin	4.4 g
	Dates, dried, 7 dates	3.0 g
Folate (Dietary folate equivalents, or DFE) to reflect food folate and added folic acid	Beef liver, braised (3 ounces)	215
	Spinach, boiled (1/2 cup)	131
	Black-eyed peas (cowpeas), boiled (1/2 cup)	105
	Breakfast cereals, fortified with folate, such as Total (3/4 cup)	100
	Asparagus, boiled, 4 spears	89
	Spaghetti, cooked, enriched (1/2 cup)	83
	Brussels sprouts, frozen, boiled (1/2 cup)	78
	Lettuce, romaine, shredded (1 cup)	64
	Avocado, raw, sliced (1/2 cup)	59
	Spinach, raw (1 cup)	58
	Broccoli, chopped, frozen, cooked (1/2 cup)	52
	Mustard greens, chopped, frozen, boiled (1/2 cup)	52
	Green peas, frozen, boiled (1/2 cup)	47
	Kidney beans, canned (1/2 cup)	46
	Peanuts, dry roasted (1 ounce)	41
	Wheat germ (2 tablespoons)	40
	Tomato juice, canned (3/4 cup)	36

NUTRIENT/PHYTOCHEMICAL	FOOD	AMOUNT
	Turnip greens, frozen, boiled (1/2 cup)	32
	Orange, fresh, 1 small	29
	Papaya, raw, cubed (1/2 cup)	27
	Banana (1 medium)	24
Iron	Cereal, fortified oatmeal (1 cup cooked)	19.78 mg
	Turkey giblets, cooked (1 cup)	14.96 mg
	Flour, wheat or white, enriched (1 cup)	10.03 mg
	Rice, white, long-grain, enriched (1 cup)	9.73 mg
	Soybeans, cooked (1 cup)	8.84 mg
	Chili with beans, canned (1 cup)	8.78 mg
	Cornmeal, enriched (1 cup)	8.41 mg
	Beans, white, canned (1 cup)	7.83 mg
	Lentils, cooked (1 cup)	6.59 mg
	Spinach, cooked (1 cup)	6.43 mg
	Oysters, raw (6 medium)	5.50 mg
	Pumpkin seeds, roasted (1 ounce)	4.24 mg
	Potato, baked, with skin (1 medium)	4.08 mg
	Turkey, dark meat, cooked (1 cup, 140 grams)	3.37 mg
	Beef, chuck blade roast, cooked (3 ounces)	3.13 mg
	Shrimp, cooked (3 ounces)	2.63 mg
	Beef, bottom round, cooked (3 ounces)	2.44 mg
	Clams, canned (3 ounces)	2.28 mg
	Beef, ground, 85% lean, cooked (3 ounces)	2.21 mg
	Cashews (1/4 cup)	2.05 mg
	Tuna, light, canned in water (3 ounces)	1.30 mg
Isoflavones (phytoestrogens) (all servings are 100 grams or 3.5 ounces)	Soy flour, full fat	178.10 mg
	Soy flour, defatted	150.94 mg
	Soybeans, dry roasted	148.50 mg
	Soy protein isolate	91.05 mg
	Natto (fermented soybeans), boiled	82.29 mg
	Miso soup mix, dry	69.84 mg
	Soybean flakes, full fat	62.31 mg
	Soybeans, boiled	54.66 mg
	Soybean chips	54.16 mg
	Tempeh, cooked	35.64 mg
	Tofu	22.70 mg
	Soy cheese, American	17.95 mg
	Soybeans, boiled (edamame)	17.92 mg
	Soy protein concentrate	11.49 mg
	Soy milk	7.85 mg
	Split peas	0.44 mg

Nutrient/Phytochemical	Food	Amount
Lycopene	Tomatoes, pureed, canned (1 cup)	54,385 µg
	Pasta sauce, with mushrooms, ready to serve (1 cup)	46,408 µg
	Tomato sauce, canned (1 cup)	34,043 µg
	Vegetable juice cocktail, canned (1 cup)	23,377 µg
	Tomato juice, canned (1 cup)	21,960 µg
	Tomato soup, canned (1 cup)	16,162 µg
	Tomatoes, stewed, canned (1 cup)	10,424 µg
	Pasta with meatballs in tomato sauce, canned (1 cup)	8,494 µg
	Tomatoes, cooked (1 cup)	7,298 µg
	Beef noodle soup, canned (1 cup)	7,147 µg
	Vegetable soup, chunky, canned (1 cup)	7,087 µg
	Watermelon (1 cup)	6,979 µg
	Papaya (1 cup)	2,651 µg
	Pink grapefruit (1 cup)	2,610 µg
Magnesium	Almonds, dry roasted (1 ounce)	80 mg
	Spinach, boiled (1/2 cup)	78 mg
	Cashews, dry roasted (1 ounce)	74 mg
	Peanuts, oil roasted (1/4 cup)	63 mg
	Cereal, shredded wheat (2 large biscuits)	61 mg
	Soy milk, plain or vanilla (1 cup)	61 mg
	Black beans, cooked (1/2 cup)	60 mg
	Edamame, shelled, cooked (1/2 cup)	50 mg
	Peanut butter, smooth (2 tablespoons)	49 mg
	Bread, whole wheat (2 slices)	46 mg
	Avocado, cubed (1 cup)	44 mg
	Potato, baked with skin (3.5 ounces)	43 mg
	Rice, brown, cooked (1/2 cup)	42 mg
	Yogurt, plain, low fat (8 ounces)	42 mg
	Breakfast cereals, fortified with 10% of the DV for magnesium	40 mg
	Oatmeal, instant (1 packet)	36 mg
Monounsaturated fatty acids	Macadamia nuts, dry roasted (1 ounce, 10–12 nuts)	16.800 g
	Hazelnuts (1 ounce)	12.940 g
	Pecans (1 ounce, about 20 halves)	11.570 g
	Olive oil (1 tablespoon)	9.850 g
	Almonds (1 ounce, about 24 nuts)	9.116 g
	Canola oil (1 tablespoon)	8.246 g
	Peanuts, oil roasted, salted (1 ounce)	7.353 g
	Cashew nuts, dry roasted, salted (1 ounce, about 18 nuts)	7.349 g
	Peanuts, dry roasted, salted (1 ounce, about 28 nuts)	6.985 g
	Peanut oil (1 tablespoon)	6.237 g
	Pine nuts, dried (1 ounce)	5.320 g
	Peanut butter, chunky (1 tablespoon)	3.930 g
	Peanut butter, smooth (1 tablespoon)	3.794 g

NUTRIENT/PHYTOCHEMICAL	FOOD	AMOUNT
	Avocado, Hass (1 ounce)	2.778 g
	Avocado, Florida (1 ounce)	1.563 g
Omega-3 fatty acids	Flaxseed oil (1 tablespoon)	7.25 g
	Chia seeds (1 ounce)	5.05 g
	Walnuts (1/4 cup)	2.5 g
	Mackerel, Atlantic, cooked (3.5 ounces)	2.6 g
	Flaxseed meal	2.0 g
	Trout, lake, cooked (3.5 ounces)	2.0 g
	Salmon, farmed, cooked (3.5 ounces)	1.9 g
	Herring, Pacific (3.5 ounces)	1.8 g
	Anchovies, canned (3.5 ounces)	1.7 g
	Tuna, bluefin, cooked (3.5 ounces)	1.6 g
	Walnut oil (1 tablespoon)	1.6 g
	Sablefish, cooked (3.5 ounces)	1.5 g
	Salmon, Chinook, cooked (3.5 ounces)	1.5 g
	Sardines, canned (3.5 ounces)	1.5 g
	Canola/rapeseed oil (1 tablespoon)	1.29 g
	Herring, pickled (3.5 ounces)	1.2 g
	Bass, cooked (3.5 ounces)	0.8 g
Potassium	Apricots, dried (1/2 cup)	1,101 mg
	Lentils, cooked (1 cup)	731 mg
	Prunes, dried (1/2 cup)	699 mg
	Squash, acorn, mashed (1 cup)	644 mg
	Raisins (1/2 cup)	618 mg
	Potato, baked, flesh only (1 medium)	610 mg
	Kidney beans, canned (1 cup)	607 mg
	Orange juice (1 cup)	496 mg
	Soybeans, mature seeds, boiled (1/2 cup)	443 mg
	Banana (1 medium)	422 mg
	Milk, 1% (1 cup)	366 mg
Selenium	Brazil nuts (1 ounce) (6–8 nuts)	544 mcg
	Tuna, yellowfin, cooked, dry heat (3 ounces)	92 mcg
	Halibut, cooked, dry heat (3 ounces)	47 mcg
	Sardines, canned in oil, drained solids with bone (3 ounces)	45 mcg
	Ham, roasted (3 ounces)	42 mcg
	Shrimp, canned (3 ounces)	40 mcg
	Macaroni, enriched, cooked (1 cup)	37 mcg
	Beef steak, bottom round, roasted (3 ounces)	33 mcg
	Turkey, boneless, roasted (3 ounces)	31 mcg
	Beef liver, pan fried (3 ounces)	28 mcg
	Chicken, light meat, roasted (3 ounces)	22 mcg
	Cottage cheese, 1% milkfat (1 cup)	20 mcg
	Rice, brown, long-grain, cooked (1 cup)	19 mcg

Nutrient/Phytochemical	Food	Amount
Vitamin B$_6$	Chickpeas, canned (1 cup)	1.1 mg
	Beef liver, pan fried (3 ounces)	0.9 mg
	Tuna, yellowfin, fresh, cooked (3 ounces)	0.9 mg
	Salmon, sockeye, cooked (3 ounces)	0.6 mg
	Breakfast cereals, fortified with 25% of the DV for vitamin B$_6$ (3/4 cup)	0.5 mg
	Chicken breast, roasted (3 ounces)	0.5 mg
	Banana (1 medium)	0.4 mg
	Marinara (spaghetti) sauce, ready to serve (1 cup)	0.4 mg
	Potatoes, boiled (1 cup)	0.4 mg
	Turkey, meat only, roasted (3 ounces)	0.4 mg
	Ground beef, patty, 85% lean, broiled (3 ounces)	0.3 mg
	Waffles, plain, ready to heat, toasted (1 waffle)	0.3 mg
	Bulgur, cooked (1 cup)	0.2 mg
Vitamin B$_{12}$	Clams, cooked (3 ounces)	84.1 mcg
	Liver, beef, cooked (3 ounces)	70.7 mcg
	Breakfast cereals, fortified with 100% of the DV for vitamin B$_{12}$ (1 serving)	6.0 mcg
	Trout, rainbow, wild, cooked (3 ounces)	5.4 mcg
	Salmon, sockeye, cooked (3 ounces)	4.8 mcg
	Trout, rainbow, farmed, cooked (3 ounces)	3.5 mcg
	Tuna, light, canned in water (3 ounces)	2.5 mcg
	Cheeseburger, double patty and bun (1 sandwich)	2.1 mcg
	Haddock, cooked (3 ounces)	1.8 mcg
	Breakfast cereals, fortified with 25% of the DV for vitamin B$_{12}$ (3/4 cup)	1.5 mcg
	Beef, top sirloin, broiled (3 ounces)	1.4 mcg
Vitamin C	Strawberries, fresh, sliced (1 cup)	98 mg
	Red pepper, sweet, raw (1/2 cup)	95 mg
	Orange juice (3/4 cup)	93 mg
	Grapefruit juice (3/4 cup)	70 mg
	Orange (1 medium)	70 mg
	Kiwifruit (1 medium)	64 mg
	Green pepper, sweet, raw (1/2 cup)	60 mg
	Broccoli, cooked (1/2 cup)	51 mg
	Brussels sprouts, cooked (1/2 cup)	48 mg
	Broccoli, raw (1/2 cup)	39 mg
	Grapefruit (1/2 medium)	39 mg
	Tomato juice (3/4 cup)	33 mg
	Cantaloupe (1/2 cup)	29 mg
	Cabbage, cooked (1/2 cup)	28 mg
	Cauliflower, raw (1/2 cup)	26 mg

NUTRIENT/PHYTOCHEMICAL	FOOD	AMOUNT
Vitamin D	Salmon, cooked (3 ounces)	447 IU
	Tuna, canned in water (3 ounces)	154 IU
	Milk, fortified (1 cup)	120 IU
	Egg yolk	41 IU
	Cereal, fortified (3/4 cup)	40 IU
Vitamin E	Wheat germ oil (1 tablespoon)	20.3 mg
	Sunflower seeds, dry roasted (1 ounce)	7.4 mg
	Almonds, dry roasted (1 ounce)	6.8 mg
	Sunflower oil (1 tablespoon)	5.6 mg
	Safflower oil (1 tablespoon)	4.6 mg
	Hazelnuts, dry roasted (1 ounce)	4.3 mg
	Peanut butter (2 tablespoons)	2.9 mg
	Canola oil (1 tablespoon)	2.4 mg
	Peanuts, dry roasted (1 ounce)	2.2 mg
	Spinach, boiled (1/2 cup)	1.9 mg
	Broccoli, chopped, boiled (1/2 cup)	1.2 mg
Vitamin K	Natto (3 ounces)	850 mcg
	Collards, frozen, boiled (1/2 cup)	530 mcg
	Turnip greens, frozen, boiled (1/2 cup)	426 mcg
	Spinach, raw (1 cup)	145 mcg
	Kale, raw (1 cup)	113 mcg
	Broccoli, chopped, boiled (1/2 cup)	110 mcg
	Soybeans, roasted (1/2 cup)	43 mcg
	Carrot juice (3/4 cup)	28 mcg
	Soybean oil (1 tablespoon)	25 mcg
	Edamame, frozen, prepared (1/2 cup)	21 mcg
	Pumpkin, canned (1/2 cup)	20 mcg
	Pomegranate juice (3/4 cup)	19 mcg
Zinc	Oysters, cooked, breaded, fried (3 ounces)	74.0 mg
	Beef chuck roast, braised (3 ounces)	7.0 mg
	Crab, Alaska king, cooked (3 ounces)	6.5 mg
	Beef patty, broiled (3 ounces)	5.3 mg
	Breakfast cereal, fortified with 25% of the DV for zinc (3/4 cup)	3.8 mg
	Lobster, cooked (3 ounces)	3.4 mg
	Baked beans, canned, plain or vegetarian (1/2 cup)	2.9 mg
	Pork chop, loin, cooked (3 ounces)	2.9 mg
	Chicken, dark meat, cooked (3 ounces)	2.4 mg
	Yogurt, fruit, low-fat (8 ounces)	1.7 mg
	Cashews, dry roasted (1 ounce)	1.6 mg
	Chickpeas, cooked (1/2 cup)	1.3 mg

Food Cures for Common Conditions

Food cures go way beyond chicken soup for colds. Try fish for allergies, pomegranates for arthritis, and oatmeal for diabetes. Here are proven food solutions for 56 common conditions.

ACNE

If you think pizza and chocolate are the bad guys behind breakouts, think again. These days, acne is blamed mostly on heredity and hormones. During puberty, a surge in male hormones called androgens (women have them, too) stimulates an increase of sebum, responsible for keeping skin moist, and keratin, needed to make hair. When too much of either clogs a hair follicle, acne can result.

Eating a cheesy pizza probably won't make much difference to your skin, but what *will* make a difference—a positive one—is eating more fruits, vegetables, and other foods that help keep hormones in balance and fight inflammation.

YOUR FOOD PRESCRIPTION

Brazil nuts

These are rich in selenium, a powerful antioxidant that appears to help improve acne, probably by protecting cells from inflammatory damage and preserving skin's elasticity. Selenium works particularly well when it's accompanied by vitamins E and A, so eat your Brazil nuts with some almonds and perhaps some red bell peppers.

Aim for: One Brazil nut delivers a full day's supply. Other foods rich in selenium are meats, fish, poultry, and whole grains.

Oysters, beans, poultry, fish,
and other foods rich in zinc

No one knows exactly why, but getting enough zinc appears to help put the brakes on breakouts. It may be that zinc helps to control the release of male hormones that kick-start acne. Zinc also helps the body absorb vitamin A, another important nutrient for healthy skin.

Aim for: The recommended amount for men is 11 milligrams; for women, it's 8 milligrams. Three ounces (85 g) of oysters has 30 milligrams of zinc, while 3 ounces (85 g) of dark turkey meat has 4 milligrams.

Helpful hint: Vegetarians who avoid animal products altogether should consider consulting a nutritionist for advice on supplementing with zinc.

Salmon, flaxseed,
and other foods rich in omega-3 fatty acids

Some dermatologists think that omega-3 fatty acids, which help keep inflammation at bay, may help keep acne under control. Fatty fish like salmon, sardines, and mackerel all boast omega-3 fatty acids, as do flaxseed and walnuts.

Aim for: At least two servings of fatty fish per week. You can also sprinkle salads with flaxseed oil, use ground flaxseed in baking and smoothies, and add toasted walnuts to casseroles and hot and cold cereals.

Sweet potatoes, carrots, cantaloupe, bell peppers,
and other foods rich in beta-carotene

Beta-carotene (found in many orange-, yellow-, and red-hued fruits and vegetables) converts in the body to vitamin A, another of the nutrients that helps to enhance selenium's benefits to skin.

Aim for: At least 1/2 cup of red- or yellow-hued vegetables a day.

Almonds, eggs, leafy greens,
and other foods rich in vitamin E

The antioxidant vitamin E helps skin heal from damage and scarring caused by acne. Good sources of E are unrefined (minimally processed) vegetable oils, nuts, and whole grains.

Aim for: The recommended daily intake of vitamin E is 15 milligrams. One tablespoon of canola oil has 2 milligrams, and 2 tablespoons peanut butter has 3 milligrams. Some physicians recommend 200 milligrams or more per day, which you'd need a supplement to get.

Helpful hint: Vitamin E is fat soluble, so eat it along with foods that contain a little fat. When you eat kale or spinach, for example, drizzle on a little olive oil.

Fruits and vegetables

When scientists looked at the diets of teens in the Kitavan Islands of New Guinea and the Ache region of Paraguay—where not one case of acne was found—they took note: The diets were rich in fruits and vegetables like yams and greens and low in refined foods like white sugar and white flour, which can cause hormones to spike. When people from a similar gene pool moved to Western regions and began to eat refined foods, they began to experience acne.

Aim for: At least five servings over the course of a day. A serving generally means one medium piece of fruit, 1 cup of raw produce, or 1/2 cup of cooked produce.

Oranges, tomatoes, melons, *and other foods rich in vitamin C*

These juicy vitamin C bombs won't cure you of breakouts, but because the vitamin strengthens cell walls, it can help protect your skin from scarring that blemishes can cause. Bioflavonoids, which often come from a C source (such as the white rind inside citrus fruits), also act as natural anti-inflammatories that can enhance the healing action of vitamin C.

Aim for: Eat enough vitamin C–rich foods to total at least 75 (women) to 90 (men) milligrams of C per day. A half cup of raw red bell pepper packs 95 milligrams of C, and 1 cup of strawberries has 98 milligrams.

NUTRITIONAL SUPPLEMENTS

A multivitamin/mineral. If your diet lacks these important nutrients, including vitamin E and selenium, you will find both, as well as other essential nutrients in most multis. **DOSAGE:** One a day.

Chromium. Some dietitians recommend chromium supplements to acne patients. There is good evidence linking chromium to better insulin use and some evidence that acne is linked with poor insulin sensitivity. Check with your doctor before taking supplements. **DOSAGE:** 50–200 micrograms per day.

OFF THE MENU

Iodized salt and other strong sources of iodine. For unknown reasons, iodized salt can cause acne flare-ups in some people. If you are sensitive to iodine, watch the amount of sodium you take in from prepared and processed foods and how much iodized salt you add from the saltshaker. Also limit shrimp and shellfish, which are high in iodine.

Refined foods. If you're serious about stopping acne, scale back on refined foods in your diet such as white bread, refined flour, french fries, and anything made with lots of sugar. They cause blood sugar and insulin to spike, and scientists suspect that those insulin spikes may contribute to acne. Diets full of refined foods and low in fruits and vegetables also come up short on magnesium, a mineral that helps to balance acne-inducing hormones.

FEATURED RECIPES

Ultimate Spiced Nuts *p. 288*
Spinach Salad with Chickpeas *p. 293*
Tropical Fruit Salad *p. 286*
Citrus Chicken Salad *p. 294*
Sweet Potato Soup *p. 297*
Three-Bean Chili *p. 306*
Baked Chicken with Tomatoes *p. 311*
Salmon Cake Sandwiches *p. 300*

ALLERGIES

When the trees bud, the grasses sprout, or the ragweed blooms, you probably reach for allergy pills and a family-size box of tissues. But if you reach for foods like fish and onions, both before and during allergy season, you may find that your sneezing has decreased and your breathing is a whole lot easier.

How can foods possibly tame hay fever? When allergens—pollen, grasses, dust mites, or molds—find their way into your nose, your body goes into attack mode if it's hypersensitive, or allergic. Immune cells release histamines, the chemicals responsible for most of your allergy symptoms. These in turn kick-start inflammation that's intended to keep the allergens from traveling into the body. The inflammation makes sinuses and nasal passages swell and eyes itch. Histamines also stimulate the nasal passages to release fluids, resulting in a runny nose and itchy throat, and cause sneezing, another attempt to send the allergens packing. Many of the foods that may help reduce allergies work by reducing inflammation or calming the immune system.

YOUR FOOD PRESCRIPTION

Salmon and other fatty fish

Fatty fish like salmon, sardines, and mackerel should be your first line of dietary defense against allergies. That's because they contain generous amounts of omega-3 fatty acids, which help minimize inflammation, a direct cause of most allergy symptoms. Several studies suggest that kids who start eating fish early in life may even be less likely to have allergies later. Eating more fish increases omega-3s in the body, which benefits the immune system and can translate into fewer allergy symptoms.

One Australian study that analyzed nearly 500 eight-year-olds found that those who ate fish at least once a week were 80 percent less likely to have ryegrass pollen allergies, a common cause of hay fever, than those who rarely ate fish. A similar study in Norway compared the fish-eating habits of more than 2,500 four-year-olds and found that those who had eaten fish in their first year of life had a significantly lower risk of developing hay fever and asthma than those who had not.

Can't get your kids to eat fish? If they're at least three years old, have them eat 1 ounce of walnuts (or 14 walnut halves) a day. Flaxseed also contains omega-3s.

Grownups should dine on fin food more often, too. One German study involving 568 adults found that high content of omega-3 fatty acids in red blood cells or in the diet was associated with decreased risk of hay fever.

Aim for: One to two servings of fatty fish such as salmon, tuna, and mackerel per week. Look to fish-oil supplements if you want to get even more omega-3s. Start your children on a fish-rich diet early in life.

Garlic

What isn't garlic good for? In the case of hay fever, the oh-so-smelly bulbs appear to work by supporting the immune system with their rich store of antioxidants. Researchers have identified a link between a higher intake of certain antioxidants and a lower incidence of hay fever.

Aim for: Use fresh garlic liberally as a seasoning. You can also cut a whole clove into several chunks and swallow them like pills for a daily dose. Your stomach acids will break them down and release antioxidants as the garlic travels through the colon.

Onions

This humble bulb packs a hefty dose of quercetin, an antioxidant that can help reduce inflammation and may help prevent the release of histamine from immune cells called mast cells. Quercetin also helps improve the body's absorption of vitamin C, another antioxidant with immunity-boosting powers. Quercetin may even work to stabilize cell membranes so they're less reactive to allergens. Other good sources are apples with skin, berries, red grapes, and black tea.

Aim for: Sprinkle raw onions on salads, stews, burritos, and other foods whenever you can.

Yogurt with live cultures
and fermented milk

The live beneficial bacteria found in yogurt and other fermented products like kefir help keep the flora and fauna in your gut—where many immune cells are located—healthy. Some experts believe that the Western diet no longer includes enough fermented foods to keep a balance of healthy bacteria in our gastrointestinal tracts and that the prevalence of allergies has risen in response. These foods stimulate the body to produce certain white blood cells and antibodies as well as various growth factors that are important for keeping the body from overreacting to allergens.

A recent Italian study found that when volunteers who regularly had bouts of hay fever ate 2 cups of yogurt daily for four months, they had half the histamine levels in their blood and fewer hay fever symptoms than those who drank 2 cups of fat-free milk daily.

Pregnant women take note: When moms-to-be eat foods that contain probiotics, such as yogurt, on a regular basis, their babies have a lower risk of developing allergies as they grow up. Studies have indicated that probiotics are especially important for infants and children, whose immune systems are still developing.

Aim for: One or 2 cups of yogurt or other fermented milk products per day. Check the label for *lactobacillus, bifidobacterium,* and *Bacillus clausii,* among other live, active cultures.

Helpful hint: If 2 cups of yogurt sounds like too much for you, vary your source of probiotics with kefir, a fermented milk product available in health food stores and many supermarkets. Substitute 1 cup of kefir for one serving of yogurt. Add it to milkshakes and fruit smoothies.

Sweet potatoes, leafy greens, wheat germ, almonds, *and other foods rich in vitamin E*

In one German study on the dietary habits of 1,700 adults with and without hay fever, those who ate foods rich in vitamin E (the equivalent of 10 to 13 milligrams per day) had a 30 percent lower incidence of hay fever than those who ate diets low in the vitamin.

Aim for: Lots of leafy greens, whole grains, nuts, and avocados. One cup of cooked spinach has 6.8 milligrams of vitamin E. One ounce (28 g) of almonds provides 4 milligrams.

Can you make the switch from ice cream to frozen yogurt? You should! Many frozen yogurts have the same live cultures that make regular yogurt so helpful in battling allergies. And frozen yogurt usually has less fat and sugar than ice cream.

Oregano, lemon balm, rosemary, *and other herbs*

All of these herbs, along with sage and marjoram, contain rosmarinic oil in their leaves. One Japanese study showed that this acid, an extract of the oil, has an anti-inflammatory effect that helps reduce the symptoms of seasonal allergies.

Aim for: Season your dishes liberally with fresh herbs to reap the most benefit. Make lemon balm tea, add chopped oregano and rosemary to pasta dishes, and use sage and marjoram on poultry and fish.

FEATURED RECIPES

Spinach Salad with Chickpeas *p. 293*
Sweet Potato Soup *p. 297*
Fish Tacos *p. 307*
Roasted Salmon with Sautéed Greens *p. 309*
Salmon Steaks with Peach Salsa *p. 308*
Tuna Kebabs *p. 306*
Almond Rice *p. 322*
Raspberry-Almond Muffins *p. 324*

NUTRITIONAL SUPPLEMENTS

Omega-3 fatty acids. If you don't like the smell or taste of seafood, you may still get hay fever relief by getting omega-3s in fish-oil supplements. **DOSAGE:** 1 to 3 grams a day. Check with your pharmacist to make sure you're buying high-quality capsules. Store them in the refrigerator.

Flaxseed oil. Flaxseed oil, an alternative to fish oil, provides substances that are converted to omega-3 fatty acids in the body. **DOSAGE:** 1 to 3 tablespoons per day. Better yet, use flaxseed meal to get the added benefit of fiber.

Probiotics. If you can't manage to eat a lot of yogurt every day, consider probiotic supplements. Look for products that contain *lactobacillus, bifidobacterium,* and *Bacillus clausii* in particular. **DOSAGE:** Take a one-billion-count capsule with *lactobacillus* and *bifidobacterium* twice daily. Both live and heat-killed varieties appear to be effective.

Vitamin C. The jury is still out on the use of vitamin C to help prevent hay fever, with some studies concluding that high doses of C can reduce symptoms and others finding no such benefits. It may be worth trying for a month or two to see if it works on your symptoms. **DOSAGE:** No more than 400 milligrams a day is currently recommended for most adults. If you experience diarrhea, cut back.

Quercetin and bromelain. If you're not eating enough apple skins, berries, and onions to get a therapeutic dose of quercetin, which appears to inhibit the release of histamine, try a supplement. Look for one that also contains bromelain, an enzyme that comes from the pineapple plant and also helps keep inflammation under control. Early studies on both of these compounds have shown promise in the treatment of hay fever, but more research is needed. **DOSAGE:** Look for a combination supplement with 200 to 400 milligrams of quercetin and up to 125 milligrams of bromelain. You can also find these two in combination with vitamin C.

Vitamin E. One of the most powerful anti-oxidants known, vitamin E may help reduce inflammation that causes hay fever symptoms. **DOSAGE:** Best to get your vitamin E with food. Some animal studies suggest high doses may increase allergic responses.

CAUTION

Honey. The honeybee harvests flower after flower for its pollen. This means if you have allergies to any of the pollens used by the bee, such as clover, you may have an allergic reaction to the honey. If this is the case, you may need to avoid unfiltered or raw honey and go for the filtered variety.

In 2012, a team of researchers at the University of Utah analyzed both raw and processed honey samples for their vitamin, mineral, and antioxidant content. They found that processing almost entirely removed the pollen from honey but did not affect nutrient or antioxidant levels. In fact, these scientists reported that processing actually increased the overall mineral content and antioxidant capacity of the honey.

Fatty red meat. Studies have shown a higher incidence of hay fever in people who consume significant amounts of arachidonic acid, an inflammatory component of fatty red meats and organ meats as well as shellfish.

"Cross-reactive" fruits and vegetables. Some people with hay fever experience similar symptoms when they eat certain fruits and vegetables, a phenomenon known as cross-reactivity. People with birch pollen allergies, for example, may notice that they get an itchy tongue when eating apples and stone fruits like peaches, cherries, and plums. People with ragweed allergies often react to melons. Although pollen allergies are seasonal, cross-reactive reactions may persist all year. Cooking the problematic fruits and vegetables often eliminates the allergic reaction.

Red wine. Some people with hay fever get headaches when they drink red wine because, along with beneficial tannins and flavonoids, the skins of red grapes contain bothersome histamines. Green grapes contain fewer histamines.

Into the Mouths of Babes

Although there is no perfect formula for preventing allergies, studies have shown that infants who have been breastfed for at least six months (and preferably longer) have a lower incidence of allergies when they get older. And, somewhat surprising, recent studies have found that offering potentially allergenic foods to babies earlier rather than later might actually prevent food allergies from developing.

For that reason, the American Academy of Pediatrics now recommends that solid foods—including those that are potentially allergenic such as dairy foods, eggs, and peanut products—be introduced as early as four to six months of age. In fact, research has shown that delaying the introduction of highly allergenic foods may increase rather than decrease an infant's risk for developing allergies. This does not apply, of course, if an infant is already experiencing allergic reactions, say experts.

ALZHEIMER'S DISEASE

Alzheimer's is a worry for many people. One in three people over the age of 80 will be its victim, and most of us sit back and hope we won't be one of them. But there *are* concrete steps you can take to lower your risk—by a lot, not just a little. In fact, recent research has found that eating a diet high in fruits and vegetables and healthful fats such as the Mediterranean and DASH diets can slow memory decline with aging. Recently, a team at Rush University Medical Center studied 960 older volunteers for five years and found that those who most closely followed a combination of these two diets—aptly called the MIND (Mediterranean-DASH Intervention for Neurodegenerative Delay) diet—had cognitive scores similar to someone 7.5 years younger in age.

While you're at it, also plan to finally keep your promise to exercise more (recent studies have found that people who exercised three or more times a week were much less likely to develop Alzheimer's), and don't forget to challenge your mind (think crossword puzzles or learning to play a musical instrument).

Alzheimer's disease often begins with what appears to be simple forgetfulness, but it wreaks much more havoc over time, destroying speech, comprehension, and coordination and causing restlessness and dramatic mood swings. Autopsies on the brains of Alzheimer's patients have revealed thick clumps of a protein called amyloid as well as tangled bundles of nerve fibers known as neurofibrillary tangles. Inflammation also plays a role, although researchers aren't sure if it's a cause or an effect of the disease.

Some of the risk factors for heart disease and stroke, such as high blood pressure, high cholesterol, and low levels of folate, may also increase the risk of Alzheimer's.

The right diet can't guarantee that you will avoid Alzheimer's, but if it lowers your risk or delays the onset of the disease, isn't a weekly salmon dinner worth it? Other steps are as simple as starting your mornings with a cup of tea, cutting out those cheeseburgers, and putting more fruits and vegetables on your plate.

A final note: If you're carrying a lot more weight than you should, here's a compelling reason to shed some of them. Research has found that people who were obese at midlife were much more likely to develop dementia and Alzheimer's disease later in life.

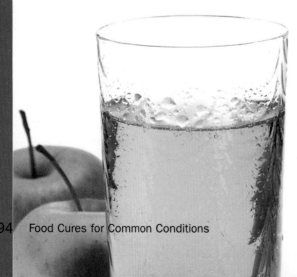

To help battle Alzheimer's, choose your drinks smartly. Have tea with your breakfast in the morning. During the day, switch from soda to natural fruit juices. Come evening, enjoy a glass of wine. All these beverages have been proven to lower the risk of the disease.

Fatty fish, nuts, and olive oil

You may know these as staples of the famously heart-healthy Mediterranean diet, but recent evidence suggests they can lower the risk of Alzheimer's, too. Eating fatty fish such as salmon, herring, or white tuna once a week may slow cognitive decline by 10 percent. Omega-3 fatty acids, especially the type known as DHA, found in fatty fish appear to be the key. Since high levels of DHA are needed for normal brain development, that makes sense. In addition, omega-3 fatty acids—including those found in walnuts, flaxseed, and canola oil—counter inflammation, which may contribute to protein buildup in the brain.

And don't forget olive oil, a rich source of monounsaturated fat, found to be a key component of the MIND diet to preserve brain function.

Aim for: At least one meal of fatty fish a week as well as several tablespoons of walnuts, olive oil, or flaxseed.

Helpful hint: Some fatty fish contain mercury, which can damage the brain. Children and women of childbearing age should avoid shark, swordfish, king mackerel, and tilefish (if it comes from the Gulf of Mexico) because of high mercury levels. Canned white albacore tuna has more omega-3s than canned light tuna, but it also has slightly higher levels of mercury. Limit your intake to 6 ounces (170 g) per week.

Broccoli, strawberries, almonds,
and other foods rich in vitamins C and E

The brain is one of the most dynamic parts of the body, with neurons firing, cells growing, and webs of electrical and chemical activity masterminding bodily functions. But the by-product of all of these chemical reactions is free radicals, unstable molecules that damage cells, possibly contributing to amyloid plaques and speeding up mental decline.

Foods that contain antioxidants neutralize those free radicals, "mopping up" the "pollution" in your brain. Research on the dietary habits of large groups of people has found that eating plenty of foods rich in vitamin C (like red peppers, currants, broccoli, and strawberries) and vitamin E (like kale, sweet potatoes, and almonds) may reduce the risk of developing Alzheimer's.

In a study conducted by researchers at the Rush Institute for Healthy Aging at Rush-Presbyterian-St. Luke's Medical Center in Chicago, people who consumed the most vitamin E from foods (averaging 11.4 IU) had a risk of Alzheimer's that was a whopping 67 percent lower than that of people who got the least (averaging 6.2 IU).

The effect of supplements is less clear, possibly because they tend to be taken in high-dose increments, unlike food that's eaten over a lifetime. Foods also contain all forms of vitamin E, whereas supplements typically contain only one type, alpha-tocopherol. The different forms of vitamin E neutralize different forms of free radicals.

Aim for: *Vitamin E:* 25 IU of vitamin E a day from foods such as 1 cup of cooked frozen spinach (5.6 IU), 1 ounce (28 g) of almonds (10 IU), or 1 ounce (28 g) sunflower seeds (11 IU). *Vitamin C:* At least 130 milligrams a day from foods like 1 cup of strawberries (98 milligrams), 1 cup of cooked broccoli (100 milligrams), or 1 cup of fresh orange juice (124 milligrams). A cup of raw red bell peppers, with 190 milligrams, or two kiwifruits, with 128 milligrams, are also terrific choices.

Tea, berries, pomegranate juice, apples, *and other foods and beverages high in flavonoids*

To defend themselves from solar radiation and hungry herbivores, plants have created an arsenal of protective chemicals called polyphenols. Flavonoids are among the toughest of these, and they also fall into the antioxidant category. Flavonoid-rich fruits include apples, blueberries, cranberries, and grapefruit. Vegetables that boast flavonoids include asparagus, brussels sprouts, cabbage, garlic, kale, kohlrabi, kidney and lima beans, onions, peas, and spinach. One study found that people who drank fruit and vegetable juices such as orange, apple, or tomato three times a week were less likely to develop Alzheimer's disease. Participants in the MIND diet study had less cognitive decline with the consumption of two or more servings of berries a week. Other studies have observed that the more flavonoids a person eats, the lower the likelihood of developing dementia.

Since there are thousands of healthful flavonoid substances in plant foods, scientists have yet to recommend an optimal intake. A half cup of fresh blueberries or green tea, for example, contains well over 150 mg of these memory boosters. One half cup of raw red cabbage has over 200 mg. Include a variety of fruits and vegetables in your daily diet and your brain will reap the benefits.

Curry powder

Cooks in India and other countries use curry abundantly, and the incidence of Alzheimer's is lower in these places than in many Western nations. Curry could be one of the reasons. A prime ingredient in curry powder is turmeric, which contains curcumin (which gives curry its yellow color). In lab and animal studies, researchers have found that curcumin is a potent antioxidant, anti-inflammatory, and anti-amyloid compound. It binds to amyloid proteins and prevents them

from grouping together to form plaque, so it may be that curcumin offers a triple blow to Alzheimer's disease. Studies have shown that people who consumed the highest amounts of curried foods actually have better brain performance.

Aim for: There's no particular recommended dosage. The best advice? Add either curry powder or turmeric to as many dishes as you can. Purchase bright yellow curry powder, which is likely to contain the most turmeric. Or take one 400-milligram turmeric capsule a day.

Helpful hint: Include up to a teaspoon of turmeric in pea soup or add it to your favorite lentil dish.

Spinach, fortified cereal,
and other foods high in folate

Doctors have known for years that deficiency of certain B vitamins, particularly folate, can make it difficult to perform some cognitive tasks. New evidence shows that even slightly low levels can have a similar effect because folate, along with vitamins B_6 and B_{12}, helps to keep homocysteine levels in check. This amino acid impairs brain function and can dramatically increase a person's risk of Alzheimer's disease (as well as heart disease). The good news is that folate from foods like dark leafy greens and dried beans may slow cognitive decline.

Aim for: The recommended daily amount of 400 micrograms. Many fortified breakfast cereals and breads provide this amount. Other good sources are cooked spinach (131 micrograms per half cup), black-eyed peas (105 micrograms per half cup), and asparagus (89 micrograms in 4 spears).

Wine

A study of 2,031 men and women in Norway reported better cognitive test scores in participants who drank up to 4 ounces (118 ml) of wine a day than those who did not.

Aim for: No more than 4 ounces (118 ml) a day for women and 8 ounces (226 ml) a day for men.

FEATURED RECIPES

NUTRITIONAL SUPPLEMENTS

DHA. Some experts recommend taking this omega-3 supplement in order to get a high dose of the most active form of omega-3 fatty acids while avoiding mercury and other contaminants found in some fish. **DOSAGE:** Up to 400 milligrams of DHA daily. Check with your pharmacist to make sure you're buying high-quality capsules.

Vitamins C and E. The Nurses Health Study, which is tracking health data on thousands of women, has found that supplementing with C and E over the long term slowed cognitive decline. A study of some 4,000 elderly Utah residents found that supplementing with these two vitamins was associated with a 72 percent lower risk of Alzheimer's. Another study found that vitamin E supplements slowed the progress of the disease in people with moderate cases, but other studies have raised doubt about this. **DOSAGE:** *Vitamin C:* 500 milligrams daily. *Vitamin E:* 400 IU of d-alpha-tocopherol daily.

Sage. As its name suggests, sage has been used since ancient times to improve memory and sharpen the mind—and for good reason, as it turns out. Some human trials have found that the herb or its oil can indeed improve memory and cognitive function, and one four-month Iranian study found the extract improved cognitive function in Alzheimer's patients more than a placebo did.

More clinical research is under way. Sage appears to work by protecting acetylcholine, one of the chemical messengers in the brain that's critical to memory and that often drops in the brains of people with Alzheimer's. It may also have anti-inflammatory benefits that help slow the progress of the disease. **DOSAGE:** 25 to 50 microliters of *S. lavandulaefolia* (Spanish sage) oil or 300 to 600 milligrams of dried sage in supplement form. You can also steep 2 teaspoons of dried sage in boiling water for a strong cup of sage tea that provides the same dosage.

OFF THE MENU

Saturated fat, trans fat, and cholesterol. Another reason to eat your chicken grilled instead of deep-fried: A diet high in these heart-wrecking fats is linked to a significant decline in cognitive function—as is a diet low in unsaturated fat (so trade that steak for a piece of salmon and that butter for olive oil or margarine made without trans fat). Thankfully, partially hydrogenated oils—the main source of trans fats in our diet—are being phased out of our food supply, according to orders by the Food and Drug Administration.

Sugar and refined grains. They may look tempting, but those store-bought muffins in the cellophane wrap are a bad idea if you're worried about Alzheimer's disease. Diets rich in sugar and refined grains (like white flour) can contribute to the risk of type 2 diabetes, a condition that in turn quadruples the risk of Alzheimer's. One theory proposes that insulin resistance, at the core of type 2 diabetes, means that cells don't get the sugar they need to function properly, and brain cells may die as a result. Another theory suggests that an insulin imbalance may lead to additional protein clumping that gums up the pathways of the brain. If you already have diabetes, keep your blood sugar under strict control to help reduce the risk of Alzheimer's.

ANEMIA

Imagine your body gasping for oxygen and pooping out like a car with a bad carburetor. That's pretty much what happens with anemia, either because there are too few red blood cells to carry enough oxygen through the body or because the blood cells lack sufficient hemoglobin, the protein that carries oxygen. Daily life becomes double the effort due to fatigue. Anemia can also lead to headaches, cold hands and feet, and pale skin (after all, it's blood that puts the blush into cheeks).

Most cases of anemia are caused by iron deficiency, often triggered by blood loss (think bleeding ulcers or heavy menstrual periods). Another type of anemia, called pernicious anemia, is caused by a deficiency of vitamin B_{12}, which is needed to make red blood cells. Older people are at risk for this because with age, the body's ability to absorb B_{12} from food tends to diminish. Folic acid is also needed for red blood cell production, so if you don't get enough, you could develop "folic acid anemia." Alcoholics, smokers, people with certain digestive disorders, vegetarians, people over 50, and pregnant or nursing women are at highest risk for folic acid and pernicious anemia.

You may need a prescription from your doctor to correct anemia, but a robust and varied diet will help keep you out of the woods once it's under control.

YOUR FOOD PRESCRIPTION

Beef, fish, shellfish,
and other foods rich in vitamin B_{12}

When your diet supplies too little vitamin B_{12}, you run the risk of developing pernicious anemia. Vegetarians are particularly vulnerable because B_{12} is most abundant in animal products like meat and fish; cheese and eggs also provide modest amounts. Many fortified cereals offer a generous dose. If you have signs of pernicious anemia, such as shortness of breath, fatigue, loss of appetite, rapid heart rate, and tingling and numbness in your hands and feet, see your doctor; you may need B_{12} supplements.

Aim for: 2.4 micrograms of B_{12} per day, the amount in 3 ounces (85 g) of light tuna.

Clams, red meat, chicken, shellfish, *and other iron-rich foods*

The body needs iron to make hemoglobin, the protein that enables red blood cells to carry oxygen. Red meat is a classic powerhouse of heme iron, the form we absorb best and that's found in animal foods. Liver is another source, but it's loaded with cholesterol. Like clams? The canned variety is one of the best sources of iron and an outstanding source of vitamin B_{12}.

Lentils, tofu, and raisins contain nonheme iron, which is less easily absorbed. To squeeze more iron from these foods, eat them with a food rich in heme iron or in vitamin C, which helps you soak up iron.

Also look to foods like oatmeal and cereal, usually fortified with iron, to "beef up" your diet.

Aim for: 18 milligrams of iron for women up to age 50; 8 milligrams for women 51 and older and adult men. This often won't be enough to correct anemia, but it should help you maintain good iron levels once the anemia is under control. You'll get 3.6 milligrams of iron from 3 ounces (85 g) of beef tenderloin, 8 milligrams from 3 ounces (85 g) of oysters, and as much as 18 milligrams from a serving of fortified cereal.

Citrus fruits, peppers, broccoli,
and other foods rich in vitamin C

Vitamin C helps the body absorb iron, so pair up half an orange and a cup of iron-fortified Cream of Wheat, or add some red peppers to your beef or chicken stir-fry. Vitamin C also helps counter the effects of phytates, substances in fiber-dense foods like wheat bran, wheat germ, nuts, barley, and oats that bind with iron. A study from Sweden showed that when vitamin C was consumed along with high-phytate foods, iron absorption increased significantly.

Aim for: At least a cup of C-rich foods per day.

Lentils, beans, cereals
and other foods rich in folate

Folate, one of the B vitamins, helps red blood cells divide rapidly, replenishing the body's oxygen carriers. Many countries, including the United States, now require manufacturers to fortify enriched breads, cereals, flours, cornmeals, pastas, rice, and other grain products with folic acid.

Aim for: 400 micrograms of folate per day. You'll get almost this much in a cup of cooked lentils, and more from a serving of fortified cereal.

NUTRITIONAL SUPPLEMENTS

Iron. Dietary iron often may not be enough to correct a deficiency. For women who have particularly heavy menstrual bleeding, or anyone with a condition that causes blood loss, supplements may be in order. Have your doctor do a blood test first to confirm iron-deficiency anemia. **DOSAGE:** Take iron only under medical supervision, at the level the doctor recommends.

Vitamin C. To help the blood absorb iron, take your iron supplements with a source of vitamin C, such as orange juice.

Vitamin B_{12}. Check with your doctor about what dosage you may need. **DOSAGE:** Doctors often recommend 1,000 micrograms of B_{12} combined with 400 micrograms of folic acid, in a form that's placed under the tongue so it's absorbed through the mouth, twice a day.

Folic acid. The body absorbs the folic acid in supplements better than the folate in foods. But take heed: If you exceed the upper limit for folic acid (1,000 micrograms), you risk a vitamin B_{12} deficiency. Take folic acid with B_{12} because a high intake of one can mask a deficiency of the other. **DOSAGE:** 400 micrograms from food (check your cereal, since grain products in many countries are fortified with folic acid) and another 400 micrograms from supplements daily.

OFF THE MENU

Tea. The tannins in tea bind with iron, blocking absorption. To avoid this problem, drink tea by itself rather than with meals.

Spinach, nuts, berries, chocolate, wheat bran and germ, tea, and other foods high in oxalates. Oxalates are compounds that bind with iron and calcium, making them hard to absorb. Don't cross these foods off your menu entirely, but if you have anemia, it's best not to overdo them until your red blood count has returned to normal. Other foods high in oxalates are rhubarb, beets, tofu, tangerines, and baked beans.

FEATURED RECIPES

Shrimp and Grapefruit Salad *p. 294*
Lentil-Tomato Soup *p. 299*
Beef in Lettuce Wraps *p. 302*
Turkey Cutlets with Grapefruit Salsa *p. 313*
Barbecued Flank Steak *p. 314*
Beef and Broccoli Stew *p. 316*

ARTHRITIS

In *The Wizard of Oz*, the Tin Man kept a can of oil handy to keep his joints from freezing up. Believe it or not, getting the right kinds of oils from foods can actually help *your* joints, too, albeit in a much different way. Evidence is beginning to mount that certain foods high in anti-inflammatory compounds—especially the oils in fatty fish—help reduce the inflammation and pain of arthritis. It's not surprising, since both osteoarthritis (the most common type) and rheumatoid arthritis, or RA (an autoimmune condition in which inflammation is triggered by an immune system reaction), result in inflamed joint tissues for which anti-inflammatory medications are often prescribed.

Although doctors don't yet fully understand arthritis, it's clear that everyday wear and tear on cartilage is hardly the whole story. Researchers now know, for example, that free radicals—unstable molecules that attack healthy cells—increase inflammation and speed up the aging process, including the deterioration of joints and cartilage, a process best slowed in anyone, but especially in people with arthritis. It's an excellent reason to add more antioxidant-rich fruits, vegetables, and tea to your menu.

YOUR FOOD PRESCRIPTION

Salmon, mackerel, flaxseed,
and other foods high in omega-3 fatty acids

For years, researchers have noticed that people with arthritis who eat plenty of oily fish seem to have less inflammation and pain than those who don't eat as much fish. Now they have an explanation: It seems that like aspirin, the omega-3 fatty acids in fatty fish boost production of a recently discovered class of anti-inflammatory fats called resolvins. In one study, both omega-3s and aspirin boosted the production of resolvins, which in turn inhibit the activity of inflammatory cells. This is good news for people with osteoarthritis and particularly for those with RA, which can inflame organs as well as joints.

Aim for: Two to three 4-ounce (113 g) servings of fish a week. If you don't like fish, aim for 1 to 2 tablespoons of ground flaxseed daily.

Helpful hint: Researchers have found that a diet plentiful in fish fights inflammation best when partnered with low doses of aspirin. However, check with your doctor before taking aspirin.

Even low doses can cause gastrointestinal bleeding in some people.

Leafy greens, peppers, broccoli,
and other foods rich in antioxidants

Need yet another reason to eat more fruits and veggies? Here it is: Colorful produce, rich in antioxidants that fight free radicals, helps protect your joints.

Researchers have suspected for some time that free radicals, those unstable molecules that attack healthy cells, play a role in causing arthritis. Now it's becoming clear how they wreak their havoc on joints. According to a Japanese study, free radicals sabotage cartilage's ability to maintain and repair itself. People with arthritis tend to have more than their fair share of free radicals and therefore should make an extra effort to get more antioxidants, especially vitamin C and beta-carotene, from foods.

In a large nine-year British study, researchers found that even a modest boost in intake of orange and yellow fruits and vegetables—as modest as adding a glass of orange juice a day—can lower the risk of RA. People who ate the most yellow/orange fruits and vegetables, full of antioxidants known as carotenoids, halved their risk of developing the disease. Think of carrots and sweet potatoes in addition to that morning glass of orange juice.

Vitamin C in citrus fruits like oranges and kiwifruit, and zeaxanthin, an antioxidant found in green leafy vegetables, lowered the risk, too. Those leafy greens (like spinach and turnip greens) also pack a fair amount of vitamin E, and some studies have shown that large doses of this vitamin from supplements may also relieve osteoarthritis pain, especially in combination with vitamin C (250 to 500 milligrams a day).

There's less research so far into the effectiveness of antioxidants for osteoarthritis, but researchers believe eating more fruits and vegetables is a smart move whatever form of arthritis you have. Although supplements are available for many antioxidants, the studies have focused on antioxidants in foods.

Aim for: 2 to 3 cups of a range of vegetables and 2 to 3 cups of a variety of fruits per day.

Helpful hint: Certain arthritis medications, such as nonsteroidal anti-inflammatory drugs (NSAIDs), can cause constipation. Many fruits and vegetables are high in fiber, which can help relieve that side effect.

Pomegranate juice

Knees ache? What about your hands or hips? Try some of this sour Persian fruit, which has both anti-inflammatory and antioxidant powers. It could actually protect your cartilage. When researchers at Case Western Reserve University in Cleveland put a pomegranate extract on tissue samples of cartilage damaged by osteoarthritis, something good happened: The juice lowered levels of an inflammatory chemical linked with overproduction of a certain enzyme. In normal amounts, this enzyme is essential for cartilage replacement, but when too much is produced—as in osteoarthritis—cartilage wears away.

Of course, you won't be pouring pomegranate juice directly on your cartilage, but it's thought that joints do absorb the juice when you drink it, so it's reasonable to believe that it may help. Although pomegranate capsules are available, it's better to just drink the juice.

Aim for: 2 to 3 tablespoons of undiluted pomegranate juice per day.

Helpful hint: To cut the juice's bitterness, add 1 tablespoon to a glass of iced green tea—also high in antioxidants and anti-inflammatory compounds—and drink it two or three times daily.

Pineapple

Bromelain, a protein-digesting enzyme in this tropical fruit, is surprisingly good at bringing down inflammation. It may be as effective for reducing osteoarthritis pain as some anti-inflammatory medications like ibuprofen, at least when it's taken in supplement form. Some studies of bromelain supplements suggest it may help reduce the pain of RA as well. Eat your pineapple between meals, not with them, or the enzymes will be used up digesting your food, and choose fresh or frozen pineapple, not canned pineapple or pineapple juice.

Aim for: Studies have found that effective doses range from 200 to 540 milligrams of bromelain a day. The amount in each serving of pineapple varies depending on the ripeness of the pineapple and its exposure to heat, but a cup a day is a good goal.

Helpful hint: Bromelain is a stomach soother, which is good to know if arthritis medications are irritating your tummy. If you develop mouth sores from NSAIDs or methotrexate, eat the pineapple dipped in honey, also a natural anti-inflammatory.

Turmeric, ginger, cloves,
and other anti-inflammatory spices

Researchers have discovered that many spices fight inflammation. Ginger and turmeric—a yellow spice that lends its color and taste to curries—contain a powerful compound called curcumin, which inhibits enzymes and proteins that promote inflammation. Several studies have found that ginger and turmeric specifically reduce pain and swelling in people with arthritis. Cloves contain an anti-inflammatory chemical called eugenol. In recent animal studies, eugenol inhibited COX-2, a protein that spurs inflammation—the same protein that COX-2 inhibitor drugs like celecoxib (Celebrex) quash. Cloves, turmeric, and ginger also contain antioxidants, important in slowing the cartilage and bone damage caused by arthritis.

Aim for: *Ginger:* 1 tablespoon of chopped fresh ginger or 1 teaspoon of powdered ginger daily. *Turmeric:* 300 to 400 milligrams three times a day, or about 1/2 teaspoon sprinkled on rice or vegetables daily. *Cloves:* 2 to 3 grams, or l to 1 1/2 teaspoons, a day.

Helpful hint: Ginger, known for soothing upset stomachs, is a great choice if arthritis medications stir up gastrointestinal problems.

FEATURED RECIPES

Tropical Fruit Salad *p. 286*
Spinach Salad with Chickpeas *p. 293*
Citrus Chicken Salad *p. 294*
Ginger Butternut Squash Soup *p. 298*
Tomato-Roasted Mackerel *p. 310*
Salmon Steaks with Peach Salsa *p. 308*
Pomegranate Ice *p. 334*
Mixed Berry Tart *p. 335*

Green tea, onions, berries, tomato juice, *and citrus fruits*

This motley crew is drawn together by one thing: quercetin. Laboratory and animal studies indicate that this chemical compound acts as a powerful anti-inflammatory and antioxidant. Early studies in animals suggest green tea may help prevent or ease symptoms of RA. And according to the Iowa Women's Health Study, women who drank more than 3 cups of tea a day were 60 percent less likely to develop RA than women who didn't drink any.

Aim for: The best bet is to drink 3 to 4 cups of tea (preferably green tea) daily and to eat a wide range of quercetin-containing foods each day.

Helpful hint: Include pineapple in your fruit salad. The bromelain in pineapple increases the body's absorption of quercetin, and its vitamin C increases quercetin's antioxidant activity.

NUTRITIONAL SUPPLEMENTS
Omega-3 fatty acids. If you're not a big fish fan—and even if you are—supplementing with omega-3 fatty acids is something many doctors recommend. Supplements come in soft-gel capsules. Because omega-3s are sensitive to heat, light, and oxygen, store the supplements in the refrigerator. Also, choose a supplement that contains vitamin E, which will help keep the omega-3s from turning rancid. Burping fish oil after taking them may mean the oil is rancid. **DOSAGE:** 1 to 2 grams per day for general health and 3 to 6 grams for relief of morning stiffness and tenderness from RA. Don't take more than 9 grams per day, and if you bleed easily, you should check with your doctor before taking these supplements.

Bromelain. Bromelain is available in tablets or capsules. A wide range of doses has been studied and used safely. **DOSAGE:** 500 to 2,000 milligrams daily, divided into two doses.

Ginger, turmeric, and cloves. Unless you cook with them a lot, it can be hard to get therapeutic doses of these anti-inflammatory spices. Talk to your doctor about whether supplements of one of them might help you. Be aware, though, that ginger supplements may irritate the stomach. Ginger and cloves also thin the blood, so check with your doctor before taking them if you take blood-thinning medication. Stop taking any of the supplements if they upset your stomach or if you see no effect after 10 days. **DOSAGE:** *Ginger:* 500 milligrams from capsules per day or 100 to 300 milligrams from an extract three times a day. *Turmeric:* 400 to 600 milligrams three times a day, always with food. *Cloves:* Although there is no established dose, a recent study found 2 to 3 grams a day effective for alleviating inflammation.

CAUTION

Fatty meats, full-fat dairy products, and trans fat. Fish counters inflammation; other foods stoke it. Saturated fat in full-fat dairy products can fan the flames of inflammation. Arachidonic acid, found in fatty meats, egg yolks, and organ meats, leads to the formation of eicosanoids, also whipping up inflammation. And definitely avoid anything made with partially hydrogenated oils, or trans fat.

Allergy triggers. Several studies have linked dairy products, corn, and wheat to increased inflammation in people with arthritis. Researchers believe that some food proteins may trigger the production of antibodies in a small percentage of people. The protein and antibodies then partner up to irritate joints. Another theory is that the antibodies attack the lining of the joints directly. The safe way to test whether certain foods such as those above act as inflammation triggers is to consult with your doctor or a registered dietitian, who can put you on an elimination diet, then add back one food at a time and observe changes in your symptoms.

Less Food, Less Burden

Excess weight is tough on joints. The foods most likely to put on weight also tend to rob you of energy (think sugar) and trigger inflammation (think saturated fats in meats, dairy products, and baked goods). The best way to lose weight is to cut out processed foods and sugar and eat fresh fruits and vegetables, whole grains, and lean proteins like fish.

These foods are not only healthier for you, they are far less dense with calories. And because they digest slower, they keep you fuller longer.

Just as important as switching to healthier, less calorie-dense foods is reducing portion sizes. Switch to smaller plates, put your fork down between bites, and take a sip of water after each bite, and you'll quickly find that you're perfectly content with your meal even though you've eaten less than you used to.

ASTHMA

We'll never tell you to reach for food instead of an inhaler. That said, studies show that nutritional therapy may help you cut down on the number and intensity of your asthma attacks.

The idea that food can soothe asthma symptoms may seem shocking, but if you understand what causes those symptoms, it makes perfect sense. During an asthma attack, an allergen or irritant—perhaps a few grains of dust or pollen—sends the immune system into full-scale attack mode. The body unleashes a barrage of histamine and other chemicals that cause inflammation in the lining of the airways. Chronic inflammation actually leads to thickening of the bronchial tubes, which means your airways are narrowed even when you feel okay. To make matters worse, the bronchial tubes begin to churn out extra mucus, which gums up the works and makes it even harder for air to make its way through, so you're left gasping for oxygen.

Inflammation is the main culprit behind asthma symptoms—and the target of many asthma drugs—so foods that fight inflammation are the natural remedies, along with those that thin bronchial mucus. Getting plenty of certain nutrients from food has also been linked with a lower risk of *developing* asthma, which is important to know (and act on) if you have kids.

YOUR FOOD PRESCRIPTION

Onions

Regularly eating onions may help you experience fewer asthma attacks. That's because onions contain several compounds that combat inflammation. One is a type of flavonoid (a class of antioxidant) called quercetin. In test tube studies, quercetin has been shown to inhibit the release of inflammatory substances from mast cells, which are involved in allergic responses. This is also how some asthma drugs work. Onions also contain mustard oils (isothiocyanates) that seem to counter asthma-induced inflammation, at least in lab animals. Pungent foods such as onions, hot peppers, and spicy mustard also trigger the release of watery fluids that help thin the mucus your body produces. (Be aware, however, that in a small percentage of people with asthma, onions actually trigger attacks.)

Aim for: There's no set amount, so just aim to get more onions in your diet.

Helpful hint: You can extract the quercetin from onion skins (where it's highly concentrated) by adding a whole unpeeled onion to a pot of soup while it's simmering. The quercetin will leach into the broth. Just be sure to remove the peel before eating the soup.

Coffee

Although it's no substitute for asthma medication, a strong cup or two of coffee, or even a cola, can help in a pinch because caffeine acts like theophylline, a drug that dilates the airways. Don't use coffee and a prescription theophylline drug at the same time, however.

Studies suggest that drinking coffee regularly may even help prevent asthma attacks, perhaps because the caffeine keeps the airways open. (If caffeine keeps you up at night, this is obviously not a good strategy for you.) Coffee also contains magnesium and antioxidants that may play a beneficial role.

Aim for: A cup or two as needed during an attack or a cup or two every day to help ward off attacks.

Green tea

Like apples and onions, green tea contains quercetin, along with extraordinary amounts of another flavonoid called epigallocatechin gallate.

Aim for: Get in the habit of drinking 2 cups a day, or less when your asthma isn't bothering you. Freshly brewed black tea also contains some quercetin.

Helpful hint: The taste of green tea may take some getting used to, although some people love it. To make sure it's not too bitter, use hot but not boiling water and don't let the tea steep for more than 2 minutes. Experiment with different brands to find one you like. Or try white tea, which is more fragrant and has a pleasant taste and even more antioxidants.

Salmon, mackerel,
and other foods rich in omega-3 fatty acids

Omega-3 fatty acids, found in fatty fish and a few other foods, have the unique power to reduce inflammation in the body, including the airways. As with antioxidants, it appears that people who take in more omega-3s have a lower risk of developing asthma than people who consume less. Getting more of these nutrients may also help if you already have asthma.

Are you wondering whether taking fish-oil supplements may help tame asthma? So are researchers. Although there is some encouraging early research, large well-controlled clinical trials are needed.

Omega-3s are also found in walnuts and ground flaxseed, but only about 20 percent are converted to usable forms.

Aim for: At least 1 gram of omega-3s a day. You can get more than this amount by eating 4 ounces (113 g) of salmon or mackerel.

Helpful hint: Like anchovies? Order them on your pizza; they're another great source of omega-3s.

Apples and berries

An apple a day may not keep the doctor away, but eating enough apples may stave off that next asthma attack. Like onions, apples are rich in quercetin, but be sure to eat the skin, since that's where most of the quercetin is. (Applesauce has only about half the quercetin of apples with the skin.) Berries are also rich in this flavonoid.

The same British researchers who showed the benefits of selenium for asthma also found that people who ate five or more apples per week reduced their likelihood of having asthma by 40 percent.

Aim for: Eat as many as you like!

food for thought . . .

"A possible contributing factor to the increased incidence of asthma in Western societies may be the consumption of a pro-inflammatory diet."

— *Journal of Alternative and Complementary Medicine,* December 2004 ∎

Foods rich in antioxidants,

especially vitamins C and E and selenium

As the airways become inflamed during an asthma attack, the body produces molecules called free radicals, which make the inflammation worse. Antioxidants such as vitamins C and E and the mineral selenium neutralize these free radicals. They may help boost lung function in people with asthma, and they definitely lower the risk of developing asthma in the first place.

Studies show that people who develop asthma tend to consume less of these antioxidants than people who don't. In fact, British researchers found that people who consumed at least 55 micrograms of selenium a day were about *half* as likely to have asthma as those who consumed 30 micrograms or less.

Antioxidants also neutralize free radicals produced in response to ozone, an air pollutant and common asthma trigger. Studies suggest they may boost lung function in people who live in polluted areas, as many of us do, and are sensitive to ozone.

Getting a combination of different antioxidants—especially vitamins C and E and selenium—is best, since these nutrients work synergistically. Eating a variety of antioxidant-rich foods will also help ensure that you get plenty of magnesium (a mineral that helps relax the airways) and other beneficial nutrients.

Aim for: *Vitamin C:* 500 milligrams daily, the amount in a cup of raw red bell peppers plus a cup each of orange juice and cooked broccoli or brussels sprouts, spread throughout the day.

Vitamin E: At least 80 milligrams daily. You won't be able to get this much from food, but get as much as you can from sources such as wheat germ, almonds, and sunflower seeds. *Selenium:* 55 micrograms daily, less than the amount in 1 ounce (28 g) of mixed nuts, a single Brazil nut, or a piece of white fish.

Helpful hint: Kiwifruit contains almost as much vitamin C as oranges or grapefruit. To eat a kiwi with minimal hassle, simply cut it in half, then spoon out the fruit. No peeling required!

NUTRITIONAL SUPPLEMENTS

Vitamin C, vitamin E, and selenium. So far, the evidence is mixed as to whether antioxidant supplements help people with asthma. For ozone-induced airway constriction, however, there does seem to be a benefit from taking a combination of antioxidant supplements. **DOSAGE:** *Vitamin C:* 250 to 500 milligrams twice a day. *Vitamin E:* 80 milligrams of a product containing both natural tocopherols (d-alpha-tocopherol) and tocotrienols. If you can't find that, look for a product with mixed natural tocopherols and take 400 IU daily. Since vitamin E is fat soluble, it's best absorbed when taken with a meal containing some fat. *Selenium:* 200 micrograms once a day. Selenium and vitamin E facilitate each other's absorption, so take them together.

Quercetin. Besides drinking green tea and eating more apples, onions, berries, and citrus fruits, you might consider a quercetin supplement. In lab animals, extracts have been shown to have anti-inflammatory and bronchodilating effects. **DOSAGE:** 400 to 500 milligrams three times a day.

Vitamin B6. One well-designed study showed this vitamin helped to improve peak flow rates (a measurement of breathing capacity) in a group of adults with severe asthma. In people with low blood levels of B6, supplements may help decrease wheezing. **DOSAGE:** 50 to 100 milligrams a day.

Magnesium. Studies are under way to determine whether oral supplements of magnesium—often

FEATURED RECIPES

Tropical Fruit Salad *p. 286*
Ultimate Spiced Nuts *p. 288*
Updated Waldorf Salad *p. 290*
Salmon Cake Sandwiches *p. 302*
Tomato-Roasted Mackerel *p. 308*
Salmon Steaks with Peach Salsa *p. 308*
Almond Rice *p. 322*
Brussels Sprouts with Caramelized Onions *p. 319*
Mixed Berry Tart *p. 335*

administered intravenously to asthma patients in the ER because it relaxes the airways—may help. The jury's still out on the benefits of taking supplements, but there's probably no harm in trying them in appropriate doses, although some forms of magnesium may cause diarrhea. **DOSAGE:** 200 to 400 milligrams of magnesium glycinate a day.

CAUTION

Food triggers. If you suspect your asthma attacks are brought on by certain foods, start keeping a detailed food diary in which you also note your asthma symptoms. Once you've identified a possible trigger, eliminate that food from your diet for two weeks and see if your asthma improves. If you dare to confirm your food trigger, reintroduce the food to see if your symptoms get worse again.

Common triggers include eggs; nuts; milk and other dairy products; sulfites (preservatives added to many foods, including dried fruit, instant soup and potato mixes, and red wine); and other food additives, such as aspartame (an artificial sweetener), benzoates, and yellow dye #5 (also called tartrazine).

Some vegetable oils, foods with trans fat, fatty meats, and full-fat dairy foods. Just as it's a good idea to eat plenty of foods that counter inflammation if you have asthma, it's also smart to cut down on foods that tend to promote it. Vegetable oils from corn, sunflower, and safflower, for example, are high in omega-6 fatty acids which some experts believe can promote inflammation. However, an intensive review by researchers in 2009 found that eating omega-6 fats did not increase inflammation. Until we have more definite guidelines, many experts say we should not eat excessive amounts of omega-6 fatty acids, especially at the expense of the well-established anti-inflammatory omega 3's.

You'll also want to avoid any food with partially hydrogenated oil listed on the label. These are a major source of trans fats, the primary culprits in inflammation.

You might also consider cutting back on fatty meat and full-fat dairy foods, since saturated

Preventing Asthma in Kids

Recent studies showed a clear link between a lower risk of asthma and the consumption of the antioxidants vitamin C, beta-carotene, and selenium. It appears that making sure your child gets plenty of these nutrients from foods like citrus fruits, carrots, squash, whole grains, and fish will significantly reduce her chances of developing asthma. If anyone in your house smokes, you should make doubly sure your kids get enough vitamin C. The research shows that kids who are regularly exposed to secondhand smoke have as much as a 40 percent lower asthma risk when they get enough C.

fat can induce inflammation. In one small study, 92 percent of asthma patients put on a vegan diet (no animal products, including dairy and eggs) experienced a significant decrease in symptoms after a year; 71 percent reported improvement after four months. All the participants were using long-term asthma medication such as cortisone at the start of the study. By the end, almost all were able to stop or drastically reduce their medication use.

ATTENTION DEFICIT HYPERACTIVITY DISORDER

Attention deficit hyperactivity disorder (ADHD) is one of the most controversial health conditions of our day, one that's long on theories and unanswered questions and short on treatments. Although it's arguably the most prevalent behavioral condition diagnosed in children, ADHD is really more a grab bag of behaviors than a single, well-defined disease. Affecting three times as many boys as girls, ADHD can—but doesn't always—include hyperactivity, distractibility, tantrums, anxiety, blue moods, impulsive behavior, and learning disabilities. It's believed to be related to a host of contributing factors, including asthma, genetic predisposition, secondhand smoke exposure, early exposure to television, and not being breastfed, although its "cause" remains murky.

That said, what *is* becoming clear is that what children eat—and don't eat—is an enormous part of the ADHD equation. Much of the research points to a likely connection between ADHD behavior and food sensitivities/allergies, along with deficiencies of key nutrients critical for brain development and function.

Most researchers are reluctant to say definitively that a child's diet causes ADHD or that eliminating food allergy triggers or correcting nutritional imbalances might cure it. Even so, consider that the first impulse is to medicate unruly kids with stimulant drugs like methylphenidate (Ritalin). Despite the drug's ability to tame bad behavior in 7 out of 10 kids with ADHD, there are concerns that in relying on it, we're making a devil's bargain. Ritalin's chemical composition is similar to cocaine's, one reason it's become the recreational street drug of choice for many teens. And it comes with a laundry list of possible side effects, including appetite loss, stunted growth, sleep disruption, tics, and heart problems. Given all the red flags, tinkering with a child's diet may be the safer place to start.

FEATURED RECIPES

Buckwheat Pancakes with Fruit Sauce *p. 286*
Lentil-Tomato Soup *p. 299*
Beef in Lettuce Wraps *p. 302*
Salmon Cake Sandwiches *p. 302*
Mac 'n Cheese Primavera *p. 304*
Tuna Kebabs *p. 306*
Chicken-Barley Bake *p. 312*

A diet that emphasizes protein and complex carbohydrates

This is perhaps the most important change you can make to your child's diet. Shifting it away from foods rich in refined sugar and flours and instead filling Junior's plate with more protein and high-fiber complex carbohydrates may eliminate some ADHD symptoms simply by stabilizing blood sugar levels. While the brain relies on blood sugar as its main energy source, too much can actually disrupt proper brain function.

Here's what happens. Sugar and other refined carbohydrates ("white foods" like rice and potatoes as well as soft drinks and juices that readily break down into sugars) are digested very quickly. That sends blood sugar levels soaring. The body overcompensates by releasing large amounts of insulin to move the sugar out of the bloodstream, making blood sugar levels plummet. The brain really rebels when blood sugar levels get too low, and that's when we start to feel tired, irritable, unfocused, and unable to concentrate. Sounds a bit like ADHD, doesn't it? Eating meals high in fiber and protein, on the other hand, slows digestion and helps level out those wild blood sugar spikes and plunges. Our brains, sated with a more continuous source of energy, function better—and it's quite possible that that can lead to better behavior.

It may be especially important to start your child's day with a good breakfast. A Tufts University study found that kids who ate oatmeal—rich in complex carbohydrates that supply sustained energy as well as being a source of protein—for breakfast performed better an hour later on memory tests than kids who ate sugary cereal or no breakfast at all.

Aim for: Fill half your child's plate with brightly colored vegetables, a quarter with lean protein, such as chicken, and a quarter with whole grains, such as barley or brown or wild rice. (Oatmeal and whole-wheat bread count as whole grains, too.)

Helpful hint: One way to wean kids off sugary breakfast cereals is to mix a handful with a healthier high-fiber brand (with no more than 2 grams of sugar) to help kids get used to the new taste. Slowly reduce the amount of sugary cereal in the mix until you can eliminate it altogether.

Lean beef, beans, lentils,
and other iron-rich foods

Iron is important for regulating dopamine, and low levels are associated with decreased attention, ability to focus, and mental activity. When French researchers looked at children with and without ADHD, they found that iron levels were markedly lower among those with ADHD. But even though a few very small studies suggest that supplements may help to reduce hyperactivity and improve behavior and scores on cognition tests, most health experts recommend getting iron from food, not supplements. Some iron supplements may be constipating, which can throw off digestion and absorption of other critical nutrients, and too much iron is dangerous.

Aim for: About 10 milligrams of iron daily for children four to eight years old.

Helpful hint: Beef is a super iron source. If you don't want all the fat and cholesterol, try almonds or pumpkin seeds. Just 1/4 cup of almonds and 2 tablespoons of pumpkin seeds can provide almost half of a child's daily iron needs.

Salmon, flaxseed, *and other foods rich in omega-3 essential fatty acids*

A deficiency of omega-3s has been linked with a variety of developmental and psychiatric disorders, such as depression and autism, so it's not surprising that it's also associated with ADHD. Studies indicate that some people with ADHD have significantly lower blood levels of key essential fatty acids; other studies show that children with low blood levels of omega-3s have more learning and behavior problems than kids with higher levels. (One way to tell if your child is deficient is to look at his skin and hair; dry skin and hair are signatures of essential fatty acid deficiency.)

It's possible that kids with ADHD are low in omega-3s either because they don't get enough in their diets or because their bodies don't metabolize what they do get very effectively. That may also help explain why ADHD affects more boys than girls: When the diet is lacking in omega-3s, estrogen helps conserve these essential fats, while testosterone has the opposite effect.

How do the omega-3 fats factor into ADHD? One theory is that they influence neurotransmitters, including dopamine and serotonin. Low levels of omega-3s are associated with low levels of dopamine, particularly in the part of the brain that's responsible for "executive functions" like planning ahead, controlling impulses, and staying on task. Ritalin works by increasing dopamine. It's possible that increasing omega-3 levels could do likewise.

Another part of this grand jigsaw puzzle is that some researchers have noticed that certain aspects of ADHD look remarkably like aspects of early bipolar (manic-depressive) disorder, leading some to wonder if much of what's thought of as ADHD may actually be an underlying mood or anxiety disorder. Researchers are still trying to fit the puzzle pieces together, but those who study psychiatric disorders have already linked low levels of omega-3s with depression and schizophrenia. It's not a big stretch to consider that insufficient omega-3s may also be a factor for ADHD children who tend to be moody or anxious.

If you can get your child to eat fish, terrific, but don't overdo it, because fish can contain mercury and other toxins. While most experts agree that any dangers of eating fish are outweighed by the benefits, children and pregnant women should take extra care by choosing canned light tuna rather than canned white albacore or tuna steaks, for instance. (For more tips on choosing safe seafood, see page 23.)

More kid-friendly omega-3 sources are sunflower seeds, pumpkin seeds, and flaxseed as well as raw refrigerated nut butters, such as those made from Brazil nuts, cashews, and sunflower seeds, and tahini, made from sesame seeds. (Be cautious with peanuts, which are a common allergen and a possible trigger for food sensitivity–related ADHD.) The body can convert the fats in these foods to the same kinds found in fish, but unfortunately, it doesn't do it very efficiently, so fish is still a preferred source.

Aim for: Two 3-ounce (85 g) servings of fatty fish a week.

Helpful hint: Whole flaxseed stays fresh longer than ground seed. Keep it refrigerated and use a coffee or spice grinder to grind it as needed, then add to yogurt, cereal, egg salad, or the batter for baked goods. You can combine flaxseed oil with soft trans fat–free margarine to make a healthier spread by melting a stick of trans fat–free margarine, adding a few ounces of flaxseed oil, and mixing together.

NUTRITIONAL SUPPLEMENTS
Essential fatty acids, especially DHA.
Children with ADHD tend to have low levels of omega-3 essential fatty acids. Does that mean that supplements can tame hyperactive kids and allow daydreamers to focus and concentrate? Given that studies of omega-3 supplements for depression have yielded some promising results, it's an intriguing possibility.

In one four-month, double-blind, placebo-controlled study of 50 children with ADHD at Purdue University, some of the kids were given a daily essential fatty acid supplement that contained a mixture of omega-3s along with a smattering of omega-6s; the rest were given an olive oil placebo. While the supplement didn't improve all of the symptoms associated with ADHD, it did improve parent-reported conduct problems and teacher-reported attention problems.

Randomized controlled studies that evaluated omega-3 supplements for children with ADHD are few and far between. A review by the American Psychiatric Association's Omega-3 Fatty Acids Subcommittee included two placebo-controlled studies that found DHA supplements alone were ineffective at alleviating symptoms of ADHD, and another three that concluded combining omega-3 and omega-6 supplements might help. While it is difficult to determine the specific benefit of omega-3 supplements for ADHD, it is clear that DHA is important for brain function. **DOSAGE:** About 200 milligrams of DHA daily.

Probiotics. Food sensitivities and allergies may be associated with ADHD behavior. Some nutritionally oriented physicians believe that when there's an overgrowth of harmful microorganisms, like bacteria or yeast, the lining of the intestines is damaged, allowing undigested food particles to leak into the bloodstream, where they can provoke an immune response or allergic reaction. Probiotic supplements, which contain billions of friendly bacteria like *lactobacillus* and *bifidobacterium,* keep these harmful microorganisms in check and therefore may help prevent these kinds of food sensitivities/allergies. There are hundreds of probiotic products on the shelves. Choose a refrigerated supplement that contains live cultures and delivers several billion live organisms per serving. **DOSAGE:** Follow the label directions for the product you choose.

A multivitamin/mineral. Researchers are studying the effects of individual nutrients, such as zinc, magnesium, and B_6, to treat ADHD, but because the data is still so speculative, parents may just want to stick with having their kids take a multivitamin/mineral supplement. Some very good double-blind, placebo-controlled studies suggest that when elementary school children are given a multi that meets even the most basic nutrient requirements, behavior and academic performance improve, particularly for kids who may have undetected nutrient deficiencies.

Researchers at California State University ran several trials with kids at two elementary schools in Phoenix. In one four-month study, 80 children were divided into two groups and given either a multi formulated at 50 percent of the recommended daily allowance or a

food for thought . . .

"For treating ADHD, nutrients are actually the most sensible place to start, rather than jumping straight for a drug [Ritalin] that really isn't as good as it's been cracked up to be."

— Alexandra Richardson, PhD, senior research fellow at the University of Oxford and author of *They Are What You Feed Them*

placebo. The vitamin takers had just under half the discipline problems compared to the placebo group. In another study with children at the same schools, the researchers gave the same type of multi to 245 children. This time they measured IQ. Although the supplements didn't produce dramatic increases in IQ for most of the children, among the students believed to eat a substandard diet, the gains were impressive, about 16 points. **DOSAGE:** Follow the label directions.

Zinc. It's not clear just how zinc factors into ADHD, but some association is likely because children with ADHD tend to be at least marginally deficient in the mineral. (An easy preliminary way to check your child's zinc status is to feel the skin on her arms. Little bumps on the outer arm may be a sign of zinc deficiency, although your pediatrician should confirm low levels with a blood test.)

Whether zinc deficiency is a direct cause of ADHD or merely a marker of the condition is still unknown, but some research suggests a correlation between low zinc levels and difficulty paying attention. It's also not certain whether zinc supplements improve attention span, but some intriguing preliminary research suggests that it might. **DOSAGE:** In some of the studies on zinc in kids with ADHD, the levels used were high—as high as 150 milligrams. But one study showed that children who were taking Ritalin and also took 15 milligrams of zinc, the amount in a good multivitamin, improved more and faster than kids who didn't take zinc. Don't give or take more than the amount in a multivitamin except under a doctor's supervision. Too much zinc can suppress the immune system.

OFF THE MENU

Refined sugar, refined flours, and other simple carbohydrates. It's a myth that sugar makes kids hyperactive. Nevertheless, you might think about helping your child cut back not only on sugary foods but also on other foods that tend to make blood sugar skyrocket, such as white rice and cereals with little fiber. In addition to affecting blood sugar, these highly processed foods are notoriously low in important vitamins and minerals (although cereal manufacturers add some of them back). Remember, steady blood sugar levels benefit the brain, whether a child has ADHD or not. But hyperactive children may have particular problems metabolizing sugar. It's worth noting that the hallmarks of low blood sugar include problems with attention and focus, moodiness, and frustration.

Nixing sugar also helps starve out the harmful fungi and bacteria in the digestive tract that thrive on sugary foods and contribute to food sensitivities/allergies and imbalanced immune function. It's interesting to note that overgrowth of harmful bacteria like Clostridia has been linked to another childhood developmental condition, autism.

Food dyes and additives. Eliminating artificial colors, additives, preservatives, and any foods that may provoke an allergic response is the cornerstone of most nutritional therapy for ADHD. Some experts believe that two-thirds of children with ADHD may have undiagnosed food allergies that may be responsible for their symptoms—although this theory isn't universally accepted. Still, for those kids who may be vulnerable to such sensitivities/allergies, removing trigger foods and additives often improves ADHD symptoms. Elimination diets have varying rates of success, with behavior improving in 10 to 80 percent of children, depending on the study cited.

Because there are literally thousands of substances that could potentially worsen ADHD symptoms, instead of driving yourself and your child crazy, start with food colors (look for names like FD&C red, yellow, green, and blue on labels). Researchers from Columbia University and the New York State Psychiatric Institute analyzed 15 double-blind, placebo-controlled trials that involved 219 children who were fed a diet containing artificial food colors and then given a diet free of dyes. They found that the children's behavior on the dye-free diet was significantly better than when they ate foods loaded with artificial colors. The researchers compared the effect of the dye-free diet to about one-third to one-half of the effect that could be expected from ADHD medication.

Artificial colors show up in many products, like vitamins, medicines, and toothpaste, so be vigilant. You may also want to consider avoiding common additives, flavorings, and preservatives. (Look for names like BHA, BHT, TBHQ, sodium benzoate, benzoic acid, vanillin, acesulfame-K, aspartame, saccharin, and sucralose.)

Food allergens. Common food allergy triggers include wheat, dairy, eggs, oranges, chocolate, apples, peanuts, and soy. Start by eliminating them for several weeks, then slowly add them back one at a time and see if there's any change in your child's behavior. (It's best to try an elimination diet with the help of a registered dietitian.) Another way to find your child's trigger foods is to think about the ones he really craves. Does he drink gallons of milk? Gorge on bread or crackers? Gobble down chocolate? A favorite food, one that he eats or drinks all the time, may be the very one he's sensitive or allergic to. Try eliminating it and see if his behavior improves.

Because there's no prescribed "ADHD diet," it may take trial and error before you home in on what sets your child off.

Caffeine. In a recent study done at the Smell and Taste Treatment and Research Foundation in Chicago, when 20 first graders were given caffeinated cola, their scores on an ADHD rating scale were much higher than when they drank decaffeinated soda, even when researchers accounted for the drinks' sugar content.

Can Breastfeeding Prevent ADHD?

We know that breastfed babies have much lower rates of all sorts of infections. They also appear to have lower rates of allergies and asthma. But can breastfeeding also protect against ADHD? A recent small study suggests that it's possible.

When Polish researchers looked at a group of 100 children ages 4 to 11—60 with ADHD symptoms and 40 without—they found that 60 percent of the ADHD kids had been breastfed for less than three months. Among the healthy children, just a third had been breastfed for that short a time. Although this is only one small study, researchers suspect that being weaned early may put some children at risk for ADHD, no doubt because breast milk is a superior source of the essential fatty acids needed for proper brain and eye development. The American Academy of Pediatrics recommends that babies be breastfed for at least 12 months. If you simply can't breastfeed—and for some women, it is a legitimate challenge either because they don't produce enough milk or because their babies have trouble latching on—look for formulas fortified with docosahexaenoic acid (DHA).

BREAST CANCER

Although women are actually more likely to develop heart disease, it's breast cancer that strikes fear in their hearts. After lung cancer, it's the most commonly diagnosed cancer in women, yet for most women, preventing it is a big mystery.

To some extent, your risk is already determined—by your age; your family medical history; when you got your first period and entered menopause; whether you had children or took birth control pills or hormone replacement therapy; and whether you carry one of the breast cancer genes, BRCA1 or BRCA2 (only 5 to 10 percent of breast cancers are BRCA-related).

Even if the breast cancer odds aren't in your favor, you can give yourself an edge. Monthly breast self-exams and annual mammograms are key, of course, to finding lumps that could be tumors. And the right diet can help prevent them. Scientists are still working to pinpoint which foods guard against breast tumors, but we do know that eating more fruits, vegetables, whole grains, and lean protein while curbing saturated fat and trans fat covers you against a lot of diseases, including cancer.

This may be because fruits and vegetables contain certain phytochemicals that have been singled out as effective cancer fighters. It's also because produce-rich diets are naturally lower in calories and fat. That's important because the one thing we do know for sure about breast cancer is that gaining weight, especially later in life, substantially increases risk.

There's much about breast cancer we can't control, but what and how much we eat is something we can. Here's where to start.

YOUR FOOD PRESCRIPTION

Broccoli *and other cruciferous vegetables*

If you're going to eat more of just one vegetable, make it broccoli. Lab studies have found that a cancer-fighting compound in broccoli called sulforaphane stops breast cancer cells in their tracks and encourages them to self-destruct. Plus, another compound in broccoli, called indole-3-carbinol, appears to inhibit estrogen's power to promote the growth of breast cancer cells. Broccoli's anticancer powers have been shown in human studies, too. In one called the Western New York Diet Study, premenopausal women who ate the most broccoli had a 40 percent lower breast cancer risk than women who didn't eat as much.

A bonus: Cruciferous vegetables like broccoli, cauliflower, and brussels sprouts, which protect barbecue lovers from colon cancer, may also shield them from breast cancer. If you're a big fan of cookouts, you'll definitely want to steam some broccoli to go with those burgers and hot dogs.

Aim for: Four 1/2-cup servings a week of broccoli and other cruciferous veggies, which include cabbage, watercress, bok choy, turnip greens, mustard greens, and collard greens.

Helpful hint: If you're not a fan of straight broccoli, sneak it into other dishes. Try adding it chopped to pasta sauces, soups, pizza toppings, and even omelets. Steam, stir-fry, or microwave (in just a bit of water) it instead of boiling it. These three cooking methods best conserve vegetables' vitamins and protective compounds.

Beans, leafy green vegetables,
and other foods rich in folate

Especially if you like to drink alcohol, even moderately, make sure you load your plate with plenty of these foods that supply folate, a B vitamin that alcohol depletes. It may protect cells from the potentially carcinogenic effects of alcohol.

The foods listed above also contain plenty of fiber, which helps lower estrogen levels and in turn breast cancer risk. (Many breast cancer tumors feed on estrogen, so reducing it may prevent tumors from developing.)

Aim for: At least one of the 2 1/2 cups of vegetables recommended each day should be from this group of foods.

Helpful hint: Spinach is one of the richest sources of folate. If you won't eat it alone, try layering it into lasagna or casseroles or sautéing it with olive oil, garlic, and sesame seeds to add other flavors.

Whole grains

Whole grains are an important source of fiber when it comes to preventing breast cancer. Think of fiber as a type of flypaper, but instead of pesky insects, what you're trapping is estrogen. Estrogen continually cycles through the digestive tract and is reabsorbed into the bloodstream. Fiber grabs it so it won't be reabsorbed, thereby lowering your body's estrogen levels.

Whole-grain foods may also help in other ways. Because fiber slows carbohydrate metabolism, foods like high-fiber cereals and whole-wheat bread may indirectly protect against breast tumors by reducing blood sugar spikes, thereby controlling insulin levels. Elevated insulin levels due to insulin resistance—a risk factor for type 2 diabetes—may play a role in the development of breast cancer.

In addition to their fiber, whole grains contain antioxidant phytochemicals called phe-nols, which can prevent and perhaps even repair damage to cells from dangerous molecules called free radicals. They also pack lignans, plant estrogens that lower natural estrogen levels in the body and actively slow the growth and spread of cancer cells.

A variety of other healthful compounds in whole grains combine to make these foods high in potential anticancer activity, says the American Institute for Cancer Research. Those substances include saponins—phytochemicals being studied for their anticancer properties and protease inhibitors that may prevent cancer cells from spreading.

Aim for: At least three servings of whole grains daily. One serving is 1/2 cup of whole-grain pasta or rice or a slice of whole-grain bread.

Helpful hint: Try mixing a cup of whole-grain cereal with 1/4 cup of dried fruit for a tasty snack that covers you for a serving of whole grains and a serving of fruit.

Fatty fish

You already know that fatty fish like salmon and tuna protect against heart disease, but could they protect against breast cancer, too? A recent analysis of 21 prospective cohort studies and 883,585 participants found that higher intakes of omega-3 fats from fish was associated with a 14 percent reduction of risk of breast cancer compared to a lower intake.

One reason for this encouraging result may be that the anti-inflammatory fats in fish help reduce the low-grade inflammation that is thought to spur tumor growth.

Not all studies have shown a protective association between the omega-3s in fish and breast cancer but recent results are indeed promising. And remember that there are plenty of other good reasons to eat fish. These marine sources of omega-3 fats are known to reduce the risk for heart attacks and stroke. Choose a salmon dinner more often than steak and you'll be cutting back on saturated fat, which, as you'll read later, is a good idea if you're worried about breast cancer.

The Soy Story

Does soy protect against breast cancer? That may depend on how old you are when you start eating it. Soy contains phytoestrogens, which are thought to lower the amount of estrogen circulating in your body and thus your breast cancer risk. But cancer specialists now believe that the reason Asian women have lower rates of breast cancer is that they grow up eating soy, unlike Western women who may start eating soy as adults.

The thought is that soy's phytochemicals may alter breast tissue as breasts are developing, making them more resistant to cancer-causing substances. Unfortunately, those phytochemicals may not protect women much once they reach adulthood.

The good news is that soy is safe for women with breast cancer, according to the latest research. Some of the studies even point to a potential benefit among women receiving certain treatments for breast cancer, says the American Institute for Cancer Research (AICR).

In addition, says the AICR, population studies do not show any harmful interactions between soy foods and anti-estrogen medications, including tamoxifen or an aromatase inhibitor. Although more studies are needed, simply eating moderate amounts of soy foods does not increase a breast cancer survivor's risk of recurrence or death.

What's a moderate amount of soy? One or two servings a day of whole soy foods such as tofu, soy milk, edamame, and soy nuts.

Aim for: It's not clear exactly how much fatty fish may protect against breast cancer. However, the American Heart Association recommends eating fish (particularly fatty fish) at least two times (two servings) a week. Each serving is 3.5 ounces (99 g) cooked, or about 3/4 cup of flaked fish. To get the most omega-3s, choose fatty fish like salmon, mackerel, herring, lake trout, sardines, and canned light tuna.

Milk and dairy foods

That milk mustache you've seen in so many ads may help prevent breast cancer—depending on your age. In the Nurses Health Study, which looked at more than 80,000 women, dairy foods seemed to have no effect for postmenopausal women, but premenopausal women who averaged two to three servings of low-fat or fat-free milk or dairy foods each day lowered their breast cancer risk by 28 to 32 percent compared to women who ate dairy just three times a month. Another study found that among more than 68,000 *postmenopausal* women, those who ate at least two servings of dairy foods a day lowered their breast cancer risk by 19 percent. A recent review and analysis of 27 studies involving more than 1.6 million participants concluded that modest to high consumption (about 2 to more than 3 cups a day) of dairy foods such as milk, cheese, and yogurt significantly reduced the risk of breast cancer compared with low dairy consumption (less than 2 cups a day).

Why dairy? It's not entirely clear. The calcium may play a role, but researchers are also focusing on vitamin D. New research suggests that the type of vitamin D used to fortify milk (known as vitamin D_3) reduces breast density, considered a risk factor for breast cancer.

Aim for: Two to three servings of milk, yogurt, or low-fat cheese a day. In addition to the vitamin D you get in milk (1 cup contains 100 IU), you may also want to think about taking a vitamin D supplement to get the recommended daily intake up to 600 to 800 IU per day. The Nurses Health Study found that premenopausal women who consumed more than 500 IU of vitamin D each day lowered their breast cancer risk by 28 percent.

Extra-virgin olive oil

It's not just how *much* fat you eat but also what *type* of fat you eat that influences your breast cancer risk. While it's generally thought that eating too much fat increases risk, one can't help but notice that that's not always the case in Mediterranean countries, where fat intake is high but breast cancer incidence is low. The key, many researchers suspect, is that people in Mediterranean cultures consume monounsaturated fat like that in olive oil rather than saturated fat like that in butter, ice cream, and meat or even polyunsaturated fat like that in corn or safflower oil. Indeed, a study of women in the Canary Islands showed that those who used at least 2 teaspoons of olive oil daily lowered their risk of breast cancer by an amazing 73 percent.

Research in this area is still unfolding, but a few theories have emerged. One is that olive oil is simply a healthier type of fat and that eating it in place of unhealthy saturated fat and trans fat lowers risk. The other piece of the puzzle is that olive oil comes from olives, fruits that contain many of the therapeutic compounds, like phenols and lignans, that we already know fight cancer. (Phenols inhibit the formation of cancer-causing compounds. Lignans convert in the body to a weak estrogen-like compound that can displace the body's own, stronger estrogen from cells.) Researchers at Northwestern University have also discovered that the oleic acid in olive oil actively suppresses a gene associated with the development of a very aggressive form of breast cancer and even improves the effectiveness of the cancer drug trastuzumab (Herceptin).

The caveat, of course, is that olive oil is high in calories, so use it sparingly—*instead of* other fats, not with them.

Aim for: 1 to 2 tablespoons a day.

Helpful hint: One reason olive oil may be so cancer protective is that it makes those veggies go down a little easier. Try sautéing vegetables in olive oil instead of butter or using olive oil in place of other vegetable oils in salad dressings.

Flaxseed

The American Institute for Cancer Research has found enough evidence to put flaxseed on its list of "Foods That Fight Cancer." Besides being an excellent source of magnesium, manganese, thiamin, and fiber and a good source of selenium, flaxseed is a rich source of lignans—plant estrogens that may be protective against breast cancer.

About half of the fat in flaxseed and flaxseed oil is ALA (alpha-linolenic acid)—the plant form of healthful omega-3 fat known for its anti-inflammatory properties. (Experts now believe that the development of tumor cells is an inflammatory process.) Flaxseed and flaxseed oil also contain vitamin E, a potent antioxidant.

Two tablespoons of ground flaxseed contain almost 4 grams of fiber. Flaxseed oil, however, does not contain fiber or some of the other nutrients—such as selenium—found in ground flaxseed.

Aim for: 1 to 4 tablespoons of ground flaxseed per day appears to be safe and potentially protective against breast cancer based on studies using those amounts, say experts. Buy it ground or grind it yourself in a coffee grinder, blender, or food processor. Store ground flaxseed in an airtight container in the fridge.

Helpful hint: Add flaxseed to your meals by sprinkling it over cereal or salads, mixing it into yogurt or smoothies, or buying flaxseed-enriched grain products like breads and waffles.

FEATURED RECIPES

Edamame Hummus with Pita Crisps *p. 288*
Broccoli Salad *p. 291*
Coleslaw with Orange-Sesame Vinaigrette *p. 290*
Spinach Salad with Chickpeas *p. 293*
Tuna and White Bean Salad *p. 295*
Brown Rice Risotto *p. 321*
Chicken-Barley Bake *p. 312*
Tomato-Roasted Mackerel *p. 308*

NUTRITIONAL SUPPLEMENTS

Vitamin D. Although vitamin D is not recommended for everyone to prevent breast cancer, some research suggests that low levels of D may increase a woman's chance for this disease. Women with healthy levels of vitamin D had 63 percent lower odds of breast cancer than women who didn't have enough of it, according to one study. Doses of 1,000 IU per day are often recommended to maintain normal vitamin D levels. Check the label to ensure you're getting D_3 (listed as cholecalciferol), which, according to a recent review of research trials, is more effective in raising vitamin D levels in the blood than vitamin D_2.

OFF THE MENU

Foods high in saturated fat and trans fat.
Already linked with so many other diseases, like heart disease, saturated fat promotes inflammation in the body, which can stimulate tumor growth. While not all studies have definitively linked fat intake with breast cancer risk, at least one suggests that women who consume more than 35 grams of saturated fat a day have double the risk of breast cancer compared to women who limit their intake to only 10 grams a day.

There's also some suggestion that trans fat, found in many packaged baked goods, snack foods, and commercially fried foods, may be linked with higher breast cancer risk. When researchers took fat samples from the backsides of nearly 700 European women with and without breast cancer, they found that the women with the highest levels of trans fat stored in their bodies also had a 40 percent higher risk of breast cancer. This is another good reason why the Food and Drug Administration has required manufacturers to eliminate partially hydrogenated oils—the major source of trans fat—from our food supply.

Researchers involved with the Women's Health Initiative Study, which followed more than 48,000 postmenopausal women, found that those who started the study with the highest-fat diets and then cut their fat intake to 24 percent of calories were able to lower their breast cancer risk by 15 to 20 percent.

That said, the jury's still out on whether reducing fat intake definitely lowers breast cancer risk. But since eating less saturated and trans fat helps with so many other conditions, it makes good sense either way.

Sugary foods and refined carbohydrates.
There is no strong evidence that directly links sugary foods and refined starches like white bread and numerous snack foods to increased cancer risk, yet there is an indirect link, say experts. When we overeat sugar, we eat more calories than our bodies can process and this can lead to excess weight and body fat. It is excess body fat that increases the risk for many types of cancer, including breast cancer. A study of more than 1,800 women in Mexico found that those who ate a lot of refined carbohydrates had double the breast cancer risk of women whose diets were more balanced.

Alcohol. There is now strong evidence that alcohol increases the risk of several cancers, including breast cancer, says the American Institute of Cancer Research. Because even small amounts of alcohol consumed regularly increase the risk for breast cancer (especially if combined with smoking), these experts recommend not to drink alcohol; if you choose to drink, limit your consumption to no more than two drinks a day for men and one drink a day for women.

Health-conscious cooks know to have a second coffee grinder just for spices, herbs, and seeds. In particular, use it to grind flaxseed, considered by some to be the ultimate food for breast cancer prevention. For maximum freshness, grind flaxseed just before you add it to your dishes.

Lose Weight, Lower Your Risk

There's one thing you can do that will surely help lower your risk of breast cancer: Maintain a healthy weight. Not only are heavy women more likely to develop breast cancer, they're also more likely to die from it. Data from the Nurses Health Study suggests that nonsmoking women who are overweight when they're diagnosed are almost twice as likely as slender women to die of breast cancer.

More body fat equals higher estrogen levels. And excess body fat, particularly around the belly, produces proteins called cytokines, which increase inflammation and cause the kind of cell damage that can lead to cancer. For that reason, "apple-shaped" premenopausal women have more than double the breast cancer risk of their "pear-shaped" counterparts. Being overweight also goes hand in hand with higher levels of the tumor-stimulating hormones insulin and insulin-like growth factor-1.

During pregnancy, it's important not to gain significantly more than the recommended 25 to 35 pounds (11 to 16 kg) and to lose that weight after giving birth. A Finnish study of more than 27,000 breast cancer patients found that gaining 40 pounds (18 kg) during pregnancy was associated with a 40 percent increase in breast cancer risk.

Gaining weight after menopause is also problematic. According to the Nurses Health Study, women who put on 22 pounds (10 kg) after menopause raised their breast cancer risk by 18 percent.

So cut calories—and get off the couch. Even apart from weight loss, exercise appears to influence hormones in a way that's protective against breast cancer.

BREAST TENDERNESS

We wish we could report that eating a pint of ice cream will banish breast tenderness. It won't. But there are plenty of other dietary tweaks that may lessen the discomfort.

Most breast tenderness can be blamed on hormone fluctuations that precede menstruation. The breasts also respond to menstruation by absorbing extra fluid, which doesn't help. Another cause is fibrocystic breast disease, in which benign lumps form in the breast tissue and can become tender, especially close to and during menstruation. Stress, pregnancy, and medications like hormones can also cause breast pain. In rare cases, breast cancer (which usually doesn't involve pain) or noncancerous tumors can cause tenderness, so letting your doctor know about breast discomfort is a good idea.

Although Ben and Jerry's won't make it all better, there are some foods you can add to your diet that may help. Subtracting certain other foods may be even more important.

YOUR FOOD PRESCRIPTION

Oily fish, flaxseed,
and other foods high in omega-3 fatty acids

With each bite of grilled salmon, you get omega-3 fatty acids that help balance eicosanoids, hormone-like substances that help control inflammation, pain, and swelling. You also get resolvins, a recently discovered class of anti-inflammatory fats, which appear to ease inflammation much the same way aspirin does.

Flaxseed offers omega-3s as well as some fiber and lignans, plant estrogens that may reduce the risk of breast cancer. To get the most benefit from flaxseed, buy whole seeds and keep them refrigerated. Grind them as needed in a coffee or spice grinder.

Aim for: 1,000 milligrams of omega-3s a day, about the amount in 2 ounces (56 g) of salmon or five walnut halves. If you're not a fish fan, aim to eat 2 tablespoons of ground flaxseed a day, added to breakfast cereal, oatmeal, smoothies, or yogurt.

Helpful hint: If you eat a lot of fatty fish or other foods high in omega-3s, you need more vitamin E than people whose diets are lower in omega-3s. Look to almonds, wheat germ, and spinach for this vitamin, which may itself help relieve breast pain, although the jury's still out.

Soy foods

The estrogen-like plant chemicals in soy and flaxseed weakly mimic human estrogen and may help assuage breast tenderness. In a small, two-month British study of women ages 18 to 35, eating soy protein containing 68 milligrams of soy isoflavones every day (about the amount in two servings of soy foods) significantly reduced breast tenderness and swelling compared to a placebo.

Aim for: About 68 milligrams of soy isoflavones daily, about the amount you'd get from a glass of soy milk and a half cup of tofu. It can't hurt to have one or two soy-based meals a week, snack on edamame (green soybeans), and pour soy milk instead of dairy milk.

Whole grains, lentils, pears,
and other foods high in fiber

One of the most important tweaks you can make to your diet to lessen breast pain is to eat more fiber. Fiber lowers estrogen levels, which helps minimize breast tenderness as well as other PMS symptoms.

Aim for: 25 to 35 grams of fiber a day. You can get there by eating a serving of bran cereal in the morning, a salad with 1/2 cup of cooked lentils at lunchtime, a pear as a snack, and a cup of winter squash with dinner.

Water

One reason breasts may get sore around menstruation is that they absorb extra fluid. Ironically, drinking plenty of water every day can decrease water retention; the more you drink, the less fluid the body feels it must hold.

Aim for: Eight 8-ounce glasses (2 l) a day.

NUTRITIONAL SUPPLEMENTS

Vitamin E. Some studies have found that vitamin E is helpful in relieving breast pain; others have not. **DOSAGE:** 400 IU daily, the dose that appeared to relieve breast tenderness in several studies.

Omega-3 fatty acids. Omega-3s come in softgel fish-oil capsules or in liquid forms such as flaxseed oil (though flaxseed oil doesn't provide any of the fiber or lignans that ground flaxseed does). Choose a supplement that contains vitamin E, which will help prevent spoilage, and store it in the fridge. **DOSAGE:** 1 to 3 grams a day. Check with your doctor before taking omega-3s if you're also taking a blood thinner such as warfarin (Coumadin).

Chasteberry extract. Women have used chasteberries for thousands of years to tame menstrual problems. Over the past 50 years, more than 30 European trials have shown that the supplements improve menstrual symptoms, including breast tenderness. **DOSAGE:** Many of the studies used 4 milligrams per day.

Vitamin B_6. According to some studies, B_6 may help relieve PMS symptoms, including breast tenderness. **DOSAGE:** 50 to 100 milligrams daily.

OFF THE MENU
Saturated fat. Put the coffee cake and butter away. Saturated fat promotes inflammation. Canola oil and olive oil are much better choices. Trans fat is a "no-no" too, so avoid products with any "partially hydrogenated" ingredients, which are being phased out of our food supply.

Alcohol. Pass on wine with dinner, at least before and during your period. Alcohol interferes with the normal hormone shifts that occur around menstruation and can increase breast tenderness.

Salt. Salt holds fluid in body tissues, adding to the swelling that increases breast tenderness.

Caffeine. Although there's no solid evidence that links caffeine with breast tenderness, some doctors still recommend dropping coffee and other caffeinated drinks, primarily because they've seen patients improve once they give them up. Try switching to caffeine-free teas and sodas for four to six months to see if you notice any difference.

FEATURED RECIPES

Edamame Hummus with Pita Crisps *p. 288*
Sweet Potato Soup *p. 297*
Ginger Butternut Squash Soup *p. 298*
Salsa Tuna Salad Sandwiches *p. 300*
Tomato-Roasted Mackerel *p. 308*
Roasted Salmon with Sautéed Greens *p. 309*
Springtime Quinoa *p. 322*

CANCER

If you think your genes spell out your risk for cancer, you're only partly right. Another part of the equation, and a big one at that, is the life you lead—in fact, a third of all cancers are directly linked to the kinds of foods people eat, how overweight they are, and how little physical activity they get. And that's regardless of whether they smoke.

When it comes to our diets, here's the hard, unpleasant truth: Just as popular American foods—cheeseburgers, french fries, super-size sodas, and the like—lead us down the garden path to heart disease, they're also tailor-made to give us cancer. Hard to swallow? Here's the good news: While you can't choose your genes, you *can* choose what to eat. In places where people consume more fish, produce, and whole grains and eat less saturated fat and fewer refined carbs, cancer rates are lower than in places where there's an abundance of processed foods, beef, and potatoes—your standard Western fare.

You don't have to move to another country to protect yourself, though. Simply fill two-thirds of your plate with vegetables, fruits, whole grains, and beans. That could probably lower your overall cancer risk by 20 to 35 percent. Better still, walk to the grocery store. Not only does physical activity help with weight maintenance, but exercise seems to independently reduce hormones believed to promote breast, colon, prostate, and uterine cancers.

YOUR FOOD PRESCRIPTION

A rainbow of fruits *and vegetables*

We really mean a *rainbow*. Don't limit yourself to the same old apples, oranges, and bananas. In one study, one group of women, all of whom were eating eight to nine servings of produce daily, were told to limit their choices to eight types of produce known to be high in antioxidants; another group was instructed to choose from up to 18 different kinds of fruits and vegetables. Blood tests later revealed that the group eating the wider variety had demonstrably less cancer-inducing DNA damage to their cells than those who cast a smaller net.

Most studies on diet and cancer—with one recent notable exception—have definitively linked higher fruit and vegetable consumption to lower risks of an array of cancers, including those of the breast, prostate, lung, mouth, esophagus, stomach, and colon. According to the most comprehensive report to date on diet,

nutrition, physical activity, and cancer, there is strong evidence that fruit and non-starchy vegetable intake can decrease the risk for digestive and other cancers. Foods containing dietary fiber (fruits and vegetables are in this category) also decrease the risk for cancers of the colon and rectum.

There is also limited evidence that a low intake of fruit can increase the risk of stomach and colorectal cancers.

It's not just the antioxidants at work. Fruits and vegetables contain other key substances, including fiber, which helps reduce hormones like estrogen that can promote cancer, and other plant compounds that actively protect our bodies from cancer.

Scientists are still working out the mystery of which compounds are most effective against various cancers. Many have already been identified, like the beta-carotene in carrots and sweet potatoes, the lycopene in tomatoes, the sulforaphane in broccoli, the folate in spinach, the sulfur compounds in garlic and onions, and the ellagic acid in berries. But researchers are still exploring the garden to discover others that may be just as potent.

What's clear is that these nutrients work best when they work together, so eating that rainbow we mentioned is far more effective than relying on supplements.

Aim for: At the very least, get 2 to 3 cups of fruits and 2 to 3 cups of vegetables a day. And don't let the big numbers deter you—you can easily get 2 to 3 cups just by eating a large salad. And you can meet your goal with raw or cooked fruit and vegetables, dried fruit, and 100 percent fruit or vegetable juices.

Helpful hint: Steam, stir-fry, microwave, or roast your vegetables. While nutrients can leach out when vegetables are boiled, these other methods help conserve them.

Broccoli *and other cruciferous vegetables*

If there's an all-star cancer fighter, it's broccoli, along with its cruciferous cousins like cauliflower, brussels sprouts, cabbage, and kale. These veggies are packed with very potent anticancer compounds, such as sulforaphane and other isothiocyanates, that not only flush out carcinogens—particularly those created when meats are grilled or fried—before they can damage cells but may also repair cell damage that could lead to tumor growth. In addition, they slow the growth of cancer cells that do develop and increase their self-destruction.

Eating more of these vegetables is associated with lower risk of breast, colon, prostate, and lung cancers. Other research has shown that these veggies also lower the risk of lymphoma and bladder cancer. And some researchers suspect that broccoli (particularly broccoli sprouts, which contain up to 20 to 50 times more sulforaphane than mature broccoli) may protect against stomach cancer by reducing levels of *Helicobacter pylori,* a bacterium that damages cells in the stomach lining.

Aim for: Four 1/2-cup servings a week.

Whole grains

There are more reasons than you can shake a stalk at to eat more whole grains. You may not think of them as a source of antioxidants, but they are. And they contain plant estrogens called lignans, which help lower estrogen levels and encourage cancer cells to self-destruct (see the Breast Cancer entry, page 114). But there's more. Because whole grains are excellent sources of fiber and complex carbohydrates, which are digested and absorbed slowly, they don't raise blood sugar as dramatically as refined carbohydrates and sugary foods do. This keeps insulin levels low. That's important because high levels of insulin, along with its cousin, insulin-like growth factor-1, encourage cells to multiply, which can ultimately cause tumors to develop and allow cancer cells to spread.

Aim for: Research suggests that eating at least four servings of whole grains (such as a slice of whole-grain bread, 1 ounce (28 g) of cereal, or 1/2 cup of rice or pasta) a week lowers overall cancer risk by 34 percent. However, to meet recommended daily fiber goals and get the protective compounds linked to overall health, it's best to eat at least three servings every day.

Helpful hint: A good way to have your pasta but avoid those refined carbs is to switch to whole-wheat pasta. Some brands and even some shapes taste better than others, so experiment until you find a kind you like. And don't forget to top it with plenty of garlic and veggies.

Water

Drinking water and noncaffeinated beverages (fat-free milk, herbal tea) may help protect against bladder cancer because fluids dilute any potential carcinogens lurking in urine. Plus, the more trips you take to the loo, the less time carcinogens are in contact with the bladder lining.

Aim for: Drink enough fluids throughout the day so that your urine is very pale. (It will have a darker yellow tinge if you're taking B vitamins.)

Fatty fish

If you're fishing for anticancer foods, you might try snaring a salmon (good luck with that, unless you're a bear). This famously heart-healthy fish, as well as other fish high in omega-3 fatty acids, such as albacore tuna, sardines, mackerel, and rainbow trout, may also help keep cancer at bay. Some studies already show an association between fatty fish consumption and lower risk of breast, colon, prostate, and lung cancers.

The research is far from conclusive, but if omega-3s do turn out to guard against cancer, it may be because they fight inflammation inside the body, which is thought to spur tumor growth. Getting more omega-3s protects against disease even more when you also reduce your consumption of omega-6 fats, which actively promote inflammation and are found in corn, sunflower, and safflower oils.

Also, let's not forget that eating grilled or steamed fish instead of steaks and burgers can help keep your waistline trim; weight gain is a significant risk factor for many types of cancer.

Aim for: The American Heart Association recommends two servings (8 to 12 ounces/226 to 340 g total) of fatty fish each week to protect against heart disease, which is also a good target for cancer protection.

Helpful hint: Worried about mercury and other toxins? Avoid swordfish, tilefish, shark, and king mackerel.

FEATURED RECIPES

Broccoli Salad *p. 291*
Spinach Salad with Chickpeas *p. 293*
Ginger Butternut Squash Soup *p. 298*
Lentil-Tomato Soup *p. 299*
Mac 'n Cheese Primavera *p. 304*
Roasted Salmon with Sautéed Greens *p. 309*
Chicken in Garlic Sauce *p. 312*
Chicken-Barley Bake *p. 312*
Brown Rice Risotto *p. 321*
Mixed Berry Tart *p. 335*

Green tea

If you want to avoid cancer, it may be time you acquired a taste for green tea, a potent source of cancer-fighting antioxidants that can protect against the DNA damage that causes cells to turn cancerous. In cell studies, one of the most important of these antioxidants, called epigallocatechin gallate (EGCG), blocked an enzyme that cancer cells need to grow.

Aim for: To get significant anticancer benefits, you'll probably need to drink 4 cups a day.

Beans *and leafy green vegetables*

Especially if you drink or smoke, consider having a green salad sprinkled with beans for lunch. Dark leafy greens like spinach, kale, and even romaine lettuce contain the cancer-fighting antioxidants lutein and beta-carotene as well as the B vitamin folate, which safeguards cells from alcohol and tobacco carcinogens. Beans are also rich in antioxidants called flavonoids, not to mention fiber.

Researchers at University College London have found that beans and other legumes, like lentils and peas, also contain a cancer-fighting compound with the tongue-twisting name of inositol pentakisphosphate, which blocks a key enzyme involved in tumor growth. It even makes some anticancer drugs work more effectively.

Aim for: At least one serving of leafy green vegetables (1/2 cup cooked or 1 cup raw) and one serving of legumes (1/2 cup) most days of the week.

Helpful hint: Sneak beans into your favorite dishes by adding rinsed canned beans to casseroles, stews, chilis, salads, salsas, and soups.

Grapes and grape juice

You know wine's good for your heart, thanks in large part to a potent antioxidant called resveratrol. The hitch is that alcohol also promotes cancer (see the Breast Cancer entry, page 118, and the Colon Cancer entry, page 137). But there's no need to toss out the baby with the bathwater. You can get resveratrol without the alcohol by eating some grapes or drinking grape juice. Laboratory studies suggest that resveratrol, minus the alcohol, protects against breast, skin, liver, and stomach cancers as well as lymphoma and leukemia.

Aim for: There's no established recommendation, but having 1/2 cup of grapes or 3/4 cup of grape juice several times a week as part of your daily 4 to 6 cups of fruits and vegetables is a smart idea.

Garlic

Whether or not garlic wards off vampires, it does seem to help ward off cancer, especially stomach and colorectal cancer. Chalk it up to garlic's powerful sulfur compounds, which flush out carcinogens before they can damage cell DNA and force cancer cells that do develop to self-destruct.

Researchers from the University of North Carolina at Chapel Hill found that people who ate an average of about five garlic cloves a week, raw or cooked, had only two-thirds the risk of colon cancer and half the risk of stomach cancer compared to people who didn't eat much garlic. The thought is that because garlic is antibacterial, along with killing cancer cells, it also kills *H. pylori,* the bacterium that damages the stomach lining, thus making it more vulnerable to cancer.

In addition, cell studies suggest that garlic works like the cruciferous vegetables in protecting cells from damage by carcinogens created when meat is cooked over open flames or high heat.

Aim for: Three to five cloves a week.

Helpful hint: Cooking deactivates garlic's therapeutic compounds. But that doesn't mean you have to eat raw garlic. One way to preserve these cancer-fighting compounds is to chop or crush the garlic and let it stand for 10 to 15 minutes before using it in cooking.

Spice Up Your Life

Who says healthy food has to be bland? When you spice things up, you also add a good dose of antioxidants and other cancer-fighting phytochemicals to your meals. Many spices in the rack, like cayenne, ginger, cumin, and oregano, are considered beneficial for their antioxidant and anti-inflammatory actions. But for cancer, turmeric, the yellow spice used in Indian cooking, is a real standout.

Turmeric contains curcumin, which not only clears out carcinogens before they can wreak havoc with cell DNA but also shuts down an inflammatory protein that encourages tumor growth. Turmeric also helps block a tumor's effort to construct blood vessels it needs to survive and spread. Research suggests that turmeric may protect against colon cancer as well as melanoma, the deadliest form of skin cancer. More research is needed to confirm these results, however.

NUTRITIONAL SUPPLEMENTS

A multivitamin/mineral. The fact is, most studies have found no connection between taking supplements and lowering your cancer risk. Indeed, some research has found that taking individual supplements of beta-carotene may actually *increase* the risk of lung cancer. Nutrition experts always advise getting your nutrients from foods because nutrients appear to work more effectively in the amounts and combinations that nature intended. That said, if you simply can't manage to eat all of the recommended servings of fruits, vegetables, and grains each day, then taking a daily multivitamin/mineral supplement to close the gap can't hurt, especially if you're over 50 and don't eat breakfast cereal or other foods fortified with vitamin B_{12}. **DOSAGE:** One a day.

Vitamin D. The sunshine vitamin may be the one exception to the "no individual supplements for cancer prevention" rule. There is a growing body of evidence to suggest that higher amounts of this vitamin—about 1,000 IU—than can be gotten from food do help reduce the risk of colon and breast cancer. Other data from the Health Professionals Follow-Up Study and the Nurses Health Study indicated that 300 IU or more of vitamin D a day lowered the risk of pancreatic cancer by more than 40 percent. **DOSAGE:** At least 400 IU daily. According to a number of studies, 1,000 IU appears to be even more protective. Check how much you're already getting from any calcium or multivitamin supplements you take, and don't forget to factor in what you may be getting from milk, fortified juice, or cereal (three servings of milk provide about 300 IU). Look at the supplement ingredient label to make sure it contains the form of D known as cholecalciferol (vitamin D_3), which is the more active form. Don't exceed 2,000 IU a day from both food and supplements without your doctor's agreement.

LESS ON THE MENU

Saturated fats. Already linked with many other diseases, like heart disease, saturated fat also promotes the kind of inflammation that damages cell DNA and permits tumors to build the blood vessel network that allows them to grow and spread. Saturated fat has been linked with cancers of the stomach, esophagus, breast, and colon.

Red meats and processed meats. Red and processed meats, which include beef, pork, and lamb, are associated with a host of cancers, not only because these meats are sources of saturated fat. It's also because grilling or frying meat creates carcinogens that have been linked with breast, colon, and other cancers. According to the latest evidence reported by the World Cancer Research Fund and the American Institute for Cancer Research, eating more than 18 ounces (510 g) of red meat a week is strongly associated with a cause of colorectal cancer. More modest amounts—less than 18 ounces (510 g) of cooked red meat a week—do not seem to increase the risk of this cancer, say researchers.

When it comes to processed meat such as ham, bacon, salami, hot dogs and sausage, all bets are off, says experts. The evidence is convincing that cancer risk, especially the risk for stomach cancer, begins with even a very low intake of these foods. This is why the expert panel advises limiting red meat and avoiding processed meat altogether.

Sugar and refined carbohydrates. Some cancer experts are branding sugary foods and the starchy, refined carbohydrates that quickly become sugar in the body as cancer promoters. When we overeat sugar, not only do the extra calories cause us to gain weight but sugar/refined carbohydrate consumption also raises levels of insulin and insulin-like growth factor-1, both of which can be considered "cancer food." Links have already been established between a diet high in refined carbohydrates and stomach, colon, prostate, and breast cancers. A diet high in sugars and refined starches, such as our typical fast fare, also increases the risk for endometrial cancer. Experts think this could be due to increased glucose and insulin levels, which lead to insulin resistance, diabetes, and obesity—factors that are associated with the development of this type of cancer.

Salty foods. Salt appears to damage the stomach lining, making it more vulnerable to cancer development, especially among people infected with *H. pylori*. Studies in Eastern Europe and Japan point to a link between high consumption of salted or smoked fish and meats and an increased gastric cancer risk of between 70 and 200 percent (depending on what was eaten and how often). Reducing your salt intake along with increasing your fruits and vegetables (and of course not smoking) can prevent as many as 75 percent of gastric cancer cases.

Alcohol. Alcohol raises the risk of several cancers, including cancers of the breast, colon, esophagus, and liver. As alcohol is metabolized, free radicals and other compounds that damage DNA are produced. Too much alcohol can also raise estrogen levels and lower folate levels, which can lead to DNA damage and disrupt the body's ability to repair it. Researchers at the University of Mississippi have also found that alcohol stimulates blood vessel development in tumors, causing them to grow and spread. One laboratory study showed that animals exposed to alcohol had tumors that were twice as big as those in the control group, and the spread of cancer cells into the blood vessels was eight times greater. For cancer prevention, it's best not to drink alcohol, say experts.

Put a plate of raw vegetables on the table with every meal. It could include carrots, celery sticks, cucumber slices, cherry tomatoes, green pepper slices, and broccoli crowns. No one is excused until the plate is empty!

CATARACTS

Get out the salad bowl and fishing lures: Fruits, vegetables, and fish appear to help stave off cataracts, cloudy coverings that can form over the lenses of the eyes as you age. Cataracts, the leading cause of blindness worldwide, occur when proteins in the lens fray, and their debris muddies the lens.

Aging is the most common culprit behind cataracts. Heredity and ethnicity (black people have a higher risk), some medications, and other eye conditions play a role, but so does a lifetime of sun exposure, smoking, and poor nutrition. Fortunately, nutrients in certain foods help protect the eye from an array of assailants. Some nutrients throw up a natural sunscreen; others fight damaging molecules known as free radicals; and still others lower blood sugar levels, which also benefits the eyes.

YOUR FOOD PRESCRIPTION

Fatty fish
and other foods high in omega-3 fatty acids

Savoring grilled salmon or tuna at least once a week may cut your risk of cataracts by as much as 12 percent, according to a long-term Harvard study. Researchers suspect that it's the omega-3 fatty acids plentiful in fish that help protect the eyes. Although scientists haven't pinpointed why these fat building blocks help, they do know that our eye membranes are awash with them and that they're essential for visual development in embryos and infants. In other words, omega-3s are clearly important to eye health.

If you hate fish, you can get some omega-3s from plant sources such as walnuts, soybeans, flaxseed, and some leafy greens.

Aim for: An average of 1,000 milligrams a day—the equivalent of a 4-ounce (113 g) serving of salmon, 1/4 cup of walnuts, or 2 tablespoons of flaxseed several times a week.

Helpful hint: No need to completely skip the mayo on your tuna salad. Previous concerns about omega-6 fats in corn, soy, and safflower oils contributing to cataracts have been put to rest by recent research. One study among 12,308 men and women in Spain, for example, found that a high intake of omega-6 fats was associated with a lower incidence of cataracts. Remember, though, mayonnaise is a fat, so a little dab—about 1 tablespoon—will do best for your eye-friendly diet.

Fruits and vegetables

Sunlight, cigarette smoke, air pollution, and infection—many of the culprits associated with cataract damage—all generate free radicals, unstable molecules that damage cells throughout the body, including those in the eyes. The antidote? Antioxidants, which neutralize free radicals. Where can you get them? Your fruit bowl and vegetable bin. A 10-year Harvard

FEATURED RECIPES

Tropical Fruit Salad *p. 286*
Spinach Salad with Chickpeas *p. 293*
Tuna and White Bean Salad *p. 295*
Sweet Potato Soup *p. 297*
Tomato-Roasted Mackerel *p. 308*
Salmon Steaks with Peach Salsa *p. 308*
Orange Beets *p. 323*
Raspberry-Almond Muffins *p. 324*

study found that serving yourself plenty of produce may cut cataract risk by 10 to 15 percent. Particularly strong protectors are the vitamin C in citrus fruits; the beta-carotene in carrots and other orange and yellow fruits and vegetables (plus spinach); and the vitamin E in nuts, seeds, and green leafy vegetables such as spinach.

Pay special attention to those leafy greens—spinach, kale, turnip greens, and collard greens. The antioxidant plant pigments lutein and zeaxanthin, found in abundance in these foods, accumulate in the eyes and provide excellent "eye armor." In one laboratory study, when lens cells were treated with these pigments and then exposed to ultraviolet radiation, a harmful component of sunlight, those cells showed 50 to 60 percent less damage than the untreated cells.

Aim for: 2 to 3 cups of vegetables and 2 to 3 cups of fruits every day.

Helpful hint: Consider freezing fruits and vegetables you don't eat immediately. It will help prevent the loss of nutrients, especially vitamin C.

NUTRITIONAL SUPPLEMENTS

Omega-3 fatty acids. Omega-3s come in fish-oil capsules and in liquids such as flaxseed oil. Buying a version with vitamin E helps prevent rancidity, as does storing the supplement in the refrigerator. **DOSAGE:** Optimal dosages aren't established, but many experts recommend 1 gram a day. If you want to take more, check with your doctor.

A multivitamin/mineral. The simplest way to get a mix of antioxidants is from a multivitamin/mineral supplement. **DOSAGE:** One a day.

OFF THE MENU

Too much alcohol. Here's another reason not to pass your glass too often. Several studies have found an association between alcohol and cataracts. In one, women who drank two glasses a week of any kind of alcohol bumped up their risk of the most common type of cataract by 13 percent, although they lowered the risk of a less common form. As usual, the message is

Sight-Saving Weight Loss

All of us know that ice cream cleaves to our waists, but now research suggests that having a bulging waistline may contribute to eye damage. In a study at Tufts University, obese women were 2 1/2 times more likely to develop a certain type of cataract than women of normal weight. It may have something to do with the effects of high blood sugar, which often goes hand in hand with weighing too much. Women with diabetes were four times more likely to have this type of lens cloudiness.

that a drink or two is probably fine, but know when to say when.

Salt and salty processed foods. Turn in the saltshaker. According to an Australian study of almost 3,000 people, liberal sprinklers who consumed more than 1 1/4 teaspoons of salt a day were twice as likely to have cataracts as people who ate about half a teaspoon. Scientists believe that excess salt bodywide may interfere with sodium levels in the eye as well. Don't forget that much of the salt we consume comes from soups, processed meats, and the many other processed foods manufacturers load with the stuff.

COLDS AND FLU

No doubt you've heard the old joke: If you treat a cold aggressively, it'll be gone in about seven days, but if you do absolutely nothing, it'll drag on for a full week.

Neither your doctor nor your pharmacy can do much to cure your cold. Don't bother begging for antibiotics—colds and flu are caused by viruses, so these drugs, which fight bacteria, won't help. (In the case of the flu, your doctor *does* have antiviral drugs that can cut it short if you start taking them right away.) But if conventional medicine has no cure for a cold, your grandma just might—if she has a good recipe for chicken soup.

That's right, chicken soup, along with other foods, drinks, and herbs, can ease symptoms and may even cut a cold short. In fact, follow our food and supplement prescriptions, and you may just sail through the next cold and flu season with nary a sniffle or ache. That's nothing to sneeze at!

YOUR FOOD PRESCRIPTION

Water, decaffeinated tea, and juices

Cold and flu bugs thrive in dried-out throats and nasal passages, but drinking plenty of fluids throughout the day can help keep your mucous membranes moist so they're better able to trap viruses. Then you can either blow them out your nose or swallow them so they're destroyed by your stomach acids before they have a chance to make you sick. Not only can this help prevent colds, but it's just as useful if you're already sick. If you find plain H_2O too boring to drink, cut up some oranges and add them to a pitcher of water for flavor. Each orange also provides 50 milligrams of vitamin C.

If you have a sore throat, sip your water hot with a bit of honey (to coat your throat) and lemon (to shrink swollen throat tissues and help kill off virus cells), or add honey and lemon to tea. Gargling with warm saltwater can also ease a sore throat by clearing away dead white blood cells and increasing blood flow to the throat, which helps your body fight the infection. Or squirt saltwater into your nose to help clear out nasal mucus. Squirt one nostril, then blow your nose. Repeat with the other nostril.

Aim for: At least eight glasses of water or other fluids each day, and more if you have a fever.

Helpful hint: Orange juice is a popular "go-to" beverage during cold and flu season. If you're planning to drink up, know this: Frozen OJ contains more vitamin C than the ready-to-drink kind. That's because more of the vitamin C in juice sold in cartons or bottles is oxidized—as much as 76 percent compared to just 20 percent of C in frozen juice—and the body doesn't absorb it as well. To get the most C from your juice, grab some frozen juice concentrate from the freezer section and drink it within a week of mixing it up.

Chicken soup

Although Grandma's favorite cold fighter hasn't yet yielded up all its healing secrets, researchers are beginning to puzzle out why it may work. For starters, hot chicken soup raises the temperature in your nose and throat, creating an inhospitable environment for viruses that prefer cooler, drier climes. Next, just like a hot, steamy shower, hot, steamy soup thins out mucus so you can more easily blow it out. Studies have proved it works better at this than plain old hot water. And finally, according to a laboratory study of both homemade and store-bought soups done at the University of Nebraska Medical Center, the soup inhibits white blood cells called neutrophils that are released in huge numbers when you have a cold. It's the congregation of these white cells that causes a cold's hallmark congestion.

Aim for: There's no prescribed "dosage" for chicken soup, so just enjoy a steaming bowlful when you're feeling sniffly and sneezy.

Helpful hint: Vegetarians don't have to miss out. In the Nebraska study, vegetable soup was just as effective for slowing neutrophil activity as soups made with chicken.

Garlic

Those pungent cloves contain allicin, a potent antimicrobial that can fend off bacteria, viruses, and fungi.

Aim for: If you can stand it, chew a clove every 3 to 4 hours. You can also cut the clove into pieces and swallow them like pills. Or simply add them to your chicken soup, along with some onions. But chop garlic first and let it stand for 10 to 15 minutes before adding it to the soup. This will allow its therapeutic compounds to form.

Helpful hint: It's totally wacky, but one way to get children to consume garlic if they won't eat it raw is to crush two cloves in a garlic press and put one in each of their socks. As they run around, the garlic will be absorbed through their skin.

Spices and spicy condiments

According to Ayurveda (traditional Indian medicine), cinnamon, coriander, and ginger promote sweating and are often used to help break a fever. You may also be able to unclog your stuffy nose by generously spicing up some dishes with cayenne, horseradish, or (for lovers of sushi) wasabi. Each of these condiments can shrink the blood vessels in your nose and throat to temporarily relieve congestion.

Aim for: As much of the spicy hot stuff as you can comfortably stand.

Helpful hint: Try this Ayurvedic fever reducer: In a cup of hot water, mix 1/2 teaspoon each of powdered coriander and cinnamon with 1/4 teaspoon of powdered ginger. Let it steep for 10 minutes, then drink.

For a double dose of healing foods, make a pot of garlicky chicken soup. Just add a few peeled cloves to the soup while it cooks. Remove the cooked garlic before serving the soup—and eat it, spread on toast.

NUTRITIONAL SUPPLEMENTS

Vitamin C. Vitamin C really doesn't seem to help prevent a cold—although people could debate this longer than which way the roll of toilet paper should go—but there's much evidence to suggest that taking high doses of C may help shorten the time you're sick by a day or so. Vitamin C acts as an antihistamine and anti-inflammatory to help dry up a runny nose. It also improves immune function. If you think of your immune system as a high-performance vehicle, vitamin C is like high-octane fuel that makes the immune cells, such as neutrophils and macrophages, better able to find and destroy viruses. By the way, being sick (or under intense physical stress) increases the body's need for vitamin C.

For added effect, look for a C supplement that contains bioflavonoids—antioxidants found in citrus fruits, tea, and other foods. **DOSAGE:** There's no consensus about how much vitamin C, if any, to take for treating colds or flu. A recent analysis of 53 placebo-controlled trials found that regular supplementation with 250 to 2,000 milligrams of vitamin C a day did not reduce the incidence of colds in the general population. However, in people under heavy physical stress (marathon runners, skiers, or soldiers), vitamin C cut the incidence of colds in half.

Taking vitamin C supplements on a regular basis has been shown to cut the duration of colds in children by 14 percent and in adults by 8 percent. Unfortunately, once you get a cold, vitamin C supplements—even in very high doses—do not seem to lessen the time you suffer with a cold. High doses of C can cause bowel problems, so if you experience gas or diarrhea, reduce your dose. And don't abruptly stop taking high doses of C. Taper off gradually to avoid "rebound scurvy," a condition that may cause gums to bleed. People who have a history of oxalate kidney stones should check with their doctors about the type of vitamin C that's best for them—a combination of buffered vitamin C and bioflavonoids doesn't appear to raise the risk of stones the way C by itself seems to.

Zinc. Getting zinc—one of the most critical minerals for overall immune function—right up against your mucous membranes seems to reduce the amount of time you have to endure a nasty cold, which is no doubt one reason why zinc lozenges are such popular cold fighters. A good stack of studies shows that taking zinc gluconate or acetate lozenges every 2 hours within the first two days of a cold can decrease its duration. (Just be sure to use them on a full stomach so they won't make you nauseated.) Alas, taking zinc preventively doesn't seem to do much to keep you from catching a cold. **DOSAGE:** Lozenges containing between 9 and 24 milligrams of zinc are most effective.

Garlic. If you just can't stomach raw garlic, don't worry: Garlic supplements seem to work just as well. A British study of 146 people found that volunteers who took a garlic supplement for 12 weeks during cold season were far less likely to get sick than those who took placebos. There were 24 colds in the garlic group compared to 65 in the placebo group. And the

FEATURED RECIPES
Quick Chicken Noodle Soup *p. 296*
Ginger Butternut Squash Soup *p. 298*
Minestrone with Fava Beans *p. 299*
Chicken in Garlic Sauce *p. 312*
Roasted Root Vegetables *p. 318*

garlic takers who did get sick recovered about four days sooner on average than the others.

If you take medications, particularly blood thinners like warfarin (Coumadin), check with your doctor before using garlic because it can increase drugs' blood-thinning effects. **DOSAGE:** 300 milligrams two or three times daily. Look for extracts standardized to contain at least 13 percent allicin.

Vitamin E. This antioxidant vitamin, another immune system booster, won't do much, if anything, to shorten a cold, but it could keep you from getting one. In one year-long, high-quality study from Tufts University, 451 adults age 65 and older were given either 200 IU of vitamin E each day or a placebo. While 74 percent of the people in the placebo group came down with at least one upper respiratory infection during the study, only 65 percent of the volunteers in the vitamin E group experienced one or more infections. **DOSAGE:** 200 IU daily.

OFF THE MENU

Caffeine and alcohol. When you're battling a cold or flu, staying well hydrated helps loosen and clear out nasal congestion, so it's better to skip caffeinated drinks like coffee, caffeinated tea, and soda, which are dehydrating. The same holds true for alcohol; although it's certainly tempting to down a few drinks to help you rest when you're feeling ill, alcohol only makes dehydration worse.

Sugary foods. Sugary foods are like Valium to your immune system. Sugar makes your white blood cells sluggish, so they're less able to hunt down and destroy viruses. In a study at Loma Linda University in California, when volunteers consumed about 100 grams of sugar (about the amount in two cans of regular soda), their white blood cell activity dropped by 50 percent and stayed low for up to 5 hours. Fruit juices may be the one exception to the "no sweets" rule because they contain good immunity-boosting and infection-fighting phytochemicals—provided they're 100 percent fruit juice, not "juice drinks."

Herbal Infection Fighters

In terms of supplements, zinc may be your best option for fighting colds, but other supplements can help, too—though not the ones you might think. A recent assessment of 24 studies on echinacea, for instance, did not show that it will shorten the time you will be sick if you take it after you catch a cold. Taking echinacea while you're well may slightly reduce your chances of catching a cold, however. More research is under way to study this plant's effects on the human immune system. And there is insufficient evidence to show whether *Andrographis paniculata*, found in products such as TriMune and Kold Kare, helps relieve cold symptoms. Ginseng is a smart choice; it's been shown to help with both colds and flu.

For flu, perhaps the supplement to try is elderberry extract, which seems to cut the severity of symptoms in half and reduce the amount of time you're sick if you take it within 48 hours after you experience your first symptoms. Elderberries contain several flavonoids, notably anthocyanidins, which help regulate immune function and reduce inflammation. In one study involving residents of an Israeli farming collective (called a kibbutz) who came down with the flu, more than 93 percent of those who took elderberry reported feeling markedly better within two days, while the majority of those taking placebos took six days to recover. For all of these supplements, follow the dosage instructions on the label.

COLON CANCER

If you live for steak, bacon, and hot dogs, it's not just your arteries and waistline that take the hit. It's also your colon—the place all that food ends up. Some people can blame their genes, in part, for colon cancer, but the wrong diet plays a major role. On the flip side, experts estimate that making even moderate diet and lifestyle changes can prevent about 70 percent of colon cancers.

Just as smoking leads to lung cancer, the endless beef-and-potatoes buffet that is the standard Western diet may nearly quadruple a person's risk of developing the growths, called polyps, in the digestive tract that lead to colon cancer. Getting a colonoscopy, which simultaneously finds and removes polyps, when you turn 50 (earlier if you have a family history) and every 10 years after that can dramatically reduce your risk. But since most colon cancers start with a polyp, preventing the darn things in the first place is a top priority. Simple steps like serving yourself some spinach salad sprinkled with beans for lunch and piling on the broccoli or brussels sprouts at dinner can go a long way.

YOUR FOOD PRESCRIPTION

Beans, lentils, peas,
and other foods high in folate

If colon cancer runs in your family, pile your plate high with these foods. Along with fiber, they also contain vast stores of folate, a B vitamin that protects cell DNA from damage. According to a Harvard study of nearly 89,000 women, those with a family history of colon cancer who consumed more than 400 micrograms of folate each day lowered their risk by more than 52 percent compared to women who consumed just 200 micrograms a day. You can get almost 300 micrograms just by eating 1 cup of chickpeas or cooked spinach. Fortified cereals are another terrific source, as is orange juice.

Of course, it pays to get more folate even if you don't have a family history of colon cancer. Several studies show it could cut your risk by 30 to 40 percent.

Aim for: 400 micrograms of folate daily. You may be getting that much already if you take a multivitamin each day or start your morning with orange juice and a fortified cereal. But you can also get there by eating at least three servings of whole grains each day along with 4 to 6 cups of fruits and vegetables. At least one of those servings should be dark leafy greens or legumes, like kidney beans, black beans, or chickpeas (garbanzo beans).

Helpful hint: Broccoli does double duty as a cancer fighter. It contains the antitumor compounds found in cruciferous vegetables as well as a fair amount of folate.

Milk and dairy foods

You know the saying "milk does a body good"? Along with building strong bones, milk can help shield you from colon cancer. Data from around the world shows that drinking at least 8 ounces (226 g) a day lowered the risk of cancers of the colon and rectum by about 10 percent. And increasing your intake of other dairy foods like yogurt and cheese lowers cancer risk even more.

Aim for: At least 8 ounces (226 g) a day.

Helpful hint: Because saturated fat is strongly linked to tumor growth, opt for low-fat varieties of milk and other dairy foods.

Cruciferous vegetables

These veggies (which include broccoli, brussels sprouts, cauliflower, cabbage, bok choy, kale, parsnips, turnips, rutabagas, and kohlrabi) are among the most powerful cancer fighters in the garden. They contain an array of compounds that flush out cancer-causing substances before they cause damage to cell DNA. Studies have consistently shown that people who eat the most crucifers have half the risk of developing colon cancer compared to those who eat the least.

If you're fond of putting steaks on the grill, you'll definitely want to serve these veggies with them. Compounds in crucifers act like little scrubbing pads to clean out the carcinogens created when meats are barbecued.

Aim for: At least four 1/2-cup servings each week.

High-fiber whole grains, fruits, and vegetables

The news on whether fiber protects against colon cancer just got more clear. The latest review of studies around the world states there is "strong evidence" that consuming whole grains and other foods that contain dietary fiber decreases the risk of colorectal cancer. Why? Fiber helps speed food through your system so any carcinogens you may have eaten don't linger long enough to cause trouble. And as it's digested by bacteria in the gut, compounds are formed that protect against carcinogenic bile acids, also produced during digestion.

It's better to get your fiber from food rather than supplements to get additional protection from the other nutrients and plant compounds in fiber-rich foods.

Aim for: Between 25 and 35 grams of fiber daily. You can get close to 25 grams with three servings of whole grains—like a sandwich made with whole-wheat bread plus 1/2 cup of brown rice—and 5 to 6 cups of fruits and vegetables.

To boost your fiber even more, add a few servings of legumes, nuts, seeds, and high-fiber cereal.

Fish and chicken

As evidence of a link between red meat and colon cancer continues to mount, you may wonder what's left to eat. The answer: fish and chicken.

Results from the EPIC study show that eating at least 10 ounces (283 g) of fish (two or three servings) weekly lowers the risk of colon cancer by 30 percent compared to eating fish less than once a week. That's not so surprising. If you're eating more fish, you're eating less meat. And if you choose fatty fish like salmon or mackerel, you're also getting more omega-3 fatty acids, which help to reduce inflammation in the gut.

If you don't like fish, flock to chicken. Studies show that unlike red meat, chicken doesn't actively promote colon cancer.

Aim for: At least two servings of fish or chicken a week.

Helpful hint: Most of chicken's fat is in the skin, so remove it before you dig in.

Turmeric

This is the spice so common in Indian food. The natural yellow pigment in turmeric, called curcumin, is considered a top anticancer agent. It's strongly anti-inflammatory, quelling inflammation that's thought to contribute to tumor growth. It also helps clean out carcinogens before they can damage cell DNA, and it may help repair any damage already done.

Aim for: There's no established recommendation; just try to use it more often in your cooking.

Helpful hint: Although the turmeric in curry powder mixes can turn your food yellow, some research suggests that several commercial curry powders don't actually contain much curcumin. It's better to use turmeric powder or, if you're using premixed curry powder, add some extra turmeric.

Garlic and onions

Garlic may not protect you from vampires, but it can help keep colon cancer away. Both garlic and onions contain sulfides, which help to clear out carcinogens and force cancer cells that do develop to self-destruct. In the Iowa Women's Health Study, women who consumed one to two cloves of garlic per week had a 32 percent lower risk of colon cancer compared to women who rarely ate garlic. And according to a study that examined fruit and vegetable consumption among more than 650 people in South Australia, onion eaters reduced their risk by 28 to 52 percent.

Aim for: Eating a couple of garlic cloves and about 1/2 cup of onions at least a few times a week may help lower your cancer risk.

Helpful hint: If you plan to cook garlic, chop or crush the cloves first, then let them stand for 10 to 15 minutes to give the therapeutic compounds a chance to form.

Black and green tea

The next time you're jonesing for a hot cup of somethin', make tea your choice. Lab studies show that the compounds in tea help disable cancer-causing agents. They also stymie the growth of cancer cells and encourage them to self-destruct.

FEATURED RECIPES

Coleslaw with Orange-Sesame Vinaigrette *p. 290*
Spinach Salad with Chickpeas *p. 293*
Simple Broccoli Soup *p. 298*
Ginger Butternut Squash Soup *p. 298*
Roasted Salmon with Sautéed Greens *p. 309*
Chicken in Garlic Sauce *p. 312*
Brussels Sprouts with Caramelized Onions *p. 319*
Brown Rice Risotto *p. 321*

Among more than 35,000 women in the Iowa Women's Health study, those who drank 2 or more cups of tea each day were almost 30 percent less likely to develop colon cancer than those who rarely drank tea. And while the participants in this study primarily drank black tea, it's worth noting that green tea contains even more of the antioxidant compounds, called catechins, that appear to work the magic.

Aim for: 3 to 4 cups a day.

Helpful hint: Brew your own tea. Commercial bottled teas generally contain less than 5 percent of the antioxidant compounds found in brewed tea.

NUTRITIONAL SUPPLEMENTS

Folic acid. If you're not getting enough folate in your diet, fill the gap with a multivitamin. The Nurses Health Study found that women who took a daily multivitamin with folic acid (the supplement form of folate) for 15 years were 75 percent less likely to develop colon cancer than those who didn't. **DOSAGE:** 400 micrograms a day, the amount in most multivitamins.

Calcium and vitamin D. These bone helpers are pretty good at protecting against cancer, too. Taking calcium supplements "probably" protects against colon cancer, according to the latest worldwide data. **DOSAGE:** For calcium, aim for 1,200 to 1,500 milligrams daily from food and supplements. With vitamin D, research suggests getting 1,000 IU from food and supplements combined is considered safe and likely to be beneficial.

CAUTION

Processed meat. When it comes to colon cancer, red meat—especially processed meats like ham, hot dogs, sausage, bacon, bologna, and corned beef—is a triple threat. The saturated fat promotes inflammation, and the high amounts of the iron, called heme iron, can aggravate the colon lining to create carcinogenic substances. Finally, grilling or frying meat over flames or very high heat creates other cancer-causing substances.

After looking at recent research, the World Cancer Research Fund (WCRF) and the American Institute of Cancer Research (AICR) concluded that "processed meat is a convincing cause of colorectal cancer." Avoid it as much as possible.

And limit your intake of red meat to 18 ounces (510 g) or less each week. Higher amounts can probably contribute to colon cancer, says the WCRF/AICR.

Sugar and refined carbohydrates. Too much sugary food—not sugar itself—puts us at an increased risk for cancer, say experts. That's because high intakes of refined carbs (such as when you wash down doughnuts or cookies with sugar-laden coffee or soda) go quickly into the bloodstream. This prompts the pancreas to secrete a load of insulin to tame the surge of sugar in the blood. It's the high insulin levels, not just the high sugar, that stimulate the growth of cancer cells, researchers now suggest.

So why does the American Institute for Cancer Research recommend we limit foods and drinks that are loaded with added sugar? To keep our weight in check (see "What's Weight Got to Do with It?" on this page) and to make room for the foods we know to be protective against cancer, such as vegetables, fruits, whole grains, and other high-fiber foods.

What's Weight Got to Do with It?

A lot. Body fat, particularly belly fat, doesn't just sit there and look bad. It produces proteins called cytokines, which crank up inflammation and lead to the kind of cell damage that encourages tumor growth. Being overweight also goes hand in hand with higher insulin levels, also linked to tumor growth. According to a study at Boston University School of Medicine, if your waist is bigger than 39 inches, you have double the risk of colon cancer. If you're also sedentary, your risk is tripled.

Alcohol. Booze depletes folate, the B vitamin that guards against colon cancer. Imbibing also makes DNA more vulnerable to damage by carcinogens. Experts also think alcohol may act as a solvent, making it easier for harmful cancer-causing agents (such as tobacco) to penetrate cells and cause damage. The risk is highest for people who have more than two drinks daily, according to the latest research.

food for thought . . .

"Filling two-thirds of your plate with whole grains, vegetables, fruit, and legumes is an easy way to protect against colon cancer."

— Karen Collins, MS, RD, CDN, nutrition advisor to the American Institute for Cancer Research ■

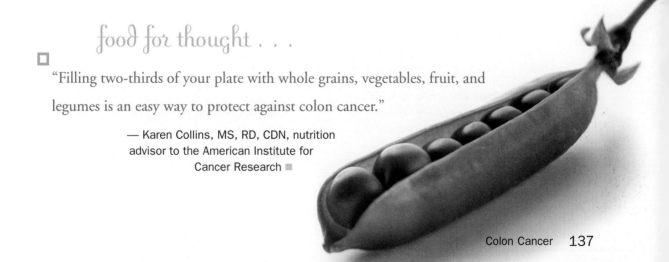

CONSTIPATION

When your "works" are all stopped up, you want relief quicker than you can say "go." If a poor diet—one lacking fruits, vegetables, and whole grains—is a major cause of the problem, better food choices and plenty of fluids are a major part of the solution. Has traveling or stress disrupted your regularity? We'll also show you some fast-acting, short-term solutions (like a handful of prunes or a cup of coffee).

If changing your diet and getting more fluids don't help, see your doctor to find out whether a condition such as hypothyroidism may be causing the problem.

YOUR FOOD PRESCRIPTION

Fruits, vegetables, beans,
and whole grains

These are full of fiber, the key to a smooth-running digestive system. As fiber travels along the large intestine, it absorbs fluids to bulk up and soften waste material. That helps stool pass more easily through the colon, where muscle contractions move it along. Fiber is particularly dense in the skin, stems, and leaves of fruit and plants, so don't peel that apple or toss those broccoli stalks.

Dark green leafy vegetables (think spinach, broccoli, and so on) can do double duty not only because of their fiber but also because of their high magnesium content (see under Nutritional Supplements on the opposite page).

Be sure to increase your fiber slowly; a sudden jump may wreak havoc with your system.

Aim for: 25 to 35 grams of fiber a day. You can get more than 8 grams just by eating 1/2 cup of cooked red beans, 5 grams from 1/4 cup of all-bran cereal, and 4.5 grams from 1/2 cup of cooked winter squash.

Helpful hint: A great way to get fiber is to start your day with a bowl of oatmeal topped with prunes rather than sugar.

Prunes

Prunes (now known as dried plums) act as a mild laxative, stimulating muscles to push waste through the large intestine. Five prunes provide about 3 grams of fiber, but because prune juice is equally effective as a laxative, researchers doubt that fiber is the key. More likely, the effect is due to prunes' high content of sorbitol, a sugar alcohol.

Aim for: 1 cup of prune juice (add 1 tablespoon lemon juice for even more effect) or four prunes a day. Stewed prunes or prunes that have soaked overnight in water may be easier to digest than the dry variety.

Helpful hint: Don't overdo it, or you may end up with diarrhea.

Coffee *and other hot liquids*

Coffee gives us that "get up and go," but it also gives us the urge to "sit down and go." Part of the reason is that hot liquids help move the bowels. Coffee may also trigger intestinal muscles to contract. It's not a good long-term solution,

FEATURED RECIPES

Spinach Salad with Chickpeas *p. 293*
Roasted Broccoli with Cheese *p. 320*
Ginger Butternut Squash Soup *p. 298*
Three-Bean Chili *p. 306*
Hearty Vegetable Stew *p. 304*
Pumpkin Streusel Bread *p. 327*
Pear Crisp *p. 332*

especially because coffee is a diuretic (so drink plenty of water as well), but in the short term, it should help do the trick.

Another alternative: hot water mixed with a tablespoon of lemon or lime juice. The juice stimulates the release of bile, and that can kick-start intestinal contractions.

Aim for: 1 to 2 cups of black coffee or 1 cup of hot water mixed with 2 tablespoons lemon juice.

Water

Fiber needs water to work its magic. When we don't drink enough water, our bodies pilfer it from our waste, leaving stools hard and difficult to pass. Make water more enticing by adding sliced seasonal fruit, like strawberries, peaches, watermelon, or citrus fruits.

Aim for: Between 8 and 11 eight-ounce glasses (2 to 3 l) a day.

Helpful hint: To help keep track of how much you're drinking, get a 1-liter bottle and put three rubber bands around it. Each time you refill your bottle, remove one rubber band.

Flaxseed and psyllium

Both help to bulk up stool. Try drinking a cup of warm milk with a teaspoon of ground flaxseed mixed in before bedtime. Sprinkle 2 tablespoons flaxseed over cereal or in a fruit smoothie in the morning. And look for cereals that list psyllium as one of the first ingredients.

Aim for: 1 to 2 teaspoons a day with plenty of water.

Salad, European-style

In Europe, many people eat their salads at the end of the meal. Adding that crunchy fiber as a finishing touch can help push the rest of the food through the digestive tract. Eating fruit an hour before or after a meal can also be helpful.

Aim for: A piece of fruit before or after lunch and a small salad at the end of dinner.

NUTRITIONAL SUPPLEMENTS

Magnesium. Magnesium is a superb laxative, as anyone who's gulped down some Milk of Magnesia can attest. While nuts, seeds, and leafy dark green vegetables are good sources of magnesium, if you're really backed up, a magnesium supplement can help. **DOSAGE:** 150 to 300 milligrams twice daily.

Fiber supplements. If you can't get the recommended 25 to 35 grams of fiber from food, psyllium-based fiber supplements such as Metamucil can close the gap. **DOSAGE:** Start with a level teaspoon once a day in 12 to 16 ounces (1/2 l) of water (you can add some fruit juice to help it go down easier), then drink another 16 ounces (1/2 l) of water. Work up to 2 tablespoons daily if necessary or follow label directions.

CAUTION

Cow's milk and other dairy products. Sometimes an intolerance to milk protein can cause constipation. An Italian study of 65 kids with chronic constipation found that when they switched from cow's milk to soy milk, constipation cleared up for 68 percent of them. If you've increased your intake of fiber and liquids and still have a problem with constipation, try cutting dairy out of your diet for two weeks to see if it makes a difference.

Excess protein. Diets very high in protein and low in high-fiber foods like beans, fruit, and whole grains can contribute to constipation.

White bread, white rice, and white pasta. "White" foods are usually stripped of their fiber and many of their nutrients in order to produce a smooth, bland food. Although many people prefer their soft texture and mild taste, refined foods lack the fiber that our bowels need to stay regular. Ditto for many packaged snack foods.

Alcohol. It's a diuretic, and if you're constipated, you need more fluid, not less.

DEPRESSION

You know the old expression "You are what you eat." Well, when it comes to mental health, "You feel what you eat" appears to be equally true. While we typically associate depression with a family history of the illness or devastating life events like the loss of a loved one, it may come as a surprise that what we eat—or don't eat—influences our emotional health as well.

Much of the current science has focused on the importance of getting the right balance of essential fatty acids—consuming more omega-3 fatty acids from fatty fish, walnuts, and flaxseed and fewer omega-6 fatty acids from vegetable oils like corn and canola oil and packaged and processed foods. Other research indicates that people with depression tend to have lower levels of certain B vitamins as well as the minerals selenium, iron, and zinc. It's still unclear, though, whether the nutrient deficiency causes depression or whether depression alters eating habits, which then leads to deficiency.

The diet connection may offer particular insight into postpartum depression. Women are more than twice as likely as men to experience depression, and researchers at the University of Pittsburgh are exploring the theory that nutrient depletion during pregnancy and breastfeeding (as nutrients are preferentially transferred to the growing baby), combined with a delay in the time it takes for a new mother's nutrient stores to return to prepregnancy levels, may be at least partly responsible for postpartum depression.

Depression can be serious and often requires professional help and sometimes medication. You should make changes to your diet in addition to, not instead of, getting the help you need. That said, increasing your intake of certain key nutrients may prevent depression, help ease symptoms, and even improve the effectiveness of antidepressant medications.

food for thought . . .

"Before 1890, the ratio of omega-6 to omega-3 essential fatty acids in the American diet was 1:1. Today, it's as high as 25:1. This radically increased intake of omega-6 essential fatty acids is thought to be behind the rise of depression in the U.S."

— "Nutrition and Depression: Implications for Improving Mental Health among Childbearing Aged Women," *Biological Psychiatry*, 2005 ■

Salmon, mackerel, tuna,
and other foods rich in omega-3 essential fatty acids

In countries where fish consumption is high, such as Japan, Taiwan, and Finland, rates of depression tend to be low. Conversely, in areas where fish consumption is low, like the United States and Europe, depression rates are much higher—as much as 10 times higher. Women who rarely eat fish have more than twice the risk of developing depression compared to those who dine on "fin food" often.

Aim for: Although it's nearly impossible to consume enough omega-3s to treat depression through food alone (you'll need between 1 and 3 grams of omega-3s a day to lift your mood), eating more fish, such as sardines, may help protect you from developing depression in the first place. Start by eating at least two fish meals a week. If you don't like fish, add a teaspoon of ground flaxseed, another good source of omega-3s, to cereal, yogurt, or salads every day.

Beans, spinach, fish,
and other foods high in B vitamins

Although all B vitamins are essential for preventing depression, most of the research has focused on folate (also known as folic acid), B_6, and B_{12} because these vitamins are often in short supply among people with depression. Harvard researchers found that between 15 and 38 percent of people with depression are deficient in folate. While it's uncertain whether low folate levels cause depression, we do know that they can interfere with antidepressant medications, delaying symptom relief.

Women who take birth control pills or hormone replacement drugs can also be low in B_6 (another possible reason why women's depression rates are twice those of men), while deficiencies of B_{12} are common among the elderly and among vegans, who don't eat any animal proteins. Studies have yet to be done on whether

Get a Whiff of This!

Sure, vanilla tastes good, but even sniffing it can help reduce anxiety, according to a study done at Memorial Sloan-Kettering Cancer Center. In the study, patients undergoing MRIs who breathed vanilla-scented air reported 63 percent less anxiety than those who breathed unscented air. Add a drop or two of vanilla to the pot before the coffee brews to fill your kitchen with the pleasing scent, or simply light some vanilla-scented candles around your home or add vanilla-scented oil to your bathwater.

eating enough B vitamin–rich foods like whole grains, lean meats, beans, and nuts can prevent or treat depression, but these foods are believed to be generally beneficial for brain health.

Aim for: *Vitamin B_6:* 1.3 to 1.5 milligrams daily. You can approach that amount with a serving (3.5 ounces/99 g) of tuna or 1 cup of chickpeas. Buckwheat flour is another good source. *Vitamin B_{12}:* 2.4 micrograms daily, which is easily gotten from a serving of beef or eggs. *Folate:* 400 micrograms daily. A cup of cooked lentils will almost get you there, and a serving of breakfast cereal (all brands are enriched with folate) will give you more than this amount. Spinach and beets are other good sources. *Thiamin:* 50 milligrams a day. Because it's not possible to get this much from food sources alone, it's a good idea to include thiamin-rich foods, like whole grains and brown rice, in your diet and get the rest from a good B-complex supplement.

Lean meats, cheese, *and bananas*

What do these foods have in common? The amino acid tryptophan. Tryptophan is critical to production of the neurotransmitter serotonin, which regulates mood. Incidentally, increasing the available serotonin in the brain is also the goal of antidepressants like fluoxetine (Prozac), which are known as selective serotonin reuptake inhibitors (SSRIs). Other sources of tryptophan are peanuts, fish, milk, dates, and even chocolate.

Because protein is a good source of the amino acid, you can help your body make its own tryptophan by eating lean meats and other good protein sources like soy and fish. Be cautious with tryptophan supplements, however. L-tryptophan supplements may be linked to a potentially fatal disorder called eosinophilia-myalgia syndrome (EMS), with symptoms that include severe muscle pain.

Aim for: It's not possible to get as much tryptophan as the British researchers used in their study from food alone, so simply aim to include more tryptophan-rich foods in your diet. Then consider talking to your physician about getting pharmaceutical-grade tryptophan from a compounding pharmacy.

Helpful hint: Gobble up some turkey. Not only is it a good source of tryptophan, but it also contains those brain-critical B vitamins along with good amounts of iron, selenium, and zinc, other nutrients being studied for their connection to alleviating depression.

Complex carbohydrates *from vegetables, fruits, legumes, and whole grains*

Carbohydrates indirectly help make serotonin. Simple carbohydrates like sugary and starchy foods and those made with white flour boost serotonin levels, too, which is why we instinctively reach for them when we're feeling blue. But these foods cause blood sugar to rise quickly and then fall quickly. When blood sugar levels fall, so do our moods. Wild swings in blood sugar that come from eating too many of these foods stress the adrenal glands, which in turn leads to fatigue and depression. By contrast, complex carbs, like those found in whole-grain products (breads, rice, and pasta), fruits, vegetables, and legumes, boost and sustain serotonin without spiking blood sugar.

Aim for: 4 to 6 cups of fruits and vegetables a day. In addition, make at least three of your grain servings whole grains. Eating a bowl of high-fiber cereal in the morning and making your sandwich for lunch with two slices of whole-grain bread will get you there.

NUTRITIONAL SUPPLEMENTS

Omega-3 fatty acids. These are essential for optimal functioning of brain cells and neurotransmitters, particularly serotonin. In addition to a healthful diet, research suggests that taking omega-3 supplements can do much to alleviate symptoms for people with depression.

The important omega-3 components for depression are EPA and DHA. A recent randomized controlled trial with 152 adults with depression showed that those who followed a Mediterranean-style diet (rich in fruit, vegetables, nuts, whole grains, and olive oil as the main cooking oil) that was supplemented with fish oil (900 milligrams DHA and 200 milligrams EPA daily) had improved mental health scores and a significant reduction in depression after following this regimen for three months. **DOSAGE:** Supplements typically contain both EPA and DHA; studies show 1 gram of EPA and DHA combined to be effective. If higher doses are needed, check with your physician.

B-complex vitamins. Studies suggest that some B vitamin supplements can help regulate mood. For instance, thiamin appears to increase general feelings of well-being, and folic acid seems to improve responses to antidepressant medications. **DOSAGE:** A good B-complex supplement daily will supply what you need. Look for formulations that contain 800 micrograms

FEATURED RECIPES

Buckwheat Pancakes with Fruit Sauce p. 286
Spinach Salad with Chickpeas p. 293
Tuna and White Bean Salad p. 295
Lentil-Tomato Soup p. 299
Tuna Kebabs p. 306
Roasted Salmon with Sautéed Greens p. 309
Brown Rice Risotto p. 321
Orange Beets p. 323

of folic acid, 50 to 100 milligrams of B_6, and at least 500 micrograms of B_{12}. Higher doses may be necessary to be therapeutic, but check with your physician.

Selenium from a multivitamin. This antioxidant mineral is a building block for glutathione peroxidase, an enzyme that protects nerves in the brain. It's also key for metabolizing thyroid hormone, low levels of which are known to cause depression. In studies in which participants ate a low-selenium diet, they experienced more symptoms of depression and hostility than when their diet had sufficient amounts. **DOSAGE:** Studies showed that compared to a placebo, 100 micrograms daily improved mood. Most multivitamin/mineral supplements contain 100 to 200 micrograms.

Iron. One of the most common nutrient deficiencies in the world, low iron is associated with fatigue, apathy, irritability, and an inability to concentrate, so it's not a big leap to consider that low levels may also play a role in depression. Research showed that postpartum depression improved among new mothers with anemia who received 125-milligram iron tablets. **DOSAGE:** Iron is a tricky supplement because too little may lead to depression, while too much can lead to heart problems. Take iron supplements only if you've been diagnosed with iron deficiency by your physician.

OFF THE MENU

Alcohol. Not only does alcohol depress the central nervous system, but it (particularly hard liquor) also depletes the body of the B vitamins that are essential for brain function.

Safflower, sunflower, and corn oils and processed foods such as chips and cookies. These oils are high in omega-6 fatty acids, as are processed foods made with them. Although we need both omega-6s and omega-3s for optimal brain function, we need them in the correct balance, and most of us get too many omega-6s, according to many experts.

Balance Your Blood Sugar

Dieters are often encouraged to eat small meals throughout the day to prevent the swings in blood sugar that can lead to cravings—and the binges that satisfy them. Keeping your blood sugar on an even keel is a good strategy for improving mood as well. To do it, never go more than a 4 to 5 hours without eating something, choose complex carbohydrates over refined grains and sugary foods, and eat some protein and healthy fats with every meal or snack (think peanut butter on whole-grain toast).

On a typical day, this might mean bran cereal topped with fruit for breakfast instead of a bagel, a sandwich on whole wheat instead of white at lunch (or a salad with beans or tuna on top instead of a sandwich), and a slice or two of roast chicken with a heap of vegetables and a half cup of brown rice for dinner instead of a big plate of spaghetti.

DIABETES

Diabetes is more tightly wound with diet than a snake in its own coil. For instance, if you have type 2 diabetes or know someone who does, you probably know that sugary foods aren't the best for a person's blood sugar. But the story doesn't end there. Refined carbohydrates (think white crackers, cookies, white pancakes, and other foods made with refined flour—foods that quickly turn into glucose, or sugar, in the body) are equal or perhaps even greater villains. Plain old eating too much, which leads to weight gain, is another trapdoor to diabetes.

Excess calories and lots of refined carbohydrates don't exactly cause type 2 diabetes—but they don't help. Studies suggest that people who eat a lot of refined carbohydrates as well as fat (particularly saturated fat) are at much greater risk for the disease than those who don't. In other words, a diet of steak and potatoes, burgers and fries, soft drinks, doughnuts, and premium ice cream lays down the type 2 welcome mat.

Fortunately, you can roll it back up by gradually tweaking your diet here and there. If you already have type 2 diabetes, eating smart and shedding a little weight if you need to can help you better control your blood sugar and possibly let you reduce your doses of insulin or other medications that lower blood sugar—or even eliminate the need for them. It's as simple as choosing slower-digesting foods—like whole-wheat bread instead of white bread and beans instead of potato chips—and eating plenty of fruits and vegetables (a key to helping many health problems). Other foods play a role, too, as you'll discover shortly.

YOUR FOOD PRESCRIPTION

Fruits, vegetables, *and other foods high in fiber and antioxidants*

Not only does a sweet, juicy orange or crunchy carrot taste great, especially when your energy seems to have leapt out the window, but these foods are full of fiber that slows digestion. What may be equally important is that they're also loaded with antioxidants.

The antioxidant vitamins E and C and carotenoids (nutrients found in yellow and orange fruits and vegetables) like beta-carotene appear to be particularly important for people with diabetes. A large European study assessed the intake of fruits and vegetables as well as the blood levels of vitamin C in 21,831 men and women. They found that as the intake of vitamin C–rich foods went up, the risk for type 2 diabetes went down, often dramatically.

And new research from Oregon State University has shown that people with metabolic syndrome (the first step toward type 2 diabetes) need significantly more vitamin E in their diets. People with diabetes are often low in both C and E.

How do antioxidants help? They neutralize unstable, cell-damaging molecules called free radicals. Research suggests that people with diabetes have more free radicals than people without the disease. Free radicals may play a role both in causing diabetes and in exacerbating its long-term effects, such as clogged arteries and blood vessel and nerve damage. Either high blood sugar or high insulin may cause a free radical invasion.

Aim for: 2 to 3 cups of vegetables and 2 to 3 cups of fruit a day. Spread out your fruit throughout the day to prevent a high intake of carbs at one time.

Helpful hint: If you have diabetes, limit your intake of dried fruits and fruit juices to very small portions. These forms are more dense in sugar than other types of fruit. Fresh whole fruit is a better choice most of the time.

Whole grains, beans, peas, and lentils

Whole grains and other complex carbohydrates deserve top billing on any antidiabetes menu. Oats, beans, and some fruits and vegetables are loaded with soluble fiber, which dissolves in water, forming a gel in your stomach. That slows digestion, which is critical for heading off blood sugar spikes. Soluble fiber also reduces cholesterol, lowering your risk of heart disease—the problem most people with diabetes ultimately die of. Insoluble fiber, which passes through the intestines intact and is found mostly in whole wheat and some fruits and vegetables, is also linked to lower diabetes risk.

Large prospective studies consistently show associations of a high dietary fiber intake (more than 25 grams per day in women and more than 38 grams per day in men) with a 20 to 30 percent reduced risk of developing type 2 diabetes. In fact, the landmark Diabetes Prevention Program study found that increasing dietary fiber in the diet along with other lifestyle changes like increased exercise and modest weight loss decreased the risk for developing diabetes by 58 percent. And a review of studies about cereal grains found that people who ate three servings of whole grains a day were 20 to 30 percent less likely to develop type 2 diabetes than those who ate less.

When it comes to diabetes, legumes—beans, chickpeas, peas, lentils, and soybeans—also pack star power. Like whole grains, legumes are digested slowly, allowing a gentle rise in blood sugar and a reduced rise in insulin levels. And legumes are a wonderful source of protein, a

Regular or Decaf

If you love your cup of joe, go ahead and indulge. A recent analysis of coffee and caffeine intake as it relates to type 2 diabetes found that the incidence of type 2 diabetes decreased by 12 percent for every 2 cups per day of coffee intake, 11 percent for every 2 cups per day of decaffeinated coffee intake, and 14 percent for every 200 milligrams of caffeine intake (what you'd find in 2 cups of coffee).

Besides caffeine, coffee is also rich in antioxidant compounds (similar to those in berries and grapes) that may help protect the insulin-producing cells in the body from free radical damage. Also, a coffee ingredient called chlorogenic acid—also found in red wine and chocolate—may help slow the absorption of sugar into cells.

good alternative if you're trying to eat less meat. They're easy to eat more of—just open a can of low-sodium lentil or bean soup for lunch and sprinkle black beans or chickpeas on any salad.

Soybeans in particular appear to shine. In a University of Illinois study of 14 men with advanced type 2 diabetes, the participants got half their daily protein from soy protein, which significantly lowered protein in the urine—a sign of kidney damage—and raised levels of HDL, or good, cholesterol. And a number of studies indicate that soy can help regulate both glucose and insulin levels.

One note of caution: Add fiber to your menu gradually, or you may end up with intestinal gas and bloating. Also, the more fiber you eat, the more liquids you should drink.

Aim for: 25 to 35 grams of fiber per day. A half cup of chickpeas has 10.2 grams, and 1/4 cup of bran cereal has 26. Three good ways to get more fiber are to have whole-grain cereal for breakfast (look for one with at least 5 grams of fiber per serving), switch to whole-wheat bread for sandwiches, and eat at least one bean-based meal per week.

Cinnamon

Care for some cinnamon on your oatmeal? Studies have found that cinnamon lowers blood sugar, cholesterol (including bad cholesterol, or LDL), and triglycerides (heart-threatening fats in the bloodstream) and boosts healthy HDL cholesterol, all factors important in fighting diabetes and heart disease. Certain compounds in cinnamon help cells take in glucose to use as energy, as insulin does, which in turn lowers blood sugar. Cinnamon also contains manganese, a mineral that appears to help the body use blood sugar.

Although the American Diabetes Association says there is not enough evidence to support routine supplementation of cinnamon to treat diabetes, it's still a healthful way to spice up your daily food. A recent analysis of 10 randomized controlled trials involving 543 patients found that up to 2 teaspoons of cinnamon a day helped lower fasting blood sugar levels but did not significantly impact A1C levels (an indicator of long-term diabetes control).

Aim for: 1/2 teaspoon a day is a good target. Work up to that amount slowly in case you are allergic to cinnamon.

Helpful hint: Can't get enough cinnamon by adding it to applesauce, oatmeal, and toast? Add 1/2 teaspoon or so to your coffee before starting the pot. You can also add it to tea. Cinnamon's also great on sweet potatoes, a smart food (in moderation) for people with diabetes.

Peanut butter and nuts

It's time for the return of the peanut butter sandwich (this time, on whole wheat). In the Nurses Health Study of more than 80,000 women with no history of diabetes, those who ate nuts five times a week lowered their risk of type 2 diabetes by 30 percent compared to women who never ate nuts; eating peanut butter five times a week cut risk by 20 percent. Researchers aren't clear why peanuts helped. It could be the magnesium, the unsaturated fats, the fiber, or a healthier lifestyle among people who grab nuts for a snack. Monounsaturated fats, which make up 85 percent of the fat in most nuts, may reduce insulin resistance, so swapping carb-rich foods such as pretzels for good-fat-rich foods such as nuts is a wise move. Replacing meats with nuts occasionally is a good idea, too.

FEATURED RECIPES

Ultimate Spiced Nuts *p. 288*
Lentil-Tomato Soup *p. 299*
Mac 'n Cheese Primavera *p. 304*
Three-Bean Chili *p. 306*
Roasted Salmon with Sautéed Greens *p. 309*
Chicken-Barley Bake *p. 312*
Roasted Root Vegetables *p. 318*
Springtime Quinoa *p. 322*
Frozen Fruit Mousse *p. 333*
Rice Pudding *p. 334*
Mixed Berry Tart *p. 335*

Aim for: About an ounce—a small handful—of nuts or about a tablespoon of peanut butter five times a week.

Helpful hint: Nuts are high in calories, with at least 150 per ounce. Subtract an ounce or two of meat or a serving of refined grains to keep your calories in balance when you add nuts.

Olive oil

One of life's great justices is that olive oil tastes wonderful *and* improves health conditions, including diabetes. A number of studies have shown that when it replaces sugary and refined starchy foods, olive oil and other monounsaturated fats lower blood sugar as well as heart disease risk. One of the most recent, a Spanish study of 772 people at high risk for heart disease, showed that people assigned a diet high in olive oil or nuts had significantly lower blood sugar levels, blood pressure, and cholesterol than those on a low-fat diet.

Olive oil is monounsaturated, which means it's a healthier fat than saturated fats like butter. It's also loaded with antioxidants.

Aim for: Enjoy at least a tablespoon a day in place of other oils.

Helpful hint: Olive oil can lose its valuable nutrients—beta-carotene, vitamin E, and other antioxidants—when exposed to light, so store it in a dark, cool place. If your oil turns cloudy, it's time to throw it away.

NUTRITIONAL SUPPLEMENTS
Vitamins C and E, zinc, and magnesium.
Antioxidants such as vitamins C and E and the mineral zinc help counter free radical damage that ups the risk of diabetes-related compli-

cations like heart disease and nerve damage. Magnesium appears to help cells use insulin. Deficiencies, which are common in people with diabetes, may promote diabetes-related eye damage. Recent research from Oregon State University suggests that people with metabolic syndrome—the hallmark of type 2 diabetes—need 30 to 50 percent more vitamin E than people who are generally healthy. Several studies have found that taking these supplements in the dosages listed below for three months significantly lowered blood sugar levels, increased "good" HDL cholesterol, and reduced blood pressure. The nutrients can also lower infection risk, which is important since people with diabetes are more susceptible to infection than those without diabetes. **DOSAGE:** *Vitamin C:* 500 to 1,000 milligrams daily. *Vitamin E:* 400 IU daily. *Magnesium:* 300 to 600 milligrams daily. *Zinc:* 30 milligrams daily. One word of caution: A recent trial found that vitamin E supplements of 400 IU per day increased the risk of prostate cancer for some men. To be safe, get this nutrient from food (see page 85) and supplement with a multivitamin that provides close to 100 percent of the recommended daily intake of vitamin E.

Calcium and vitamin D. A 20-year study by Boston researchers of almost 84,000 nurses, none of whom had diabetes at the study's start, found that women who took 1,200 milligrams of calcium and 800 IU of vitamin D per day had a 33 percent lower risk of developing type 2 diabetes than women who consumed much lower amounts.

Not all calcium supplements are equally well absorbed. The body absorbs the calcium from chewable supplements better than from pills. **DOSAGE:** *Calcium:* Boston researchers found that 1,200 milligrams daily lowered the risk of

There's more to peanut butter than just sandwiches. Peanut butter can be the central ingredient in all types of sauces and glazes, including some particularly yummy Asian-style dips. It's an ingredient in many muffin, soup, and cookie recipes as well.

Is a Glass of Wine Fine?

A systematic review of 12 observational studies found that moderate alcohol consumption was protective against type 2 diabetes for men and women. Best to know the meaning of moderate, however—no more than one drink a day for women, two or less for men. Moderate amounts of alcohol also lower the risk of heart disease. We're not suggesting you become the new life of the party, but if you drink, a small amount is best. Drinking alcohol by itself increases the risk of low blood sugar, so be sure to eat a meal with that glass of red or white or that beer, and include the alcohol in your calorie count. And skip those high-calorie, high-carbohydrate "umbrella-sporting" cocktails.

type 2 diabetes. To improve absorption, divide it in two doses, one in the morning and one at night. *Vitamin D:* 400 to 800 IU daily.

CAUTION

Sugar and refined grains. If the food on your plate looks as white as snow, it's time for a new, more colorful menu. Refining grains strips them of nutrients and often fiber. Foods made with white flour and/or sugar digest too quickly, spiking blood sugar. In fact, researchers believe that diets high in these foods lay the groundwork for type 2 diabetes by putting on weight and increasing the risk of insulin resistance and metabolic syndrome. You don't have to deny yourself all these foods all the time, but try to cut back, slowly switching to more whole grains and higher-fiber foods. Limit yourself to one or two small desserts a week, dividing a portion with a friend. If you typically slurp down sugary sodas or fruit juice, switch to water or other calorie-free drinks.

High-fat dairy products, red meats, margarine, and other foods high in saturated fats or trans fat. Next time you have steak for dinner, take a look at your plate after the trimmings cool. The congealed saturated fat isn't any lovelier in your arteries, upping your risk of heart disease, a risk already high for people with diabetes. Recent research suggests that the harm to your heart from saturated fats is especially increased when your diet is swimming in sugar and other refined carbohydrates. Best bet—cut the excess sugar and replace some of your butter and bacon with sources of monounsaturated fats such as olive oil, nuts, seeds, and avocados.

Regardless of heart disease risk, saturated fat is just plain bad for people with diabetes. Studies show that it increases insulin resistance by increasing inflammation and making cell membranes less flexible so insulin has more trouble getting blood sugar into cells.

Trans fat is just as bad or worse. That is why the FDA ordered foods made with partially hydrogenated fats—the main source of trans fats—to be removed from our food supply.

Should You Kiss Meat Goodbye?

According to the American Diabetes Association (ADA), a variety of eating patterns are acceptable for the management of diabetes, including those that restrict animal foods. A dinner of tabbouleh, sliced fresh tomatoes, and marinated chickpeas sounds tasty—and the fact that it doesn't contain meat may help control your diabetes. In a study published by the ADA, 74 people with type 2 diabetes were randomly assigned to eat either a vegetarian diet or a conventional diet for diabetes. Both diets were low in calories. After six months, the vegetarian group had lost more weight and had a 30 percent improvement in insulin sensitivity while the other group had a 20 percent improvement in this indicator of diabetes control. The vegetarian group also showed less oxidative stress—a sign that their bodies had less of the inflammation that is associated with diabetes, obesity, and heart disease—than the non-vegetarian group.

Other studies have shown that vegetarian diets can be very effective at managing blood sugar levels in people with diabetes. And they tend to be more protective against kidney damage since plant-based proteins from beans, grains, and vegetables are thought to place less stress on these organs than proteins from animal sources.

Maybe you won't scrape your plate of all animal products today—a big change from the typical Western diet—but these studies do drive home the importance of whole grains, vegetables, and other plant foods.

DIARRHEA

When you eat, food passes through the stomach and the small intestine, accumulating liquid as it goes so that by the time waste reaches the large intestine, it's quite watery. Much of that liquid is then absorbed through the large intestine. But when triggers like bacteria or viruses interrupt that process, the intestinal walls can become inflamed, making it difficult for them to absorb liquid. The result: diarrhea.

Diarrhea usually clears up pretty quickly. To baby your bowels in the meantime, choose foods that are easy to digest and "binding" foods that help reverse the problem. Even more important is replacing lost fluids.

YOUR FOOD PRESCRIPTION

Apple juice, water, herbal tea,
and other clear fluids

Diarrhea can deplete the body of fluids and lead to dehydration. Water replenishes lost liquids, as do other clear liquids like apple juice and broths, which also help replace salts and minerals lost to diarrhea. Avoid citrus, pineapple, tomato, and other juices that you can't see through because the acid in them can irritate already inflamed intestines.

Aim for: Start with sips of clear liquid and work your way up to drinking a cup every half hour.

Black tea, blackberry tea, raspberry-leaf tea, and red tea

Tannins in tea bind the mucous membranes in the intestines and help the body absorb fluids while calming inflammation in the intestinal tract. Blackberry and raspberry-leaf teas are particularly helpful. Be sure to choose those that contain real leaves rather than just flavoring, and opt for decaffeinated teas, since caffeine is dehydrating. Red teas, now becoming more commonly available, can calm spasms in the colon.

Aim for: 3 to 4 cups a day.

Rehydration solutions

When diarrhea continues for several days, it can disrupt the balance of electrolytes, especially sodium and potassium, in the body. Without these minerals to influence the proper distribution of fluids, the body is vulnerable to dehydration, which can be serious, particularly in children. Sports drinks like Gatorade replenish electrolytes, but they pack a wallop of sugar, which can worsen diarrhea. Better choices are oral rehydration solutions, sold over the counter at pharmacies (try Pedialyte for children). You can also make your own rehydration solution:

  1 quart water
  1/4 teaspoon salt
  1/4 teaspoon baking soda
  2 tablespoons sugar or honey

Place the ingredients in a pitcher or other container and stir until the salt, baking soda, and sugar are completely dissolved.

Aim for: Use rehydration solutions as directed. Sip homemade solutions frequently for a total of 3 quarts or liters daily.

White rice

Foods such as white rice and those made with white flour, which are generally lacking in fiber, tend to constipate people who eat them a lot, which is why they'll work well for you now.

Aim for: Eat 1/2-cup portions until diarrhea is under control.

Bananas

A ripe banana is often a baby's first food because it's bland and easy to digest, which also makes it a perfect snack when your "waste management system" is out of whack. Bananas also have plenty of the electrolyte potassium, which can be depleted by diarrhea.

Aim for: One or two a day while diarrhea persists.

Unsweetened applesauce

Part of the BRAT (bananas, rice, applesauce, and toast) diet recommended for diarrhea, applesauce contains pectin, a fiber that helps counteract the runs by soaking up extra fluid in the intestine. Avoid raw apples, which won't do the trick.

Aim for: 1/4 to 1/2 cup every hour or so.

Yogurt with active cultures

Brands that contain active cultures of beneficial bacteria can help prevent and treat diarrhea caused by "bad" bacteria. If your diarrhea is a side effect of antibiotics, which kill both good and bad bacteria, it's especially important to replenish the "good guys." Avoid those with added sugar, however; it can aggravate diarrhea.

Aim for: 1/2 cup twice a day.

NUTRITIONAL SUPPLEMENTS

Probiotics. If you don't tolerate the lactose in yogurt, consider taking probiotics to fortify the "good" bacteria in your gut that can help keep diarrhea at bay. **DOSAGE:** Take no more than one to two billion live organisms once a day. Higher doses sometimes cause intestinal discomfort.

***Saccharomyces boulardii* (SB).** Studies have shown that this yeast can help prevent traveler's diarrhea and diarrhea caused by infections and antibiotics. **DOSAGE:** 500 milligrams four times a day.

When Water Is a Risk

If you're traveling to a developing country where water supplies may not be clean, follow these tips to avoid bacteria that cause diarrhea.

• Never drink tap water or use it to brush your teeth. Drink sealed water, juices, and sodas or boiled drinks.

• Avoid ice, raw fruits and vegetables, and salads. You can eat fruits and vegetables that you have peeled yourself.

• Avoid raw or rare meat or fish and make sure cooked meat or fish is hot when served to you.

• Don't buy food from street vendors.

• Avoid unpasteurized milk and cheeses.

Carob powder. Rich in tannins that help bind the mucous membranes in the intestinal tract, carob, a legume sometimes used as an alternative to cocoa, is particularly effective for young children with diarrhea. **DOSAGE:** For children, 1 gram for every 1.5 pounds of weight, up to 15 grams, divided into three equal doses and mixed with applesauce or yogurt. For adults, a total of 15 to 20 grams per day.

OFF THE MENU

Doughnuts, ice cream, french fries, and other foods with a lot of fat or sugar. Fat can be difficult to digest, and sugar can make diarrhea worse by feeding diarrhea-promoting bacteria.

Foods and chewing gums that contain sorbitol. Too much sorbitol, a sugar substitute used in some foods, mints, and chewing gums, can cause diarrhea.

Milk and other dairy foods. If you can't digest lactose, you probably develop diarrhea and bloating when you eat dairy. The sugars in milk can also worsen existing diarrhea from other causes.

Alcohol and caffeine. Both are diuretics.

Vitamin C supplements. High doses (several thousand milligrams) can trigger diarrhea.

DIVERTICULOSIS

Imagine a bicycle inner tube freckled with weak spots that can give way, bubbling out like air-filled blisters. The same thing can happen to your large intestine, a.k.a. colon. The weak spots in this case can give way to marble-size protruding pouches called diverticula. If you have them, you have diverticulosis.

Scientists aren't sure what causes it, but they do know the condition is more common with age. It's also more common in Western societies, where people tend to overdose on low-fiber foods like white bread and shy away from high-fiber foods like fruits, vegetables, and whole grains. In fact, diverticulosis barely existed prior to 1900, when highly refined flour was a thing of the future.

Fiber is a colon's best friend. It bulks up and softens stool so it can make a timely, smooth exit. Low-fiber diets, on the other hand, create hard, dry, small stools akin to rocks that pile up and stay put. The effort to move them out causes pressure that can damage the intestine's walls by causing those nasty pouches to form. If stool or bacteria get caught in them, trouble's knocking. You may need antibiotics or even surgery.

Rest assured, you don't have to start eating twigs and berries (well, the berries are a good idea). If you have diverticulosis, you can help prevent painful symptoms by doing something as simple as changing your breakfast cereal, snacking on fruit, and eating beans more often. You might as well take the plunge, because these are the same habits that are key to just about every other aspect of good health.

YOUR FOOD PRESCRIPTION

Whole grains, fruits, vegetables, *and other foods rich in fiber*

You may have rolled your eyes whenever your mother mentioned the benefits of "roughage," but fiber is remarkably critical for keeping you and your colon in good health. It can help prevent diverticulosis and, if you have the condition already, help prevent painful inflammation of the diverticula.

There are two different types of fiber, and both help. Insoluble fiber, found in most fruits, vegetables, and whole grains, absorbs water to bulk up and soften stools so they can pass easily. Soluble fiber, found in oatmeal, eggplant, lentils, apples, pears, and blueberries, dissolves in water, becoming soft and sticky in the intestine. Recently, doctors have found that it too can help prevent constipation, although they aren't sure how. It's also the kind of fiber that helps lower cholesterol.

If you're not eating much fiber now, you can easily "swell" your daily servings by switching to a breakfast cereal that contains at least 5 grams of fiber per serving; eating bread with a first ingredient listed as "whole"; switching to whole-grain pasta and brown rice; and eating more fruits, vegetables, and beans. To get the most fiber from fruits and vegetables, eat the skin on those apples and potatoes. Just make sure you clean them with fresh water. An easy way to boost your vegetable and fiber intake is to eat a salad every day.

Aim for: 25 to 35 grams of fiber per day. Get there by eating 2 cups of fruit, 2 1/2 cups of vegetables, three 1/2-cup servings of whole grains, and 1 cup of legumes (beans and peas).

Helpful hint: Don't add heaps of fiber to your diet all at once, or you may induce new intestinal outcries: gas and bloating. Aim to make one change a week. Start by adding an extra serving of fruit or vegetables to the menu. The following week, swap your white bread for whole wheat, and so on.

Water, juice, *and other fluids*

As you increase the amount of fiber in your meals, it's important to also increase the amount of fluids you drink. Fiber absorbs the fluid and, as a result, it bulks up and softens stools. Without enough water, fiber can cause constipation.

Aim for: Eight 8-ounce glasses (2 l) a day.

NUTRITIONAL SUPPLEMENTS

Fiber. Supplements that have concentrated natural fibers like psyllium husk or wheat dextrin can be useful if dietary fiber isn't doing the trick for you. Be sure to drink plenty of water when taking them so they can work properly, and don't take them for more than seven days without a physician's guidance. **DOSAGE:** Follow the label directions. Some of these supplements come in capsule form, and others are powders to be added to beverages or soft foods.

CAUTION

Refined grains and sugary foods. If fiber is your colon's best friend, foods that fall short on fiber, like white bread, cookies and most baked goods, packaged snack foods, and most sugary cereals, are ones you shouldn't spend much time with. Even fruit juices aren't perfect because they lack the fiber of whole fruit. It's still important to consume plenty of liquids, but after one small glass of juice, favor water or herbal tea the rest of the day.

A Questionable Nut

For years, doctors suspected that nuts and seeds could easily lodge in the pouches that line the large intestine of people with diverticulosis and cause infection. But there is no scientific evidence to support that theory, and few doctors subscribe to it anymore. In fact, nuts and seeds, including popcorn hulls, sesame and poppy seeds, and almonds, all contain fiber that may actually help people with diverticulosis. That said, each person reacts differently to foods. If you experience bloating or pain after eating certain foods, including nuts, be sure to chew them thoroughly before swallowing. If that doesn't help, avoid them.

FEATURED RECIPES

ECZEMA

Most of us take our birthday suits for granted, but for people with eczema, skin can be a constant source of itching and irritation. Eczema often targets babies and children, but anyone can have it. Areas on the face, wrists, hands, and inner creases of the knees and elbows dry, flake, swell, and sometimes blister. The itching is relentless, and over time, itchy patches can thicken and turn a grayish brown.

Eczema appears to have a genetic link and also seems to stem from an oversensitive immune system that produces a response just short of a true allergic reaction. That response is often to certain foods that trigger eczema or make it worse. Avoiding those foods is key, of course, but so is getting more of other foods that seem to bring relief.

YOUR FOOD PRESCRIPTION

Salmon, herring, anchovies,
and other foods rich in omega-3 fatty acids

Go figure: The very creatures that sport the ultimate scaly skin are those that offer some of the best protection from eczema. Salmon and the other foods above are good sources of the omega-3 fatty acids that our bodies need to grow new skin, prevent inflammation, and stave off conditions like eczema. They're particularly rich in a key component of omega-3s known as EPA, which helps reduce skin inflammation. Studies on relieving the symptoms and causes of eczema have focused more on fish oils than on fish itself, but the evidence has convinced plenty of dermatologists to emphasize the importance of fish in the diet.

Tired of salmon? Try canned sardines, which are excellent sources of omega-3s. Sauté some onion and garlic in olive oil and add sardines canned in tomato sauce. When they're heated, pour over whole-wheat pasta and toss with lemon juice and grated Parmesan.

Aim for: Two to three servings of fatty fish a week. Dine on fish for dinner once or twice a week, enjoy a sandwich of canned tuna or salmon, or stuff a tomato with tuna salad.

Helpful hint: Some people have allergic reactions to fish that may worsen rather than relieve the symptoms of eczema. If you're prone to allergies, work with your doctor or a registered dietitian to determine whether fish is among your problem foods.

Oolong tea

A staple in Chinese pantries, oolong tea tastes like a cross between robust black tea and more bitter green tea. In a month-long study in Japan, people with eczema who drank 3 cups of oolong tea felt relief from their itching in just

FEATURED RECIPES

Tuna and White Bean Salad *p. 295*
Open-Faced Sardine Sandwiches *p. 300*
Tuna Kebabs *p. 306*
Fish Tacos *p. 307*
Salmon Steaks with Peach Salsa *p. 308*

one week, and 63 percent of the 118 volunteers continued to improve over the next three weeks. The researchers suspect that polyphenols (a class of antioxidants) in the tea may help repair skin. Other studies have shown that the astringent tannins in tea may also work to reduce inflammation.

Aim for: 3 cups daily, made by steeping the tea in hot water for at least 3 minutes.

Yogurt with live cultures

The beneficial bacteria in these yogurts (and other fermented foods such as kefir) benefit the immune system, especially the many immune cells located in the intestinal tract. The "good" bacteria (a.k.a. probiotics) seem to affect inflammation and stimulate the body to produce certain white blood cells and antibodies as well as various growth factors that are important for keeping the body from overreacting to allergens. Studies have indicated that probiotics are especially important for infants and children, whose immune systems are still developing. Two of these bacteria, *Lactobacillus acidophilus* and *bifidobacterium,* also help your body to better absorb nutrients, including "good" fats that help ward off eczema.

Aim for: 1 to 2 cups per day.

NUTRITIONAL SUPPLEMENTS

Probiotics. A number of studies have looked closely at how probiotics may offer protection from eczema for pregnant women and infants. In Finland, researchers who studied 230 babies with eczema first removed cow's milk from the diets of the babies and their nursing mothers. They then gave half of the babies daily probiotic supplements and the rest placebos. All the infants improved, but those given the probiotics experienced a 30 percent greater improvement than those given the placebo. Researchers suspect that the beneficial bacteria help to establish a strong immune system early in a child's development. Probiotics have also been found to be effective in older children. **DOSAGE:** For babies, check with your pediatrician about supplementing formula or breast milk with a probiotic powder. Pregnant and nursing mothers should take a one-billion-count capsule containing *lactobacillus* and *bifidus* twice daily.

Omega-3 fatty acids. Especially for kids who won't eat fish, fish-oil capsules may be the best way to get enough of the omega-3s, especially EPA, that help keep skin inflammation at bay. In one study, EPA-rich fish-oil capsules taken over three months by people with eczema eased itching and inflammation by 30 percent. **DOSAGE:** For adults, four 1-gram fish-oil capsules a day (be sure they contain EPA). You may have to take the oil for at least 12 weeks before noticing an effect. For children, look for fish oil in a liquid or chewable tablets formulated for kids. They're flavored, making them a much easier sell. Follow the dosage directions on the label.

CAUTION

Cow's milk, eggs, wheat, soy foods, and nuts. These common trigger foods may cause reactions in children prone to allergies and may worsen eczema. The best way to determine if certain foods are making things worse is to follow an elimination diet in which you cut out the most likely allergens for two weeks and then reintroduce them one by one to see how your body reacts. It's best to enlist the help of a physician or registered dietitian to get the clearest results and make sure you don't end up scratching foods from your diet for no good reason.

Coffee. Some adults with eczema experience more dramatic symptoms when they drink coffee. It may be that the body sees coffee as an irritant. One explanation is that coffee can promote acidity in the body, which in turn can promote inflammation. Try eliminating it for three weeks to see if it helps.

Red meat. Because red meat contains fatty acids that promote inflammation, you may find it helpful to limit burgers, pot roasts, and the like during flare-ups.

FATIGUE

If walking to your mailbox or making it through the day without a nap seems beyond your current energy level, you may be suffering from fatigue. It has many causes, including stress, medications, overwork, sleep difficulties, or illness. If your fatigue is chronic or extreme, ask a doctor to check you out. But once you're certain that your tiredness doesn't stem from a medical problem, it may be time to reconsider your diet. Plenty of all-too-common eating habits sap energy—and plenty of relatively simple fixes can inject more oomph into your day.

YOUR FOOD PRESCRIPTION

Fish, meat, dairy products, beans, *and other foods high in protein*

If you're someone who eats salads with no meat, fish, or beans for lunch and then craves an afternoon nap, snubbing protein may be your problem. Studies have shown that people who skip protein at breakfast, for instance, are more apt to be depressed, stressed, and less physically fit than those who regularly add protein to their plates. Amino acids, which make up proteins, are the body's building blocks, growing and repairing everything from blood vessels to hair. Amino acids also help increase levels of neurotransmitters that in turn boost mood and alertness. And eating protein at every meal helps ensure steady blood sugar levels—and steady energy.

Aim for: A good rule of thumb is simply to eat some protein with every meal. If you'd rather go by the numbers, you need 0.36 gram of protein per pound (.45 kg) of body weight. For example, if you weigh 150 pounds (68 kg), you need 54 grams of protein. One serving of beef tenderloin has 32 grams of protein; 1 cup of black beans, 15 grams; and 1 cup of milk, 8 grams.

Red meat, molasses, beans, *and other foods high in iron*

Iron isn't just strong; it offers strength. It's essential to red blood cells, combining with protein and copper to make hemoglobin, the part of red blood cells that carries oxygen. Iron deficiency is the most common cause of anemia, leading to a low volume of red blood cells that results in fatigue. Symptoms include weakness, pallor, fatigue, and brittle nails. If you suspect anemia, check with your doctor. Most cases are caused by blood loss (for example, from a bleeding ulcer or heavy menstrual flow).

Aim for: The recommended amount of iron is 8 milligrams per day for men and menopausal women and 18 milligrams for menstruating women. One 3-ounce (85 g) serving of beef has 3.2 grams, and a cup of soybeans provides 8.8.

Helpful hint: Our bodies absorb iron much better from meat than from plant foods. If you get most of your iron from vegetarian sources like beans and peas, eat them with foods like citrus fruits that are high in vitamin C, which aids iron absorption.

FEATURED RECIPES

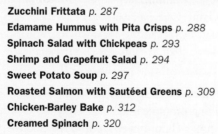

Zucchini Frittata *p. 287*
Edamame Hummus with Pita Crisps *p. 288*
Spinach Salad with Chickpeas *p. 293*
Shrimp and Grapefruit Salad *p. 294*
Sweet Potato Soup *p. 297*
Roasted Salmon with Sautéed Greens *p. 309*
Chicken-Barley Bake *p. 312*
Creamed Spinach *p. 320*

Whole grains, fruits, vegetables,
and other complex carbohydrates

Carbohydrates are the body's primary energy source, but many of us eat too many "simple" carbs that digest quickly, sending blood sugar on a wild ride that saps energy. Choose complex-carb foods like brown rice over white, an orange over a glass of orange juice, and raisin bran cereal over sugar pops to get a steady supply of energy instead of a candy-bar burst followed by a slump. In a British study of 142 people who ate high-fiber cereal at breakfast for two weeks, the volunteers had more energy, mental clarity, and less emotional upset than they did when they went back to eating to their usual breakfasts.

Another reason to get your fill of whole grains: They're a good source of B vitamins. Run low on Bs, and you're apt to slump. They have many functions, including the breakdown of carbohydrates, fats, and proteins into glucose, the fuel our bodies run on. They're also involved in the production of red blood cells.

Aim for: In addition to the recommended 4 to 6 daily cups of fruits and vegetables, aim to get at least three carbohydrate servings from whole grains like whole wheat or brown rice. A serving of bread is one slice; a serving of rice is 1/2 cup.

Pumpkin seeds, spinach,
and other foods high in magnesium

Popeye's spinach habit wasn't for naught. One of its nutrients, magnesium, is essential for the production of a molecule called adenosine triphosphate, the end product of food's conversion to energy. Magnesium also relaxes muscles and aids sleep. If we don't have enough, we feel tired and weak.

Aim for: 400 to 420 milligrams of magnesium daily for men; 310 to 320 milligrams for women. A quarter cup of pumpkin seeds has 185 milligrams; a cup of cooked spinach has 157.

Eat and Drink Often

Sometimes fatigue is simply a signal that you're hungry and thirsty. Eating small meals throughout the day, or three meals and two smart snacks like nuts and fresh fruit, helps keep your blood sugar stable, which fends off fatigue. Choose fresh fruit over dried, which has more concentrated sugar. Unsweetened yogurt's a great snack, too, full of protein and carbs without lots of sugar and calories.

Water is also crucial. Without it, your body works at keeping a fluid balance instead of producing energy molecules. The Institute of Medicine suggests that women consume at least 11 cups of fluids a day and men 16 cups (about 20 percent of those fluids come from food).

Citrus fruits, peppers, broccoli,
and other foods high in vitamin C

When 17th-century sailors swooning with scurvy sipped lemon juice, their lethargy vanished. Present-day studies have found that vitamin C deficiency is associated with fatigue. C is necessary for a healthy adrenal system, which helps prevent fatigue from physical or emotional stress. It also helps fight off infections and helps us absorb iron.

Aim for: The recommended amount is 75 milligrams a day for women and 90 milligrams a day for men, but more is better in this case. One red bell pepper has about twice that amount; a cup of broccoli also provides more than the quota.

Helpful hint: Cooking reduces vitamin C by about 25 percent, so eat some fruits and veggies raw.

Sweet potatoes, carrots,
and other foods high in beta-carotene

Add color to your plate, and you'll add energy to your step. Beta-carotene, the vitamin A precursor that puts the color in carrots, sweet potatoes, and spinach, helps boost a depressed immune system, often at the root of chronic fatigue. By promoting healthy cell membranes, beta-carotene boosts protection from viruses, bacteria, fungi, and allergies. It also ups the activity of T cells, which fight infections, and it's necessary for healthy red blood cells.

Aim for: Make five of your daily produce servings leafy dark green vegetables and yellow or orange fruits and vegetables.

Helpful hint: Lightly steaming (not overcooking) foods like carrots and spinach can help your body absorb their beta-carotene.

Spinach, avocados, squash,
and other foods high in potassium

Run short on potassium, and you risk muscle weakness and exhaustion. Studies have shown that people low on potassium have weaker hand grips than people with enough of the nutrient. In studies of chronic fatigue, potassium and magnesium supplements have returned lost zip. Potassium helps transport nutrients to cells, maintain water balance, regulate muscle contraction, and maintain a healthy nervous system and heart rate.

Aim for: 4,700 milligrams of potassium per day. One cup of cooked spinach has 839 milligrams; an avocado, 875; and a cup of winter squash, 896.

Helpful hint: Potassium decreases the excretion of calcium, so boosting your potassium intake also helps keep your bones healthy.

NUTRITIONAL SUPPLEMENTS

Iron. Pregnant women and women of childbearing age, infants, toddlers, teenage girls, and people with kidney failure are most likely to benefit from iron supplements, because they either need more iron than most people, run low on the mineral, or absorb it poorly. However, because excess iron can cause organ damage (children are especially susceptible to overdose), take supplements only under medical supervision. The doctor will probably do a blood test to determine whether you could benefit from supplements. Ferrous iron salts are the best absorbed form. **DOSAGE:** The upper limit set by the Institute of Medicine is 45 milligrams per day.

B-complex vitamins. Most multivitamins contain the dosages of B vitamins you need daily. **DOSAGE:** One multivitamin a day.

Vitamin C. People who have frequent colds or infections, who smoke, or who suffer from stress can benefit from vitamin C supplements. Vitamin C boosts the immune system and helps get rid of toxins. High doses (5,000 milligrams or more) can cause diarrhea. The National Academy of Sciences has set an upper tolerable level of 2,000 milligrams a day. Higher doses may not be safe. **DOSAGE:** The recommended daily amounts are 75 milligrams for women, 90 milligrams for men, and 100 milligrams for smokers. Studies show that 1,000 milligrams a day may shorten a cold and lower markers of stress, such as levels of the stress hormone cortisol and high blood pressure, as well as subjective feelings of stress.

Magnesium. People who have digestive problems like diarrhea, malabsorption, or ulcerative colitis may need to take magnesium supplements. Physical stressors such as colds, trauma, and surgery can also lead to a magnesium deficiency, as can alcoholism and kidney disease. Chelated forms like magnesium citrate are better absorbed than nonchelated forms like magnesium oxide. **DOSAGE:** The amount varies depending on the cause of the deficiency. Check with a doctor if you suspect you are deficient. Signs include loss of appetite, nausea, and fatigue.

OFF THE MENU

Sugar, caffeine, and alcohol. A dip in blood sugar may send you for a sugary pick-me-up or a caffeinated soda. Neither will do you any good in the long run. Sugar gives you a brief burst of energy, but afterward, you may feel even more tired than before.

But what about caffeine? Anyone who's awakened with their eyelids drooping by their nose would swear by it. Caffeine wakes you up by stimulating your central nervous system and increasing your heart and breathing rate. But its effect wears off, leaving you needing more. And if you consume it too late in the day, it can keep you up at night. Cut it out for a month to see if you have more energy.

Finally, how about a drink in the evening? Despite alcohol's initial boost to your spirits, it's a depressant that eventually puts you to sleep—but only for a while. You wake up later on as it withdraws from your system. The result: The life of the party drags the following day.

The Power of Breakfast

By the time you lift your head off the pillow, your tank is on empty. Without a healthy breakfast like cereal, milk, and fruit that combines whole grains, protein, and a little fat, you'll be nodding off before noon. A number of studies show that people who eat breakfast concentrate better and are more productive than those who go without. They also tend to have better control over their weight because they're not ravenous by lunchtime.

For the typical adult, a healthy breakfast should fall between 300 and 400 calories. That's not a lot of food—and that's a good thing, particularly for those people who have a false notion that it's not a real meal if it doesn't involve cooking or serious preparation. A healthy breakfast often takes just a minute to put together, and just a few minutes to eat. So no excuses for skipping it! Here are some great options:

• A bowl of high-fiber, multigrain cereal, lots of strawberries, and low-fat milk.

• A granola bar, an apple, and a glass of cold milk.

• A cup of nonfat yogurt with fresh bluberries mixed in, and a slice of whole-wheat toast with fruit spread.

• A scrambled egg, a whole-wheat roll, fresh fruit salad, and a cup of low-fat milk.

FOOD ALLERGIES AND SENSITIVITIES

For most people, food is a source of great pleasure. But for others, nature's bounty is more of a minefield of edible hazards—foods that trigger unpleasant side effects (usually due to a food intolerance) or even life-threatening reactions (usually due to a food allergy). The answer, of course, is to avoid the offenders while filling your plate with equally nutritious foods. But oftentimes that's easier said than done. The following advice should help.

First, let's clear up the difference between food allergies and food intolerances. If you're allergic to a food—say, nuts or shellfish—trouble usually starts almost as soon as you put down your fork (although some allergic reactions are delayed by 24 to 72 hours). You may feel your mouth and tongue itch or your tongue and throat swell. You may have trouble breathing. In the most serious scenario, you may develop a severe and sometimes fatal form of shock called anaphylaxis.

Food allergies involve an immune system reaction by antibodies called immunoglobulin E (IgE) or by immune cells called lymphocytes in the GI tract. The antibodies and immune cells are designed to protect the body from foreign invaders—in this case, particular foods.

If the immune system's not involved, you have a food intolerance or sensitivity, often caused by a problem in the metabolism or digestion of the food. Although food intolerances can affect your health, they don't pose an immediate threat to life.

Sometimes food sensitivities and allergies are hard to distinguish since symptoms overlap. Both can cause gastrointestinal trouble, including cramps, diarrhea, and nausea. Some foods, like dairy products, can elicit both true allergic reactions and nonallergic ones. The most common food allergies and sensitivities are those to wheat, gluten, dairy products, soy, eggs, peanuts, nuts, fish, and shellfish.

For both allergies and sensitivities, it's important to see a doctor for testing to confirm what you're reacting to (see "Protecting Yourself" on page 165). And obviously, part of the treatment will involve eliminating the foods that cause a reaction without sacrificing essential nutrients. Unfortunately, food allergies can't always be prevented or cured, but some, like milk or egg allergies in children, diminish or even vanish with age. The good news is that most foods that cause reactions have tasty substitutes that may even broaden your palate. Who knew that millet and buckwheat could be such delicious substitutes for wheat, or that soy milk could actually boost the flavor of breakfast cereal when milk's not an option? Read on for some suggestions to keep both health and taste on your plate.

FOR PEOPLE WHO CAN'T EAT WHEAT:

Corn, rice, millet, barley, oats,
and all other grains except wheat

Relatively few people have an IgE-mediated wheat allergy beyond a very young age; many more have celiac disease and must live a gluten-free life, which means no wheat, rye, barley, or spelt (see the entry on gluten avoidance below). If you do have a wheat allergy, know that it's one of the most powerful food allergies. The first step is to stop eating wheat and any food containing it, such as wheat starch or soy sauce. To replace wheat, a good source of whole grain, choose whole, unprocessed wheat substitutes like cornmeal, brown rice, or millet, which offer the same B vitamins and fiber.

Aim for: Six to eight 1/2-cup servings daily.

Helpful hint: Spelt and kamut, lesser-known grains, are ancestral cousins of wheat that are hazardous for people with an IgE-mediated wheat allergy or celiac disease.

FOR PEOPLE WHO CAN'T EAT GLUTEN:

Ancient grains, flaxseed, arrowroot, beans, rice,
and all grains that don't contain gluten

For people who are intolerant of gluten, a protein found in wheat, barley, kamut, rye, spelt, and triticale, baked goods are verboten. One serious form of the intolerance, celiac disease, can damage the small intestine or even be life threatening. The disease is also associated with an itchy, blistery skin rash called dermatitis herpetiformis. Even oats, which contain no gluten, can be a problem if they came in contact with gluten-containing grains during milling or storage. Fortunately, people with gluten allergy needn't go grainless. Buckwheat, which is not a wheat, regardless of its name, corn, quinoa, amaranth,

and other grains make excellent flours full of fiber and B vitamins. Make sure any grain you use is stored and processed in a gluten-free place.

Aim for: Six to eight 1/2-cup servings daily.

Helpful hint: Read the food label on every purchase you make. If you're still unsure whether a product contains gluten, don't eat it, and contact the manufacturer for information.

FOR PEOPLE WHO CAN'T EAT DAIRY:

Rice, almond, and soy milk,
and other dairy substitutes, plus calcium-rich foods

Milk doesn't always do a body good. It can provoke both allergies and intolerances. People with allergies react to casein or whey, which are milk protein fractions. Those with intolerances react to lactose, a sugar in cow's milk. Most of us produce enough of an enzyme called lactase to avoid a reaction to lactose, but for those who don't, lactose heads to the large intestine, where trouble begins.

In either case, the symptoms aren't pretty: Lactose intolerance causes gas and diarrhea; milk allergy can cause those GI symptoms as well as a skin rash and asthma, and it may take as long as two days for the reaction to hit, although the effects are usually more immediate. As with other foods, eliminating dairy isn't as simple as it sounds. Dairy products can lurk in unexpected places, such as breath mints, nutrition bars, and salad dressings. The less processed food you eat, the easier the job of eliminating dairy. For many of us, dairy foods are also our main source of

FEATURED RECIPES

Buckwheat Pancakes with Fruit Sauce *p. 286*
Corn, Tomato, and Quinoa Salad *p. 292*
Roasted Salmon with Sautéed Greens *p. 309*
Brown Rice Risotto *p. 321*
Springtime Quinoa *p. 322*

calcium, an essential nutrient for strong bones as well as for many body functions, such as blood clotting and nerve transmission. Although drinks like rice, almond, and soy milk taste great in place of milk over cereal or in coffee, they aren't nutrient-to-nutrient matches with milk. (And some people who react to cow's milk also react to soy and goat's milk.) So you'll want to "bone up" on foods high in calcium, such as dark leafy greens and bony sardines, as well as calcium-fortified orange juice. If you are lactose intolerant, yogurt is also an option, since its good-for-you bacteria produce the very enzyme needed to digest lactose.

Aim for: 1,000 to 1,200 milligrams of calcium daily, the amount in 3 to 4 cups of calcium-fortified soy milk or 2 cups of tofu made with calcium sulfate.

Helpful hint: Processed soy foods like soy hot dogs and sausage (but not tofu) often contain added dairy proteins, so be sure to read the label before eating any of those foods.

FOR PEOPLE WHO CAN'T EAT EGGS:

Fish, chicken, soybeans,
and other low-fat proteins

Egg allergies are common in young children but are frequently outgrown. As with other food allergies, proteins are the culprits. More than half of the egg white is made of the primary protein allergen called ovalbumin; a reaction to egg

yolks involves other proteins. Reactions to either part of the egg can range from mild to severe.

Eggs provide exceptional low-fat protein. Luckily, fish, chicken, and soybeans and other legumes do as well. To replace the binding, tenderizing, and leavening qualities that eggs add in baking, try ground flaxseed (it turns egg white–like when liquefied with 1/4 cup water or other liquid in a recipe), bananas, tofu, prunes, and egg replacements (if they don't contain egg whites).

Aim for: 5 to 6 ounces (142 to 170 g) of protein per day.

Helpful hint: Eggs can show up not only in baked goods but also in noodles, sauces, pretzels, tartar sauce, and even wine. As always, read labels and don't eat anything you're unsure of.

FOR PEOPLE WHO CAN'T EAT SOY:

Meat, fish, legumes,
and other substitutes for soy

Soy has its own problems: A handful of different proteins in soy may cause allergic reactions. To add confusion, some soy foods may cause reactions, while others may not. Soybean oil, for instance, does not contain proteins and thus may not trigger symptoms. Reactions to soy include a rash, asthma, gastrointestinal symptoms, and anaphylactic shock.

If you have to give up soy, you can still get more than your fair share of protein from fish, chicken, meat, nuts, and dairy products. One thing you

food for thought . . .

"Up to 25 percent of adults believe they have a food allergy. Scientific studies and testing, however, find that only 1 to 2 percent of adults have a true food allergy."

— *The New Nutrition* by Felicia Busch, MPH, RD, FAD ■

can't easily get elsewhere is soy's phytoestrogens, called isoflavones, which may help protect against heart disease as well as certain cancers and perhaps osteoporosis. Other beans and peas offer only a small fraction of the isoflavones soybeans do, but a healthy diet full of whole grains and plenty of fruits and vegetables also provides protection against these diseases.

If you can't drink soy milk *or* cow's milk, look to almond-, oat-, and rice-based drinks as possible substitutes.

Aim for: 5 to 6 ounces (142 to 170 g) of nonsoy protein per day and 3 cups of legumes weekly.

FOR PEOPLE WHO CAN'T EAT FISH OR SHELLFISH:

Chicken, flaxseed, walnuts,
and other substitutes for shellfish and fish

Nothing's fishy about an allergic reaction to fish or shellfish: It's straightforward, severe, and can even cause anaphylaxis. Seafood allergies tend to predominate in countries where people eat a lot of seafood and in people who work in the seafood industry. Unfortunately, these allergies tend to last a lifetime, and reactions can sometimes worsen with each incident. (Sufferers can sometimes become sick simply from inhaling the steam from fish as it cooks.) The reactions, which occur from 2 to 24 hours after exposure, are the classic allergy symptoms: itching, swelling, trouble breathing, upset stomach, or systemic shock.

Seafood is a delicious, low-fat source of protein. Fortunately, most people with a fish allergy can still eat shellfish, and most people with a shellfish allergy can still eat fish—and even some types of shellfish. (Some must avoid all shellfish, but most need to avoid either only the crustacean category, which includes shrimp, crab, and lobster, or only the molluscan category, which includes clams, oysters, abalone, and squid.)

Chicken, beans, and eggs can make up for the loss of protein from seafood. But fatty fish like salmon and tuna are also the best food sources of omega-3 fatty acids, powerful anti-inflammatories with heart-protecting effects. Look for these in flaxseed, walnuts, and soybeans.

Aim for: 5 to 6 ounces (142 to 170 g) of protein per day and 1,000 milligrams per day of omega-3 fatty acids (the equivalent of two to four servings a week of walnuts or flaxseed).

Helpful hint: Processed foods that appear to be fishless may in fact contain seafood. Check all labels.

FOR PEOPLE WHO CAN'T EAT PEANUTS OR TREE NUTS:

Fish, chicken, beans, *and*
other substitutes for peanuts and tree nuts

Peanut and tree nut allergies are nothing to sneeze at. The most prevalent life-threatening allergies in children, they are caused by a reaction to proteins in the nut. Even a trace of nut dust can set off a reaction in a few highly sensitive individuals. Some children outgrow it, but for most, the allergy is lifelong. New research now shows that introducing peanuts earlier, rather than later, in a child's diet, may actually decrease his or her risk of developing an allergy to this food.

Although reactions to peanuts are most common, many people who are allergic to peanuts are often also allergic to tree nuts such as cashews or almonds. Symptoms include itching, shortness of breath, swelling, and possibly anaphylactic shock.

Nuts are an excellent source of protein, healthy monounsaturated and polyunsaturated fats, and fiber. Low-fat dairy foods and chicken can replace lost protein. Fish provides both low-fat protein and healthy fats. Olive oil is also a healthy fat replacement. You can get more low-fat protein plus fiber from a plateful of beans and other legumes.

Aim for: 5 to 6 ounces (142 to 170 g) of protein per day, two servings of fish per week, and 25 grams of fiber per day (about 2 cups of kidney beans).

Helpful hint: A nut isn't always a nut. Nutmeg comes from the seed of a tree, and water chestnuts are plant roots. Both are safe.

NUTRITIONAL SUPPLEMENTS

Calcium. Scientists are still researching the optimal amount of calcium necessary to slow bone loss. For now, the National Academy of Sciences recommends taking the amount below. Calcium supplements also often include vitamin D, which helps the body use calcium. **DOSAGE:** *Calcium:* 1,000 to 1,200 milligrams daily. *Vitamin D:* 400 IU daily.

Omega-3 fatty acids. Omega-3s come in fish-oil capsules or in liquids such as flaxseed oil and cod-liver oil. Buying a version with vitamin E helps prevent rancidity, as does storing the supplement in the refrigerator. People allergic to fish should not take fish-oil capsules or cod-liver oil. **DOSAGE:** Optimal dosages aren't established, but the FDA considers 1 to 3 grams daily in capsule or liquid form safe.

OFF THE MENU

Wheat and gluten. Wheat and gluten allergies put the kibosh on wheat by any name: durum, semolina, kamut, rye, barley, bran, couscous, or spelt. But wheat can appear in many products without being obvious, including broth and soup bases, some candies, imitation bacon and seafood, marinades, processed meats, self-basting poultry, soy sauce, communion wafers, herbal and malt supplements, medications, and Play-Doh (a problem if it's handled).

Dairy. Milk and other dairy products show up in more places than a Kardashian: breath mints, coffee whiteners, fortified cereals, protein powders, nutrition bars, and salad dressings all contain some form of dairy product. Dairy products are often used to flavor processed

Sometimes, it's not natural foods that cause a reaction, but the chemicals and additives that packaged-food makers add to them. Monosodium glutamate, a flavor enhancer, is well known for causing asthma-like reactions in some people. Sulfites and benzoic acid (both preservatives) also can cause reactions, as can some artificial colorings. So stick to fresh foods.

meats. Also, just because a product is labeled "lactose-free" doesn't mean it's dairy-free. And dairy-free doesn't necessarily mean casein- and whey-free.

Soy. Soy too shows up in unexpected places: baked goods containing soy flour, cereals, processed vegetables with sauce or breading, fruit drink mixes and sauces, coffee, coffee substitutes, hot chocolate, processed meats, canned soups, candies, butter substitutes, salad dressings, and condiments. Soy oil is safe. Vitamin E capsules often contain oil derived from soybeans. Like soy oil, it's probably safe, but it has not been tested.

Eggs. Eggs, alas, are omnipresent. If you're allergic, be wary of baked or battered foods, noodles, salad dressings, egg substitutes, marshmallows, some fat substitutes, and even some wines. If you have any doubt about a product's ingredients, call the manufacturer.

Fish and shellfish. Even "imitation" seafood contains fish. The basis for imitation crab, for example, is pollock, also used in imitation beef and pork products. Caesar salad dressings and steak sauces may contain anchovies, as can a delicious Italian relish called *caponata*. Producers sometimes use fish gelatin to clarify wine and coffee, but fish gelatin is clinically proven to be safe for people with fish allergies.

Peanuts and tree nuts. Removing peanuts and tree nuts from your diet can *drive* you nuts. Avoid all nut butters; artificial nuts (which may be peanuts reflavored with another nut); peanut or arachis oil that's been cold pressed or expeller pressed (other peanut oils are safe); Asian and African foods, which are often flavored with nuts; barbecue sauces; cereals; crackers; and a type of cold cut called mortadella (which may contain pistachios). Also avoid anything processed in the presence of nuts, such as sunflower seeds and foods sold in bakeries, ice cream parlors, and candy stores. Beanbags and other filled bags may be stuffed with nut shells. Even some cosmetics, skin creams, and craft materials may contain nuts.

Protecting Yourself

Food sensitivities are at the least discomforting and at the worst life threatening, so knowing how best to protect yourself is important. The first step is to see a doctor or an allergist to confirm what you are sensitive or allergic to. The doctor may do a blood test called the radioallergosorbent test (RAST), which measures the amount of various antibodies in your blood, each of which indicates an allergy to a certain food. He may also give you a relatively pain-free skin test, placing a tiny amount of several allergens on your skin to see if the skin reacts.

If it's still unclear what you're reacting to, your doctor may ask you to keep a food diary, tracking foods and reactions. The doc may also ask you to eliminate probable suspects and then add them back to your plate one at a time.

Once you know which food is the villain, a nutritionist can help you figure out how best to rearrange your diet so you don't miss out on any nutrients, what hidden dangers may lurk, how to read and understand a food label, and what substitutions work best in cooking and baking. If your allergy is severe, the doctor may give you an epinephrine injection kit to carry in case of a reaction. Epinephrine, a hormone most of us know as adrenaline, reverses the effects of a severe reaction, reducing swelling in the throat and airways and keeping blood pressure steady.

GALLSTONES

In medieval times, health was thought to depend on the four "humours," or vital fluids of the body, including bile. Too much of the liquid was believed to produce a violent temperament. Today, we know that bile doesn't make you a nasty person, but if there's too much cholesterol in your bile, you may be headed toward a nasty gallstone.

Bile is made in the liver, stored in the gallbladder, and used in the small intestine to digest fat. When you eat a greasy hamburger, the gallbladder contracts and pushes bile through a duct that connects with the small intestine. There the bile helps break down and digest the fat in that burger. But too much cholesterol in the bile can turn into trouble in the gallbladder, hardening into stones that range from the size of sugar granules to the size of plums. Some stones linger benignly in the gallbladder. But when a stone tries to pass through a duct, it can cause inflammation, intense pain, and a dangerous blockage that may require surgery.

If too much cholesterol in the gallbladder can cause stones (heredity also plays a role), it makes sense that foods that lower your cholesterol can help you dodge them. Eating smaller meals throughout the day can also help because it keeps the gallbladder contracting regularly so there's no time for the bile to form stones.

YOUR FOOD PRESCRIPTION

A breakfast cereal that contains psyllium

At Brandeis University in Massachusetts, when hamsters were fed diets that included psyllium, a fiber found in many natural laxatives and some breakfast cereals, they were much less likely to have gallstones. The researchers suspect that psyllium increases the amount of bile released from the gallbladder, making it less likely to build up and form stones. Psyllium is also a great source of cholesterol-lowering soluble fiber.

Aim for: 1/2 cup every morning. If nothing else, this should help you stay regular.

Avocados, olive oil, canola oil, fish, and nuts

All fats stimulate the gallbladder to contract, but it's saturated fat from burgers and bacon that raises cholesterol and your risk of gallstones.

The fat in avocados, olive and canola oils, fish, and nuts is unsaturated, so it's healthy for your gallbladder and may actually help prevent stones by stimulating the gallbladder to contract and keep bile moving.

Aim for: Try to replace most of the butter and lard in your diet with olive and canola oils, have fish or nuts in place of meat, and trade the cheese in your sandwich for a slice or two of avocado.

Fruits, vegetables,
and whole grains high in fiber

In the Nurses Health Study, which monitors tens of thousands of women across the United States, the women who ate the most fiber had a 35 percent lower risk of developing gallstones. Foods that offer insoluble fiber—whole-grain bread and most fruits and vegetables, for instance—appear to be particularly helpful. One study showed that people who followed vegetarian diets had a lower risk of gallstones.

Aim for: 25 to 35 grams of fiber daily. Eating 2 cups of fruit, 2 1/2 cups of vegetables, and three servings of whole grains every day will help you hit your goal.

An evening glass of wine

Many recent studies have shown that moderate amounts of wine can help lower cholesterol and help decrease the risk of gallbladder attacks.

Aim for: One to two glasses per day (the higher amount is for men).

Coffee

In the large National Health and Nutrition Examination Survey, women with gallstones who regularly drank between 1 and 4 cups of coffee per day reported fewer symptoms than women who passed on java.

Aim for: 1 to 4 cups a day. If you're sensitive to caffeine, drink your joe before 3:00 in the afternoon, or cut back.

Turmeric

The spice that gives curry its yellow hue, turmeric has been shown to help decrease inflammation in the gallbladder. Some scientists also suspect that it helps stimulate the movement of bile. If you have active stones (particularly larger ones), use turmeric with caution because it can stimulate contractions.

Aim for: A tablespoon per day. Use it in curry dishes and add it to butternut squash, pea soups, stews, and casseroles.

NUTRITIONAL SUPPLEMENTS

Vitamin C. Vitamin C may help break down cholesterol in bile. One study showed that women who had higher blood levels of vitamin C were 13 percent less likely to develop gallstones. **DOSAGE:** 200 to 500 milligrams per day. Higher intakes may increase your risk for kidney stones.

Omega-3 fatty acids. Omega-3s can lower triglycerides in the bloodstream, and that can in turn lower cholesterol and the risk of gallstones. **DOSAGE:** Up to 4 grams per day if you have high triglycerides and your doctor orders this therapeutic dose.

CAUTION

Fatty meat and fried foods. Foods high in saturated fat can trigger gallstone attacks. The same goes for trans fats, although most are now banned in our food supply. Eat these foods less often and in smaller portions.

Extreme dieting. Rapid weight loss is one of the most common causes of gallstones. Skipping meals may also cause a shift in the balance of cholesterol and bile salts in the gallbladder.

Sugar. In some people, a diet packed with sweet baked goods, candy, soda, and ice cream can change their bile in a way that makes them more susceptible to gallstones. For sweet treats, look to dried fruits and fruit desserts.

Colas. Most dark-colored sodas contain phosphoric acid, which could soften and move gallstones. This may be dangerous if a stone moves into the duct. In general, it's smart to avoid colas. Note, however, that some natural medicine doctors believe in dissolving the stones with a "flush" of cola combined with apple juice, which contains a different type of acid. If you consider trying this, do so only under expert supervision.

FEATURED RECIPES

Ginger Butternut Squash Soup *p. 298*
Salsa Tuna Salad Sandwiches *p. 300*
Curried Chicken Salad Sandwiches *p. 301*
Hearty Vegetable Stew *p. 304*
Roasted Salmon with Sautéed Greens *p. 309*
Turkey Ragu with Spaghetti *p. 314*
Pear Crisp *p. 332*

GOUT

Many of us associate gout with excess; we think of plump kings downing steins of beer and gobbling fatty haunches of lamb. But gout is actually one of the most painful forms of arthritis, affecting rich and poor alike. Fortunately, there are medications that effectively control gout symptoms—and the right dietary changes can help, too.

Characterized by severe joint pain and tenderness, especially in the big toe, gout is caused by a buildup of uric acid, which forms crystals that nestle into the joints and inflame them. Uric acid results from the breakdown of purines, compounds in body tissues and in many foods, especially red meats and alcohol. Yes, you'll want to cut back on these to avoid gout flare-ups. However, dealing with gout doesn't have to be about nixing steak dinners and fine wines; there are also foods that offer relief.

YOUR FOOD PRESCRIPTION

Fresh cherries

If Little Jack Horner had had gout, he would have been better off sticking his thumb in a cherry pie. According to a USDA study at the University of California, women who ate two servings (about 1 1/2 cups) of bing cherries after fasting had significantly lower levels of uric acid in their blood and higher levels in their urine than they had before eating the cherries. The researchers found that the cherries also cut markers of inflammation. Blueberries and strawberries may also be beneficial.

Aim for: 1 1/2 cups a day.

Helpful hint: Although the California researchers used bing cherries, earlier research found black, yellow, and red sour cherries to be effective, too.

Fresh or frozen pineapple

Slice open a pineapple and enjoy a sweet, juicy snack. Bromelain, a protein-digesting enzyme in the fruit, can help reduce the pain and inflammation of a gout attack.

Aim for: The amount of bromelain in each serving of pineapple varies depending on the ripeness of the fruit and its exposure to heat (we don't recommend canned pineapple for this reason). Aim for at least one serving—a half cup—a day when gout flares. To get even more bromelain, which is more plentiful in the fruit's stem, take bromelain supplements. A typical dose for gout attacks is 500 milligrams twice a day between meals.

Helpful hint: Eat your pineapple between meals, not with them, or the enzyme will be used up digesting your food.

Tofu, edamame, soy milk,
and other soy foods

People with gout should limit animal protein, which contains purines, but soy foods are a different story. Several studies show that soy reduces uric acid, making it a terrific way to get protein and combat gout.

Aim for: Eating soy foods once or twice a week in place of meat or poultry is a smart idea.

Tomatoes, bell peppers,
and other foods rich in vitamin C

In a two-week study at Tufts University, people who ate two bowls a day of gazpacho containing tomatoes, green bell peppers, and other vegetables high in vitamin C had significantly lower levels of uric acid than they did prior to the study; acid levels were reduced by 18 percent in men and by 8 percent in women. These foods are also rich in lycopene, an antioxidant found in red fruits and vegetables that may lower levels of uric acid.

Aim for: At least 72 milligrams of vitamin C daily, the equivalent of 2 cups of gazpacho, one orange, or half of a red bell pepper.

Olive oil, canola oil, avocados,
and other foods rich in unsaturated fats

Several studies suggest that unsaturated fats, found in these foods, may lower uric acid levels (notice we didn't list fish, which contains purines). In a South African study, after patients with gout replaced saturated fats with unsaturated ones, their blood levels of uric acid dropped 17.5 percent after 16 weeks. Getting more of your calories from unsaturated fats may also lower insulin levels, which indirectly helps protect you from gout attacks.

Aim for: Up to 30 percent of your calories should come from fat, and at least 20 percent of that should be unsaturated.

Helpful hint: Replace butter and creamy salad dressings with olive oil.

Water *and other nonalcoholic liquids*

Drinking plenty of fluids helps wash the uric acid out of your system.

Aim for: At least eight glasses a day.

Cabbage, kale, leafy greens, celery, and carrots

These vegetables are low in purines, and because they're also low in calories and high in fiber, filling half your plate with them will help keep your weight down. A wide waistline and high levels of uric acid seem to go hand in hand.

CAUTION

Red meat and seafood. These are high in purines, the compounds that break down into uric acid. Organ meats like liver and sweetbreads and game meats like goose are especially packed with purines. So are fatty fish like anchovies, sardines, mackerel, and herring, as well as scallops and mussels.

Although other meats and fish, such as chicken, salmon, crab, and shrimp, have only moderate levels, you should scale back. A 12-year study of more than 47,000 men found that those who ate the most meat were 40 percent more likely to have gout; those who ate the most seafood had a 50 percent higher risk. Eat only small servings of low-fat meats and seafood, no more than 5 to 6 ounces (142 to 170 g) a day. Or, consider a vegetarian diet.

Purine-rich vegetables and grains. Asparagus, beans, peas, and cauliflower contain moderate amounts of purines. Limit them to a 1/2-cup serving a day. Whole-grain cereals, wheat germ, oatmeal, and wheat bran also contain purines; limit yourself to three servings a day.

Alcohol and yeasty foods like bread and beer. Most alcoholic drinks don't contain many purines (beer is the worst offender), but because of the way alcohol is processed in the body, all alcohol raises uric acid levels. Yeast, an ingredient in beers and many breads, does, too.

Sugar. Research from the University of Florida shows that large amounts of table sugar and corn syrup increase uric acid levels.

FEATURED RECIPES

Tropical Fruit Salad *p. 286*
Edamame Hummus with Pita Crisps *p. 288*
Roasted Cherry Tomatoes in Parmesan Cups *p. 289*
Coleslaw with Orange-Sesame Vinaigrette *p. 290*
Corn, Tomato, and Quinoa Salad *p. 292*
Sweet Potato Soup *p. 297*
Hearty Vegetable Stew *p. 304*
Carrot Cake with Cream Cheese Glaze *p. 332*

GUM DISEASE

Oysters are rumored to help steam up a romance, but did you know they help protect your gums, too? Or that a squirt of lime juice now and then can help your mouth battle bacteria?

Many factors contribute to gum disease, and poor diet is one. The mildest form is gingivitis, a buildup of bacteria in the plaque that continuously forms on teeth. The result is inflamed, bleeding gums. Usually, a professional cleaning and better brushing and flossing take care of it. Let it go, however, and the bacteria-laden plaque descends below the gumline, triggering an inflammatory response that breaks down tissues. The gums pull away from the teeth, those pockets become infected, and eventually, infection can even destroy the bone. This kind of gum disease also boosts the risk of heart disease by 15 percent. Fortunately, many nutrients that protect our gums—vitamins C and E, zinc, and folate—protect our hearts, too.

YOUR FOOD PRESCRIPTION

Lean beef
and other foods rich in zinc and vitamin B_6

We're not advising you to gobble down whole sides of beef; after all, animal fat is bad for your heart. But oysters, beef, and lamb are high in zinc, a mineral with anti-inflammatory, antioxidant, and immunity-boosting powers that can battle gum disease.

Vitamin B_6, plentiful in beef as well as seafood, also fights gum disease. In a one-year study at Pennsylvania State University, older adults with low intakes of vitamin A and vitamin B_6 had persistent problems with tooth decay and gum disease.

Aim for: *Zinc:* 8 milligrams for women, 11 milligrams for men (roughly what you'd get from a roast beef sandwich). *Vitamin B_6:* 1.3 to 1.5 milligrams for women and 1.3 to 1.7 milligrams for men. One 3-ounce (85 g) serving of tuna has 0.88 milligram; a medium potato with skin, 0.62 milligram; a banana, 0.55 milligram; and 3 ounces (85 g) of top sirloin, 0.53 milligram. Many fortified cereals give you most or even all of the B_6 you need in one serving.

Helpful hint: Drink up that milk in your cereal bowl! After the cereal soaks, many of the vitamins, minerals, and other nutrients with which cereals are fortified end up in the milk.

FEATURED RECIPES

Tropical Fruit Salad *p. 286*
Broccoli Salad *p. 291*
Sweet Potato Soup *p. 297*
Beef and Broccoli Stew *p. 316*
Mac 'n Cheese Primavera *p. 304*
Orange Beets *p. 323*
Creamed Spinach *p. 320*
Springtime Quinoa *p. 322*

Whole-grain cereal with milk and an orange

Consider this the ultimate breakfast for a healthy smile. That milk on your cereal is rich in calcium, which protects your gums. In a long-term study of 13,000 people, those who ate only half the recommended servings of calcium-rich foods doubled their risk of gum disease. Scientists speculate that calcium keeps the jawbone stronger, helping it fight invading bacteria. (Get your calcium at lunchtime, too, by eating a cup of yogurt.)

The cereal adds its own benefits. Canadian researchers have found that people who ate multiple helpings of whole grains daily were 15 percent less likely to develop gum disease, probably because whole grains tend to keep blood sugar levels lower than refined grains (like most rice and corn cereals and white bread) do. Limiting blood sugar spikes may in turn limit the production of destructive compounds called AGEs (advanced glycation end products), which inflame soft tissues like the gums.

And trade that glass of OJ for a whole orange. Besides being rich in vitamin C, whole fruit is rich in fiber, which helps to clean the teeth when we munch, says the American Dental Association.

Aim for: Start each day with whole-grain cereal, milk, and a piece of fruit, then aim to get five to six servings of whole grains per day (a serving is a cup of whole-grain cereal, a half cup of whole-grain pasta or rice, or one slice of whole-grain bread) and 1,000 to 1,200 milligrams of calcium daily, the equivalent of one glass of fat-free milk, plus 1 cup of yogurt, and one serving of spinach and canned salmon (also good calcium sources).

Fruits and vegetables high in antioxidants

Forget eating spinach for strong muscles—eat it for strong gums. Its beta-carotene, which converts to vitamin A in the body, is a powerful antioxidant and immunity booster. Other good sources are other dark leafy greens (including beet greens), sweet potatoes, carrots, winter squash, and yellow fruits such as cantaloupe and apricots. To drive infections off, also look to vitamin C, which is abundant in citrus fruits, bell peppers, and broccoli, not to mention the orange juice we already mentioned.

Aim for: 2 to 3 cups a day of vegetables, especially yellow vegetables and dark leafy greens, and 2 to 3 cups of fruits, especially those mentioned above.

NUTRITIONAL SUPPLEMENTS

A daily multivitamin. A healthy diet should give you all the nutrients you need to protect your gums, but a multivitamin may be smart insurance. Fruits and vegetables provide plenty of vitamin C, but if you smoke, you'll need more of it and other antioxidants (look for a high-antioxidant multi). Meats and fortified cereals provide zinc, but if you're undereating, drink alcohol to excess, or have a digestive disease, you may need help from the zinc in a multi. Many older Americans and people with poor diets have low levels of vitamin B_6 and should consider a supplement if they can't boost their levels by eating more fortified cereals, beans, or meat. The easiest and best way to get B vitamins is from a multivitamin. **DOSAGE:** One a day.

Calcium. If you skimp on dairy foods and dark leafy greens, calcium can help you meet your goal. **DOSAGE:** A total of 1,000 to 1,200 milligrams daily from food and supplements.

OFF THE MENU

Sugar. Sugar is bacteria's friend, and bacteria are at the root of gum disease. The bacteria in plaque seize on sugar, using it to increase acid production and creating a welcome mat for more bacteria. And sugar lowers the ability of white cells to fight bacteria.

Take aim at sugary drinks. A long-term study of almost 14,000 people found that among young adults 18 to 34, those who were obese were 76 percent more likely to have gum disease than those of normal weight. Researchers suspect that sugary drinks were the culprits. Drink water instead.

HEARTBURN

When you think of heartburn and food, your Uncle Edgar's famous five-alarm chili may come to mind. In fact, though, you'd be better off avoiding pizza, since fatty and acidic foods (think tomatoes) are actually more likely than spicy ones to trigger that searing sensation. And while you're avoiding foods that ignite heartburn, you'd do well to add some that douse the flames.

As you swallow food and liquids, muscle contractions in the throat force them down the esophagus. Think of this long tube as a chute with a trapdoor at the bottom. When you swallow food, the trapdoor—known as the lower-esophageal sphincter (LES)—swings open for a few seconds, allowing your meal to enter the stomach, then closes quickly.

Some foods and beverages cause heartburn through direct contact as they pass through the esophagus. But many others create chemical changes in the gastrointestinal tract that relax the LES after a meal, causing it to open for long periods. That allows stomach contents and digestive acids to splash upward, or "reflux," scorching the tender lining of the esophagus. In some cases, food may back up all the way into the throat, which may make you cough or taste acid and have bad breath. Foods that increase stomach acid can make heartburn worse.

The foods that fan the flames vary from one person to the next. To identify your triggers, doctors recommend eliminating potentially troublesome foods from your diet one at a time for a week or two. See a doctor or nutritionist for details.

Chronic heartburn, known as gastroesophageal reflux disease, or GERD, is a serious matter. Not only is it a painful nuisance, but frequent acid baths can produce scar tissue that may make it difficult to swallow or, in rare cases, cause cell damage that results in cancer of the esophagus. Whether heartburn is an occasional woe or a daily hassle, choosing the right foods can help you chill out.

FEATURED RECIPES

Edamame Hummus with Pita Crisps *p. 288*
Curried Chicken Salad Sandwiches *p. 301*
Pork Chops with Dried Fruits *p. 316*
Roasted Root Vegetables *p. 318*
Pear Crisp *p. 332*

YOUR FOOD PRESCRIPTION

Whole-grain bread
and other high-fiber foods

Your doctor has probably been telling you for years to add more fiber to your diet. Now there's one more reason to follow her advice. Recent research suggests that eating a lot of roughage appears to protect against heartburn. Swedish researchers found that people who ate high-fiber whole-grain bread every day had half the risk of GERD compared with people who preferred low-fiber white bread.

How does fiber help? There are several possible explanations. Some foods (such as cured meats) contain substances called nitrites, which the body may use to produce nitric oxide. This gas can cause the LES to relax, allowing caustic stomach acid to sear the lining of the esophagus. Fiber soaks up nitrites, which blocks the production of nitric oxide. Fiber also forces us to chew our food more thoroughly, and chewing releases saliva, which helps protect the esophagus. Fiber helps us to feel full with less food so we don't overeat at one sitting, which helps prevent heartburn because overeating is a common trigger.

Aim for: Many health experts and organizations recommend 25 to 35 grams of fiber per day, which you can get by eating 2 to 3 cups of fruit, 2 to 3 cups of vegetables, and at least three servings of cereal and grain foods (a serving is a slice of whole-grain bread, 1/2 cup of brown rice, or about 3/4 cup of most cereals) each day.

Helpful hint: If your diet has been relatively low in roughage until now, suddenly adding huge servings of fiber may cause a decidedly unwelcome side effect: flatulence. Increase your fiber intake gradually.

Dishes containing ginger, turmeric, chiles, and cinnamon

Yes, that's right, we're recommending spices for heartburn. Researchers have discovered that not only do spicy foods (at least ones that aren't greasy) *not* usually contribute to heartburn but also that certain spices can actually help. Many of them, especially ginger and turmeric (found in curry powder), combat inflammation and kill bacteria. Be sure to add the spices during cooking rather than at the end to release their full healing potential. A bonus: Spices can often take the place of seasonings high in sugar and salt and help you get more enjoyment out of low-fat foods. Spicy foods don't have to be greasy.

Of course, if a food diary or elimination diet reveals that certain spices do aggravate your heartburn, cut them out.

Slippery elm tea

Slippery elm is also recommended for sore throats, and for the same reason: It coats mucous membranes like those in the throat and digestive tract, thanks to its mucilage. The slick stuff is a form of soluble fiber—after all, slippery elm is made from the bark of a tree. You can buy slippery elm tea bags in health food stores.

Aim for: A cup when your heartburn flares.

Gentian root tea

The dried root used to make this tea has been used for many years as a digestive bitter. You can find tea bags in health food stores.

Aim for: A cup before or after meals.

Water

It's a simple trick, but drinking a glass of water helps wash the acid in your throat back into your stomach, where it belongs. It also dilutes your stomach acid a bit.

Aim for: A small glass of water (4 to 6 ounces/ 113 to 177 ml) when heartburn strikes.

What causes heartburn?
Fatty foods. Salty foods. Acidic foods. Alcohol.
Eating too fast. Eating too much. The path to prevention?
That's simple: Eat healthy meals, in healthy amounts,
at a healthy speed.

NUTRITIONAL SUPPLEMENTS

DGL tablets or wafers. Deglycyrrhizinated licorice, or DGL, is licorice with a certain blood pressure–raising compound removed. It soothes and coats the stomach, preventing that burning feeling. **DOSAGE:** One or two chewable tablets or wafers before each meal.

Calcium. Many popular antacids are simply calcium supplements. While some antacids use other minerals, such as magnesium or aluminum, to neutralize stomach acid, calcium protects your bones as it battles heartburn. Take a calcium supplement, or any antacid, following a meal you suspect may trigger an attack of acid indigestion or when you feel heartburn symptoms arising. If heartburn wakes you at night, popping an antacid before bed may be wise, too. **DOSAGE:** Follow the label directions. 2 to 3 500-milligram tablets per day is typical. Don't exceed the recommended dose; taking too much calcium to treat heartburn may cause other GI problems, such as constipation, bloating, gas, and flatulence. (Look for a calcium supplement that also contains magnesium to sidestep the constipation problem.) It may also set you up for something known as rebound reflux. Besides, if you need frequent relief, you may require more serious medicine. Talk to a doctor if you take antacids for heartburn more than a few times a week.

CAUTION

Tomatoes, onions, and orange juice. Acidic foods, such as the tomatoes used to make marinara and pizza sauce, may inflame the lining of the esophagus on contact as they pass through. This explains why your favorite Italian takeout place has a Rolaids dispenser by the counter. That doesn't mean you need to ban tomatoes, which are especially good for men, but you may need to cut back. The same holds true for some juices, such as orange, grapefruit, and pineapple. (The fruits themselves shouldn't bother you—in fact, they contain digestive enzymes that help break down animal protein at a meal—but the juices are too concentrated.) Don't worry too much about lemons and limes; they are actually weak acids and may do more good than harm. But avoid lemonade; all the sugar may be irritating, and it feeds bacteria.

Finally, high acidity is the reason many heartburn sufferers find themselves repeating the same mantra—"Hold the onions!"—when they dine out. In one study, people with persistent heartburn were able to eat plain hamburgers without incident, but eating burgers with onions consistently produced acid indigestion and reflux. You may have better luck with cooked onions—and skip the ketchup.

Fatty foods. Studies show that people who consume diets high in total fat and saturated fat (the kind in dairy foods and meats) have a higher risk of GERD. Eating a juicy steak, or even a bag of peanuts, causes the body to release the hormone cholecystokinin, which

It's proven: Excess weight raises the odds of developing chronic heartburn. In fact, studies show that severely overweight people have double the risk of GERD. So if heartburn is an issue, don't just avoid trigger foods —shed a few pounds!

makes the LES go slack, allowing stomach acid to slosh upward and burn the esophagus.

Swap fatty meats for fish, which actually counters inflammation, or choose the leanest cuts, such as London broil steaks, extra-lean ground beef, and skinless chicken breasts. For flavor without added fat, grill meats instead of frying or sautéing.

Dairy products, including full-fat milk, are notorious heartburn triggers. (Ironically, until the early 1970s, many doctors instructed patients to drink milk as a way to *prevent* heartburn.) They appear to increase production of stomach acids, and they prolong the length of time that acid clings to the lining of the esophagus. Opt for fat-free milk and low-fat cheese and yogurt (buy a brand that's not overly sweetened and add your own fruit to increase the fiber). Feta and goat cheese are typically less fatty than hard cheese.

Alcohol, caffeine, and chocolate. Not surprisingly, alcohol, a relaxant, loosens the LES. Caffeine appears to have a similar effect; although a few studies have exonerated coffee and tea, some heartburn sufferers say that just a few sips of hot brew—even decaf—can set off an attack. (If you still want your coffee, drink it after a meal, never on an empty stomach.) Chocolate contains fat and caffeine, so your beloved bonbons may also be causing your digestive misery.

Salty foods. A 2005 study found that people who reported eating salty foods more than three times a week increased their risk of GERD by 50 percent. In the same study, people who said they always sprinkle extra salt on their food were 70 percent more likely to have reflux after meals than people who never added salt. It's not clear if salt is linked to heartburn, or if salt lovers may simply have other diet habits that make them vulnerable. However, there's no harm—and plenty of benefits—in eschewing the saltshaker.

Peppermint. Even freshening your breath after dinner could be perilous; the menthol in peppermint causes the LES to relax.

To Beat Heartburn, Learn to Walk and Chew Gum

Your body produces its own natural antacid: It's called saliva. The stuff that keeps your mouth moist is full of bicarbonate, a chemical that neutralizes acid. (That's why bicarbonate is an ingredient in many heartburn-relief products.) Keeping your esophagus well lubed with saliva may be enough to stifle acid indigestion. Chewing sugarless gum is one way to do it, although the sugar alcohols these gums contain make some people bloated. Other options include sucking on sugar-free lozenges or hard candy. Several studies have shown that chewing gum after a meal prevents or reduces heartburn symptoms; in one, subjects with frequent reflux who took a 1-hour stroll while working their jaws gained modest additional relief.

Need another reason to give up cigarettes? Smoking dries up saliva.

HEART DISEASE/ HIGH CHOLESTEROL

Would you believe that eating just half a serving of fish a week can help keep you from dying of a heart attack? The catch (and we don't mean the fish): You have to actually *do it* to get the benefits!

It's pretty easy to ignore your risk of heart disease. You can't feel many of the problems that contribute to it, and if nothing hurts, the temptation to assume (or pretend) everything's fine can be overwhelming. It often takes the sudden death of a friend or relative from a heart attack to instill the fear that moves you to act. But remember, heart disease takes many years to develop, and you can't reverse it overnight. So why not start now?

If diet is one of the biggest contributors to heart disease, *changing your diet* is one of the best ways to prevent it. The big changes are fairly obvious, like laying off the bacon cheeseburgers and eating more fish, fruits, vegetables, and whole grains. But you don't have to make them all at once. Tackle a few you think you can handle, then tackle a few more. *Eating just one fruit or vegetable at every meal can significantly lower your risk of a heart attack.*

Even if you already have heart disease, the right diet can help you reverse it—something no cholesterol-lowering pill will do—by improving your cholesterol readings and taming high blood pressure, steadying blood sugar, dousing inflammation, and even taking off extra pounds. Many studies have proved it. For instance, the Lyon Diet Heart Study showed that when people with heart disease follow a Mediterranean-style diet that eschews red meats and processed foods in favor of produce; whole grains; and good fats from fish, olive oil, or nuts, they are 50 to 75 percent less likely to have repeat heart attacks compared to patients who stick with standard Western fare.

Fish anyone?

food for thought . . .

"Almost 80 percent of cardiovascular disease could be prevented by lifestyle changes, and among the most important of these are dietary changes."

— Guy Reed, MS, MD, chief of cardiovascular medicine at the Medical College of Georgia in Augusta ▪

Fatty fish

Salmon may be the first food that comes to mind when you envision a heart-healthy diet, and for good reason. Salmon and other fatty fish, such as mackerel, sardines, and tuna, contain now-famous omega-3 fatty acids, particularly compounds known as eicosapentaenoic acid (EPA) and docosahexaenoic acid (DHA).

Consider these nature's heart medicines. According to a recent study, consuming small quantities of fish—just half a serving a week—lowers the risk of dying from cardiovascular disease by 17 percent and the risk of a nonfatal heart attack by 27 percent. Each additional weekly serving reduces the risk of dying from cardiovascular disease by another 4 percent.

Eating food with fins benefits your heart and its "plumbing" in a number of ways. Having fish for dinner once a week probably means one less meat-based meal, and that in itself helps—for instance, by keeping your cholesterol under control. But the fats in fish are themselves beneficial. They help stabilize heart rhythms to prevent arrhythmias (irregular heartbeats that can lead to heart failure, blood clots, and stroke); lower cholesterol and triglycerides; and reduce inflammation in the arteries, which was recently discovered to play a major role in heart disease. Fish eaters have levels of C-reactive protein (CRP), a marker of inflammation, that are up to 33 percent lower than those of people who don't eat fish. Because high levels of CRP have been found in heart attack patients whose cholesterol levels were normal, some heart specialists believe it may be even better than cholesterol for predicting who will develop heart disease.

Aim for: At least two servings of fatty fish (8 to 12 ounces/227 to 340 g total) a week. Since mercury contamination is a concern, opt for fish lower in mercury, such as salmon or canned light tuna, and steer clear of fish known to be higher in mercury such as shark, swordfish, king mackerel, and tilefish (see "Choosing Safe Seafood" on page 23).

A rainbow of fruits and vegetables

Most of us have nothing against fruits and veggies per se; we just don't make the effort to eat enough of them. But this statistic may send you straight to the salad bar: Research from a major survey that analyzed the connection between disease risk and fruit and vegetable consumption in more than 9,000 healthy adults showed that eating a fruit or vegetable at every meal cut the risk of dying from cardiovascular disease by 27 percent.

Need more reason to serve yourself a helping of spinach or have an apple snack? According to research from the Nurses Health Study and the Health Professionals Follow-Up Study, which looked at the eating habits of well over 100,000 men and women, people who ate eight or more servings of fruit and vegetables each day had a 30 percent lower risk of developing cardiovascular disease than people who ate fewer than two servings a day.

Fruits and vegetables are among the best sources of fiber, which lowers cholesterol and helps reduce the low-grade inflammation in our bodies that contributes to heart disease. Opt for brightly colored fruits and vegetables; they contain the most antioxidants, which counteract the damage free radicals do to arteries and help prevent the breakdown of LDL ("bad") cholesterol that leads to plaque buildup. You can't rely on supplements for your antioxidants, since they don't seem to have the same effects as food.

Aim for: At the very least, get 4 to 6 cups of raw or cooked fruits and vegetables each day.

Helpful hint: Start one meal a day with a salad or add a side of steamed spinach. If you're already eating about five servings of green vegetables a day, adding a sixth lowers heart disease risk by another 23 percent.

Oatmeal, oat bran, legumes, beans, and peas

The secret ingredient in these foods is soluble fiber, the kind that reduces cholesterol by soaking it up so it's flushed out of the body as waste. Studies show that eating 5 to 10 grams of soluble fiber a day can reduce the bad LDL cholesterol in the blood by at least 5 percent, which in many cases may be enough to get you into the target range.

Aim for: 25 to 35 grams of fiber each day. Of that, at least 10 grams should be soluble fiber.

Helpful hint: Registered dietitians call beans "soluble fiber superstars." One cup of cooked beans (black, red, white, or pinto) contains 8 to 10 grams of soluble fiber. And oats are higher in soluble fiber than other grains. Count on 2 to 3 grams in 1 cup of cooked oatmeal.

Virgin olive oil

Low-fat diets have been shown to prevent and even reverse heart disease. The problem is, they can be hard to stick with. So how can you enjoy some fat in your diet and protect your heart, too? By swapping saturated fats (like butter) for olive oil, particularly virgin olive oil.

Olives and olive oil are mainstays of the famously heart-healthy Mediterranean diet. They contain monounsaturated fat, which is healthier for the heart than saturated fat. But olives—which are fruits, after all—and their oil also contain antioxidants called polyphenols, which, research suggests, help reduce inflammation in the blood vessels and help improve cholesterol and triglyceride levels.

It's important to opt for virgin olive oil; because it's minimally processed, it retains many of the polyphenols that are stripped from more heavily processed olive oils.

Aim for: Limit yourself to no more than 1 to 2 tablespoons of oil or 5 to 10 medium olives daily. And remember, olives and olive oil are meant to replace other fats in your diet, not be added to them.

Walnuts, almonds, and peanuts

Eating nuts in place of other fatty foods can potentially lower your risk of heart disease by up to 39 percent, according to research done at Pennsylvania State University. Although nuts contain a lot of fat, it's the monounsaturated and polyunsaturated varieties, which lower cholesterol and protect against heart disease. Nuts also seem to lower CRP and fibrinogen, both of which are markers for inflammation. Plus, they're good sources of fiber and protein as well as vitamin E, the B vitamins, magnesium, and potassium, all of which are essential for good heart health.

Aim for: 1 ounce (28 g) of nuts at least five times a week.

Helpful hint: Almonds and walnuts lower cholesterol, but don't leave peanuts out of the mix. As sources of antioxidants go, peanuts are on a par with blackberries and strawberries. They contain good amounts of vitamin E as well as vast stores of antioxidant polyphenols. Roasted peanuts contain even more of them.

Tofu, edamame, and soy milk

Soy foods aren't the cure-alls we once thought; they lower cholesterol only a little bit, according to reviews of recent studies. But there are still plenty of good reasons to rotate them into your diet, especially in place of meats and full-fat cheeses. The fact is, like other beans, soy is an excellent source of protein with none of the saturated fat of meat. It also contains hormone-like compounds called isoflavones that seem to help fight certain cancers.

Tasteless chunks of tofu are not your only option—although tofu really is good in stir-fries because it takes on the flavor of the sauce. You can add it to beef stir-fries to cut down on the amount of meat you use or add it to lasagna in place of some of the cheese (you won't notice it's there). But one of the simplest and tastiest ways to enjoy soy is by stocking the freezer with soybeans (also called edamame), either in or out of their shells. They make a fun, satisfying snack when you squeeze them out of their pods (thaw them first), or you can sprinkle shelled soybeans on salads or into soups.

Aim for: There's no official recommendation, but you can do your heart good by occasionally eating soy foods instead of meats and dairy products. When you eat tofu, choose the low-fat variety.

Special margarines *and other foods enriched with plant sterols or stanols*

Sterols and stanols are natural compounds found in vegetables, nuts, and seeds and often added to margarines and other foods because they lower cholesterol by reducing how much you absorb from food. Swapping regular salad dressing, milk, cheese, yogurt, margarine, and orange juice for the same foods fortified with plant sterols or stanols can lower LDL cholesterol within just a few weeks.

Finnish researchers split a group of 164 adults with mild to moderately high cholesterol into two groups. Half ate a range of low-fat dairy foods with these compounds added, while the other half functioned as the control group. After six weeks, the people eating the enriched dairy foods lowered their total cholesterol by 6.5 percent and their LDL cholesterol by more than 10 percent.

Aim for: If you need to lower your cholesterol, aim for approximately 2 grams of plant sterols/stanols daily. In general, eating plant sterol/stanol-enriched foods in place of foods like butter or high-fat salad dressing that actively raise cholesterol is a good idea.

Helpful hint: Pay attention to the serving sizes listed on the labels, because the enriched margarines and salad dressings are often still high in calories. These sterols/stanols are best absorbed with a little fat, so if you opt for orange juice, drink it with a meal.

Wine, beer, and spirits

Red wine gets all the attention in terms of heart health, but the fact is, other types of alcohol also protect against heart disease when consumed in moderation. In general, moderate intake of alcohol increases HDL ("good") cholesterol, lowers LDL ("bad") cholesterol, and in some cases, reduces fibrinogen and CRP, the

The More Heart-Healthy Foods, the Better

All of the foods in this entry help protect against heart disease, but some provide even more protection when they're eaten together. For instance, the combination of soy protein, almonds, oats, barley, and plant sterols—dubbed the Portfolio Diet by researchers at St. Michael's Hospital in Toronto—reduced LDL cholesterol in people with high cholesterol by an amazing 28 percent when eaten regularly as part of a diet low in saturated fat. By comparison, the people who followed a regular diet low in saturated fat and took a statin drug saw their cholesterol drop only slightly more (31 percent).

Another diet, dubbed the Polymeal Diet, focuses on wine, fish, dark chocolate, fruits, vegetables, almonds, and garlic, all known to lower the risk of heart disease, mainly by reducing cholesterol levels and lowering blood pressure. Data from the Framingham Heart Study and Framingham Offspring Study suggests that when these foods are eaten every day (except for fish, which is recommended just two to four times a week), they collectively lower the risk of cardiovascular disease by 76 percent.

inflammation markers. A recent study done at the University of Florida found that older adults who have one alcoholic beverage a day were 30 percent less likely to develop heart disease. Another study of cardiac patients hospitalized after heart attacks found that study participants who averaged two drinks a day were 32 percent less likely to experience fatal heart attacks.

Red wine does offer some added benefits from plant compounds found in grape skins, such as flavonoids, which help prevent blood clots, and resveratrol, which helps lower cholesterol.

Aim for: One to two drinks a day (the higher number is for men) is the amount considered generally safe and beneficial to the heart.

Helpful hint: Not sure what constitutes a drink? It's 4 ounces (118 ml) of wine, 12 ounces (355 ml) of beer, or 1.5 ounces (44 ml) of hard liquor.

Tea

You may think of fruits and vegetables when you think of antioxidants, but tea is an even better source of these disease fighters. Green tea is associated with reduced cholesterol levels and lower rates of artery blockages. But both black and green teas contain significant amounts of flavonoids, antioxidants that appear to protect against heart disease by slowing the breakdown of LDL cholesterol, preventing blood clots, and improving blood vessel function.

People who drink a cup or two of tea a day have a 46 percent lower risk of developing narrowed arteries. Upping that to 3 cups a day lowers the risk of having a heart attack by 43 percent and of dying from a heart attack by 70 percent. It can even help prevent a second heart attack. In a study of 1,900 patients recovering from heart attacks at Beth Israel Deaconess Medical Center in Boston, the death rate among patients who drank at least 2 cups of tea a day was 44 percent lower than among non-tea drinkers.

Aim for: 2 to 5 cups of green or black tea daily.

Helpful hint: Choose decaffeinated tea if you're looking for a beverage low in caffeine.

Cranberry juice

Women have long relied on cranberry juice for fending off urinary tract infections. Now research suggests that the juice, one of the richest sources of antioxidants, can also raise levels of HDL cholesterol. In a three-month study of 19 volunteers with high cholesterol, three servings of cranberry juice a day boosted their HDL cholesterol levels by 10 percent, which in turn lowered their risk of heart disease by 40 percent.

Aim for: Three 4- to 6-ounce (113 to 177 ml) servings a day.

Helpful hint: Opt for low-sugar cranberry juice to avoid drinking excess calories.

Apples

An apple or two a day really may keep the cardiologist away! Apples contain bushels of antioxidants that, like statin drugs, stimulate the liver to remove harmful LDL cholesterol from the blood. In addition, the antioxidants in apples and apple juice delay the breakdown of LDL cholesterol by about 20 percent. The longer it takes for LDL to break down, the less plaque there is in the arteries.

Aim for: Two apples or 12 ounces (340 g) of 100 percent apple juice a day.

Helpful hint: Go for red-skinned apples. Compared to other types, they contain the most antioxidants. And be sure to eat the skin, which contains five times more antioxidants than the flesh. Buy organic apples if you're concerned about pesticide residues in the skin.

Red grapefruit

It's great with breakfast, and it can lower your cholesterol and triglyceride levels, too. In an Israeli study of 57 men and women who had had bypass surgery and whose cholesterol levels weren't responding to statin medications, those who ate a red grapefruit a day for 30 days along with their regular meals lowered their total cholesterol by more than 15 percent, their LDL cholesterol by more than 20 percent, and their triglycerides by more than 17 percent. Because grapefruit can interact with certain medications, check with your doctor first if you're taking one or more prescription drugs.

Aim for: 1 cup of fresh grapefruit or 1/2 cup of 100 percent grapefruit juice a day.

Garlic

Fresh cloves contain an antioxidant compound that gives garlic its characteristic aroma, which may explain why garlic may be helpful for reducing blood clots and artery plaque and modestly lowering cholesterol. When eaten daily along with other heart-healthy foods (see "The More Heart-Healthy Foods, the Better" on page 179), garlic can help lower heart disease risk by 76 percent.

Garlic's blood-thinning properties are helpful, but if you're already taking a blood-thinning drug such as warfarin (Coumadin), or you have a blood or platelet disorder or are going into the hospital for surgery or to have a baby, talk to your doctor before consuming large amounts of garlic.

Aim for: Some experts suggest eating as many as two to four cloves a day.

Helpful hint: Although cooking can deactivate garlic's therapeutic compounds, chopping or crushing the cloves and letting the garlic stand for 10 to 15 minutes before cooking will help preserve them.

Tomato sauce

Could eating spaghetti be good for your heart? It's possible, provided you pour on the tomato sauce. Tomatoes contain lycopene, one of the more potent antioxidants in the carotenoid family that appears to protect against heart disease by preventing the oxidation of LDL cholesterol. When researchers at the University of North Carolina at Chapel Hill looked at fat samples from nearly 1,400 men who'd had heart attacks and compared them with samples from healthy men, they found that the men who had more lycopene in their fat had about half the risk of heart attack compared to those with less lycopene.

Aim for: 1/2 cup twice a week.

Helpful hint: Cooking releases lycopene from tomatoes, which is why you'll get more of this nutrient from tomato sauce than from raw tomatoes.

Get a handsome, large mason jar—one that your hand can fit into—and fill it with a mix of roasted nuts, dark chocolate chips, and raisins. A fistful (but not more!) is not only a scrumptious afternoon snack or dessert but also a powerhouse of heart-healthy ingredients.

Dark chocolate

Yes, you can have your wine—and chocolate—on a heart-healthy diet. Dark chocolate is full of the same antioxidants found in red wine and green tea. In fact, it contains more flavonols (a subclass of flavonoids, in case you're paying attention to the technical stuff) than tea or red wine and has about four times the catechins in tea. These compounds prevent blood clots, slow the oxidation of LDL cholesterol (making it less likely to stick to artery walls), improve blood vessel function, and reduce inflammation. Another plus for chocolate: It gives good cholesterol a slight boost.

Of course, chocolate's high in fat, but a third of that fat is stearic acid, a particular type of saturated fat that doesn't raise cholesterol, while another third is a type of monounsaturated fat that lowers cholesterol.

Aim for: Some research suggests that 1.5 ounces (42 g) a day may reduce the risk of heart disease by 10 percent. Look for dark chocolate that contains at least 60 percent cocoa.

Helpful hint: Choose dark chocolate over milk chocolate. Dark chocolate, which has a higher cocoa content, contains more flavonoids, and although milk chocolate contains some, the milk actually prevents their absorption. Dark chocolate also tends to contain less sugar.

FEATURED RECIPES

NUTRITIONAL SUPPLEMENTS

Omega-3 fatty acids. Along with eating fish twice a week, if you have heart disease, the American Heart Association recommends taking fish-oil supplements with EPA and DHA (the two main components of omega-3 fatty acids). These have been shown to reduce LDL cholesterol and triglycerides while also increasing HDL cholesterol. They also combat inflammation. **DOSAGE:** 1 gram daily if you have cardiovascular disease; 2 to 4 grams daily (under a doctor's supervision) if your triglycerides are elevated. Taking the supplements with food can help reduce the burping often associated with fish oils, as can choosing a fish-oil supplement that contains citrus essence.

Coenzyme Q10. This naturally occurring chemical boosts energy in all of the body's cells, including those in the heart muscle, which is why it's thought to protect against heart failure. Because statin medications deplete CoQ10, people taking statins should talk to their doctors about also taking CoQ10 supplements. **DOSAGE:** It will depend on which statin you're taking and at what dosage.

Plant sterols/stanols. The same LDL cholesterol–lowering plant sterols/stanols used to fortify some "heart-healthy" margarines can also be taken as supplements to lower cholesterol. There's no need to take them if your cholesterol is in the normal range. **DOSAGE:** 1 to 3 grams daily from food and/or supplements.

Garlic. Along with using fresh garlic in food, taking garlic supplements may also improve cholesterol. One study done at Pennsylvania State University showed that when men with high cholesterol took garlic supplements, they lowered their total cholesterol by 7 percent and their LDL cholesterol by 10 percent compared to volunteers taking placebos. **DOSAGE:** 600 to 900 milligrams a day is considered safe.

CAUTION

Fatty meats and full-fat dairy. Although recent studies have shown that lean cuts of beef (4 to 5 ounces/113 to 142 g day) can lower total and LDL cholesterol levels, saturating your diet with higher-fat meats (prime rib, for example) can be a true heart breaker.

According to a Cleveland Clinic study, eating even one meal that's high in saturated fat interferes with artery elasticity and encourages plaque deposits. And recent research from 73,147 women involved in the Nurses Health Study and 42,635 men who were in the Health Professionals Follow-Up Study found that a high intake of the most commonly consumed saturated fatty acids—lauric, myristic, palmitic, and stearic acid—was associated with an 18 percent increased relative risk of coronary heart disease. Replacing just 1 percent of your daily intake of these fatty acids with polyunsaturated fats, whole-grain carbohydrates, or plant proteins could reduce your risk for coronary heart disease by an estimated 6 to 8 percent.

Sugar and refined, processed carbohydrates. Sugary foods and drinks have something in common with starchy foods like potatoes and refined carbohydrates like white bread and white rice. All of them are quickly broken down into sugars in the body, raising blood sugar and insulin levels. Over time, this can lead to weight gain and insulin resistance, both contributors to heart disease.

Cutting Calories Cuts Heart Disease Risk

Can cutting calories turn back the cardiological clock? It appears so. When researchers at Washington University School of Medicine looked at 25 people who cut 600 to 1,000 calories from their daily diets (most Americans eat between 2,000 and 3,000 calories a day) for six years, their hearts looked 15 years younger than their chronological age. The people in the study were also leaner and had lower levels of inflammatory markers, cholesterol, triglycerides, and blood pressure. The study participants cut their calories by eating nutrient-dense foods and limiting empty calories from refined and processed foods and sodas.

HEMORRHOIDS

Hemorrhoids are a real pain in the ... well, you know where. Essentially varicose veins in an extremely inconvenient spot, hemorrhoids—some of which bleed and some of which don't—typically occur with chronic constipation, the result of repeated straining to go to the bathroom. (Diarrhea can aggravate hemorrhoids.) Hemorrhoids are more common with age as the muscles that help propel blood through the veins tend to weaken—especially if we become overweight and sedentary. They're also common in pregnant women because of the extra pressure the baby puts on abdominal veins and because pregnancy hormones relax blood vessels, both of which cause veins to swell.

Many of us who aren't pregnant can probably blame the problem on the typical Western diet—and the typical Western lack of exercise. What's the solution? Eat plenty of fruits, vegetables, and whole grains—foods that promote regularity—along with foods that strengthen blood vessels. Why not cook dinner tonight? You can sneak in plenty of these foods and get out of your chair for a while (sitting for long periods also contributes to hemorrhoids).

YOUR FOOD PRESCRIPTION

Water

If you don't drink enough water, fiber becomes a plug instead of a broom. The other thing you can do with water is sit in it, preferably with some Epsom salts added, since salt literally pulls fluid from the blood trapped in a varicose vein or hemorrhoid to reduce swelling and inflammation.

Aim for: Between 8 and 11 eight-ounce glasses, or 2 to 3 liters, a day.

FEATURED RECIPES

Broccoli Salad p. 291
Spinach Salad with Chickpeas p. 293
Lentil-Tomato Soup p. 299
Chicken-Barley Bake p. 312
Raspberry-Almond Muffins p. 324
Frozen Fruit Mousse p. 334
Mixed Berry Tart p. 335

Foods that help prevent constipation

Because hemorrhoids are mainly associated with constipation, you'll want to follow all the advice in the Constipation entry (see page 138), such as eating more fruit (particularly prunes), vegetables, and whole grains. Fiber is nature's laxative. It helps hold water in waste to bulk it up, and then it works like a broom to move it through the colon. The better the broom sweeps, the less pushing you need to do.

Fiber is helpful even when hemorrhoids require medical treatment. Danish researchers studied 92 people whose hemorrhoids were treated with a procedure called rubber band ligation (in which rubber bands are used to cut off circulation to the hemorrhoid) every 2 weeks for up to 10 weeks. Some of the patients were instructed to eat bran twice a day, while others received standard care. Not only did the bran eaters need fewer treatments to heal their hemorrhoids, but only 15 percent of them experienced recurrences compared to 45 percent of their no-bran counterparts.

Aim for: At least 25 grams of fiber a day, though 35 is preferable.

Berries

The darker the berry, the sweeter the fruit—and the more flavonoids it contains. Flavonoids, found in many berries but also in citrus fruits and onions, help to reduce inflammation and strengthen blood vessel walls. Some research suggests they may also reduce the pain, bleeding, itching, and even the recurrence of hemorrhoids. In fact, finely ground, highly purified flavonoids called diosmin and hesperidin are the active ingredients in the French prescription hemorrhoid drug Dalfon.

Berries do double duty by helping to prevent constipation, since they're also good sources of fiber.

Aim for: Include 3/4 cup of your favorite berries, like blackberries, red raspberries, blueberries, strawberries, and even cherries, among your daily fruits and vegetables.

Kale, spinach,
and other foods high in vitamin K

Vitamin K is key for helping blood clot, and eating more of these foods may benefit people who have hemorrhoids that bleed.

Aim for: The recommended amount of vitamin K is 65 micrograms for women and 80 micrograms for men, an amount that's easily gotten in a serving of bitter greens like kale, spinach, and turnip greens, as well as broccoli and even green tea.

Tea Time?

We don't mean it's time to drink it. Tea's astringent tannins reduce inflammation, so try soaking a compress in cold black tea and applying it to the problem area. Or apply a paste made from ground elderberry and water.

NUTRITIONAL SUPPLEMENTS

Vitamin C. Vitamin C can be helpful for bleeding hemorrhoids associated with constipation. It promotes healing by reducing inflammation, helping build connective tissue around the hemorrhoids, and improving the overall tone of veins. **DOSAGE:** Start with 1,000 milligrams and gradually increase the dose until stools loosen, then scale back (or you may end up with diarrhea).

Magnesium. Magnesium's a good laxative because it helps keep water in the stools, making them softer. See Constipation on page 139 for more details. **DOSAGE:** 300 to 600 milligrams daily.

Psyllium. Getting 25 to 35 grams of fiber each day is ideal for preventing constipation and thus hemorrhoids. But if you don't seem to be able to consume the seven servings of fruits and vegetables and three servings of whole grains that will get you there, then fiber supplements like psyllium can help close the gap. For more information, see Constipation on page 139. **DOSAGE:** 1 to 3 tablespoons daily dissolved in water.

Do you have an all-day water glass? You should! At the start of each day, get out a large, clean glass, fill it up with water, and sip from it throughout the day, refilling it every time it gets empty. No excuses if you are on the go—just use a portable water bottle instead.

HERPES

Like a sleeping giant, the herpes virus can awaken at any time. Once it's in your system, it remains there, hibernating in nerve cells until something—stress, fatigue, sun exposure, or another trigger—rouses it. Scientists have discovered that certain foods are among those triggers, nourishing the beast, while a few other foods starve it, helping to keep it dormant—the ultimate goal.

You also want to eat foods that help keep your immune system strong. That's because when you get sick, you're especially vulnerable to a herpes outbreak (either a cold sore or genital herpes), adding insult to injury. Foods that help boost the immune system also help shore up your defenses against herpes.

YOUR FOOD PRESCRIPTION

Dairy foods, meat, fish,
and other foods high in lysine

Scientists have discovered an interesting phenomenon. Foods that contain an amino acid (a building block of protein) called arginine seem to feed the herpes virus (we'll tell you about these foods in the Off the Menu section on the next page). But adding foods that contain another amino acid, lysine, to your diet can help by blocking the action of arginine. Keeping a high ratio of lysine to arginine in your system may help keep herpes under control.

Aim for: Up to 3,000 milligrams of lysine, spaced throughout the day. See the table below for the lysine counts of specific foods.

FOODS RICH IN LYSINE

FOOD	LYSINE (MG)
Chicken (3 ounces/85 g)	1,800
Steak (4 ounces/118 g)	1,640
Flounder (3 ounces/85 g)	1,500
Shrimp (3 ounces/85 g)	1,500
Cottage cheese (4 ounces/118 g)	1,200
Plain yogurt (1 cup)	706
Fat-free milk (1 cup)	663
Muenster cheese (1 ounce/28 g)	606

Garlic

Because it's full of antioxidants, especially immunity-boosting selenium, and has antiviral power, garlic is something you'll want to eat liberally to boost your defenses against ailments like the common cold that wear you down and make you more vulnerable to a herpes outbreak.

Aim for: Use garlic liberally raw and in cooking. Cut a clove into pieces and swallow them like pills throughout the day. Stomach acids will break down the garlic and release its antioxidant power as it travels through the intestines.

Helpful hint: When using garlic in recipes, chop it and let it stand for 10 to 15 minutes before cooking. The waiting period allows the garlic's active compounds to develop.

Plain yogurt with active cultures

This type of yogurt is full of beneficial bacteria that help keep the body strong by keeping the population of "bad" bacteria in check. Plus, research has found that yogurt with active cultures boosts immune cell activity. While yogurt won't directly prevent herpes, it can help keep your body healthy, making it less vulnerable to outbreaks.

Aim for: 1 cup per day. Be sure to choose yogurt with live, active cultures (look on the label for *lactobacillus, bifidus, Streptococcus thermophilus,* and *acidophilus,* among other active cultures).

Licorice

Here's an old-fashioned remedy with some science behind it. Purchase real licorice from a health food store (not the five-and-dime variety found in candy stores). Cut it into very thin slices and place them directly on herpes sores for 10 minutes. The licorice will diminish the pain and help speed healing. An antiviral compound in licorice called glycyrrhizinic acid (GLA) is probably responsible. You can also find topical creams and ointments that contain GLA in natural foods stores.

Aim for: Apply fresh slices several times a day.

NUTRITIONAL SUPPLEMENTS

Lysine. In a study at the University of Missouri, volunteers with a history of herpes outbreaks who took 1 gram of lysine per day for six months developed significantly fewer lesions than in the six months they didn't take the supplements. **DOSAGE:** Studies have suggested that taking between 1 and 3 grams a day is safe and effective in keeping herpes at bay. Take 1 gram three times a day without food. *Caution:* If you have high cholesterol, check with your doctor before taking lysine supplements over the long term. Some animal studies suggest that a high lysine-to-arginine ratio can raise cholesterol levels. Lysine also comes in creams you can apply directly to a cold sore. Look for them in natural foods stores.

A multivitamin/mineral. You are most vulnerable to herpes outbreaks when your immune system is stressed, which can happen to anyone who is under stress, exhausted, or undernourished. Anyone under stress may be taxing their stores of vitamin C and the B vitamins. Also, as people age, they often have difficulty absorbing certain nutrients, such as zinc and vitamin E—nutrients that keep the immune system

Prevent Shingles at the Farmers' Market

Herpes zoster, the virus that causes chicken pox, can cause shingles later in life. This painful rash of blisters can leave you feverish and put you out of commission for weeks. If you're vulnerable to shingles, make a weekly stop at the farmers' market. A study in London showed that people who ate more than three servings of fruit a day had three times less risk of getting shingles than those who ate less than one piece per week. The researchers suspect fruit's vitamins and other nutrients help fend off shingles by keeping the immune system strong.

robust—from food. A multivitamin/mineral can help close the gap. **DOSAGE:** One per day. Alternatively, choose a multi that's designed to be taken two or three times a day, which means it will deliver a continuous supply of nutrients as the body needs them. Take it with food for best absorption.

OFF THE MENU

Chocolate, nuts, seeds, and gelatin. These are rich in arginine, the amino acid that competes with more beneficial lysine in the herpes battle. Legumes (including soybeans) and whole grains are also rich in arginine, but we'd be remiss in suggesting you avoid these healthy foods. Instead, consider limiting them when you have a herpes outbreak.

FEATURED RECIPES

Mac 'n Cheese Primavera *p. 304*
Thai Roasted Shrimp *p. 310*
Baked Chicken with Tomatoes *p. 311*
Chicken in Garlic Sauce *p. 312*
Barbecued Flank Steak *p. 314*

HIGH BLOOD PRESSURE

High blood pressure usually creeps up with no warnings and no symptoms. If you don't go to the doctor very often and never check your own blood pressure, you could go for years without knowing you have it. But just because you don't feel "ill," that doesn't mean high blood pressure (a.k.a. hypertension) isn't doing harm. Doctors call it the silent killer for good reason: It's the biggest risk factor for stroke and a major contributor to heart attacks and kidney failure, as well as erectile dysfunction and even blindness.

Age, stress, and the foods we eat all conspire to raise our pressure. Fortunately, one of the easiest ways to control it is by making very simple changes to your diet—namely by eating more fruits and vegetables instead of fast food, junk food, and processed foods. That helps to naturally increase your intake of key nutrients like magnesium, potassium, and calcium, all of which lower blood pressure, and to reduce sodium consumption, which raises it. Keep your pressure in the normal range, and you lower your risk of stroke by up to 40 percent and of heart attack by up to 25 percent.

YOUR FOOD PRESCRIPTION

Bananas, potatoes, raisins,
and other foods rich in potassium

Of course, you've heard that eating less salt can help reduce high blood pressure (and in case you haven't, see Caution on page 190). But what's equally important is increasing the amount of potassium you consume. When researchers looked at the biggest factors contributing to high blood pressure among people in five countries, they found that low potassium consumption accounted for 4 to 17 percent of hypertension risk. Other epidemiological studies have found that in communities where potassium consumption is generally higher, blood pressure levels are generally lower.

If you can manage to increase your potassium while also decreasing your sodium—which will happen quite naturally when you eat more fruits and vegetables and fewer processed foods—you're doing even better. In one study, people who ate a diet that was low in sodium and high in potassium reduced stress-related spikes in blood pressure by 10 mmHg.

Aim for: 4,700 milligrams of potassium a day. You can get that much by eating the recommended 4 to 6 cups of fruit and vegetables, particularly if you focus on those listed on page 188 as high in potassium.

Helpful hint: Baked potatoes are especially rich in potassium, with more than 1,000 milligrams each. Skip the butter or sour cream and use a margarine-like spread fortified with plant sterols and/or stanols. You'll lower your blood pressure and your cholesterol.

Fruits and vegetables

It's likely that you can lower your blood pressure if you do nothing else but swap some of the junk food you eat for more fruits and vegetables. That was the finding of the landmark study of nutrition and blood pressure known as Dietary Approaches to Stop Hypertension, or DASH (see "Doing the DASH" on page 191). When people in the study stuck to a typical Western diet and simply increased their fruit and vegetable intake, they were able to lower their systolic blood pressure (the top number) by 2.8 mmHg (millimeters of mercury) and their diastolic blood pressure by 1.1 mmHg. Lowering your blood pressure by even a few points can substantially reduce your risk of heart attack and stroke.

Aim for: 4 to 6 cups of fruit and vegetables daily. That includes fresh, cooked, frozen, dried, or juiced produce as well as beans and legumes.

Helpful hint: It's easier than you think to work extra fruits and vegetables into your meals. Try adding a banana or a half cup of strawberries to your morning cereal, starting dinner with a salad, and tossing a cup or two of vegetables

into soups or pasta sauce. Even 1/2 cup of fruit or vegetable juice counts as a serving.

Soy foods, beans, nuts, and seeds

Now's the time to grab a bag of edamame from your grocer's freezer and start using it. People who eat more vegetable-based protein like soy (as well as beans, legumes, nuts, and seeds) tend to have lower blood pressure compared to people who get most of their protein from animal sources like meat.

Soy contains plant estrogens that are thought to help lower blood pressure, but it's also possible the benefits come as much from what soy displaces from your diet—like meat that's high in fat and calories—as from the soy itself. Weight gain tends to raise blood pressure.

Aim for: About four servings of soy foods (about 25 grams) daily. A serving is a glass of soy milk, a cup of soy yogurt, one-fifth to one-quarter of a package of tofu, or about 2.5 ounces (71 g) of edamame (young soybeans still in their pods).

Low-fat and fat-free dairy foods

A glass of low-fat or fat-free milk is good for the ol' bones, but did you know it's good for your blood vessels, too? Experts don't completely understand why dairy foods lower blood pressure, but they suspect that their calcium, potassium, and magnesium—all of which relax arteries and improve blood flow—play a role. Recent research suggests that people who eat more low-fat dairy products like yogurt, cheese, and low-fat or fat-free milk have lower systolic pressure as well as a lower overall risk of hypertension. The DASH studies showed that diets rich in produce and fat-free dairy foods help lower blood pressure, and another study done in Spain found that people who ate more low-fat and fat-free dairy foods had half the risk of developing hypertension compared to those who didn't eat as much.

Aim for: Two to three servings daily. A serving is a cup of low-fat or fat-free yogurt or fat-free milk.

NUTRITIONAL SUPPLEMENTS

Magnesium and calcium. Magnesium is known to relax the arteries and improve blood pressure, but it's less clear whether supplements have the same effect as food sources like black beans, pumpkin seeds, spinach, and even halibut—all of which contain more than 100 milligrams a serving. But if you have high blood pressure and can't seem to get enough magnesium in your diet, you might consider a supplement. When Japanese researchers gave 60 people with high blood pressure magnesium supplements for eight weeks, their systolic blood pressure dropped by about 2.7 mmHg, while their diastolic reading dipped by 1.5 mmHg.

Calcium is also beneficial. If you find that you're not getting the recommended two or three servings of low-fat dairy foods each day, consider taking a calcium supplement. If you want to limit the number of pills you take, buy a calcium/magnesium combo. **DOSAGE:** 500 milligrams of magnesium and 1,000 milligrams of calcium daily from food and supplements combined.

Omega-3 fatty acids. Some research suggests that omega-3 fatty acids, particularly DHA, found in fatty fish like salmon, tuna, and mackerel, can modestly lower high blood pressure.

Researchers don't generally recommend taking fish-oil supplements just for blood pressure, mostly because other diet changes produce more substantial results. But if you're already taking fish oil for some other reason (to lower your triglycerides, for instance), you may find that your blood pressure also drops a bit. **DOSAGE:** At least 1,000 milligrams daily. The American Heart Association currently recommends 2 to 4 grams daily to help lower triglycerides. If you wish to take more, talk with your doctor.

CAUTION

Sodium. Reduce your sodium (a component of salt), and you can substantially lower your blood pressure. Both the American Heart Association and the National Heart, Lung, and Blood Institute recommend limiting salt to no more than 1 teaspoon (which contains about 2,300 milligrams of sodium) each day.

A tall order? You bet. But data from studies on the DASH Diet proves it's worth it. Reducing sodium intake to 2,300 milligrams a day can lower blood pressure by 2.1/1.1 mmHg. Cut back even more—to about 2/3 teaspoon daily—and you can drop your blood pressure by 6.7/3.5 mmHg.

Make raisins a secret ingredient in your cooking. They go well with sautéed vegetables—just add a handful near the end of cooking. Or toss into roasts of chicken, beef, or pork. They'll plump up and soften if cooked in liquid, adding both sweetness and visual surprise to your meals. And their high potassium levels can help reduce your blood pressure.

The good news is that the salt you sprinkle on after food is prepared isn't that much of a concern—provided, of course, that you're not dumping a whole shaker into every dish. It's processed foods that are the big problems; they account for about 75 percent of the sodium we consume. Many foods that you wouldn't even think of as "salty," like some cereals, contain more sodium than potato or corn chips! The best way to curb your sodium intake is to steer clear of these high-sodium processed foods. You can also follow this rule of thumb: When you check the calorie and sodium content per serving on product labels, the number of milligrams of sodium should be less than or at most equal to the number of calories.

Alcohol. Whether alcohol should be "off the menu" or not largely depends on how much you drink. Light to moderate drinking is considered heart healthy because it raises HDL ("good") cholesterol and makes blood less likely to form artery-blocking clots, so one drink daily for women and two drinks for men are generally considered safe. But heavy drinking will increase blood pressure—and raise your stroke risk by as much as 69 percent.

Coffee and other caffeinated drinks. Your morning cup of java could be giving you more of a jolt than you bargained for. Although the antioxidants in coffee may help lower the risk of heart disease and cancer, if your blood pressure is on the high side, the caffeine could make it worse. Some research done at Duke University Medical Center suggests that for some people, drinking 4 to 5 cups a day boosts stress hormones like adrenaline by about 32 percent, which in turn increases blood pressure. According to these studies, blood pressure can rise within an hour of having your morning cup of joe, and levels stay high all day. Even so, the research is far from definitive. Data from more than 155,000 women in the Nurses Health Study found no connection between coffee drinking and hypertension, though it did find a link with regular and diet sodas.

Doing the DASH

Following the DASH (Dietary Approaches to Stop Hypertension) Diet can lower your blood pressure by 5.5/3 mmHg. That alone is enough to reduce your heart disease risk by 15 percent and your stroke risk by 27 percent. Follow the DASH Diet and cut your salt intake to less than a teaspoon a day, and you could lower your blood pressure by 8.9/4.5 mmHg. That's the kind of reduction blood pressure medication can produce. Here's what it takes to do the DASH.

Grains: Six to eight servings a day, such as a slice of bread or 1/2 cup of rice, pasta, or cereal.

Fruits and vegetables: Four to five servings a day, such as 1/2 cup of chopped fruit or cooked vegetables, a cup of leafy vegetables, 1/4 cup of dried fruit, or 1/2 to 3/4 cup of fruit or vegetable juice.

Low-fat/fat-free dairy: Two to three servings a day, such as a cup of milk or yogurt.

Lean meat, poultry, or fish: 6 ounces (170 g) a day.

Nuts, seeds, and legumes: Four to five servings a week, such as 1/2 cup of beans, 1/3 cup of nuts, or 2 tablespoons of peanut butter.

Sweets and added sugars: Less than five servings a week, such as a tablespoon of sugar or jam or 1/2 cup of sorbet.

IMMUNE WEAKNESS

Are you one of those people who seem to catch whatever bug is going around? Do colds and other upper respiratory infections seem to drag on and on and bring you down lower than they should? It's true that our immune systems tend to weaken with age; that's why older people generally don't respond as well to vaccinations as younger people, and why the flu can be fatal in elderly folks. But no matter what your age, it's well within your power to boost your defenses.

The various elements of the immune system are often likened to troops in an army that protects your body. And as the Emperor Napoleon once said, "An army marches on its stomach." When we don't eat well enough (or we don't get enough sleep and exercise, or we feel stressed), that army gets sluggish. Perhaps not weak enough to sound any serious alarms, but just enough to allow bacteria, viruses, and parasites to slip through the defenses. Even minor deficiencies of key micronutrients like zinc, selenium, and iron can hamper your body's ability to fend off disease and infection.

Before the next cold and flu season comes along, consider giving your diet a "shot in the arm." That can be as simple as brightening your plate with colorful produce, enjoying a delicious shrimp dinner now and then, spicing up your meals with more garlic, and cutting back on the fatty and sugary foods that work against you.

YOUR FOOD PRESCRIPTION

Chicken, fish, beans, eggs, yogurt, *and other foods high in protein*

Protein is the building block for many of the immune system's key players, like antibodies and the white blood cells that search out and destroy germs and cancer cells. Many protein foods are also great sources of zinc, iron, and many B vitamins, all of which are essential for strong immune function.

The typical Western diet isn't lacking in protein, but elderly people and vegetarians in particular need to be sure they get enough. If you eat meat, pass on the greasy burgers and fried chicken and choose lean beef and skinless chicken; as you'll read later on, saturated fat and fried foods promote the kind of low-grade inflammation in the body that can be a slow drain on your immune resources.

Aim for: 3 to 4 ounces (85 to 113 g) of protein—the amount in a serving of meat or fish the size of a deck of cards or in a half cup of peas—twice a day; have more if you're larger or more active than average.

Helpful hint: Sardines can be triply protective. Not only are they lean proteins but they also contain anti-inflammatory omega-3 essential fatty acids along with good amounts of zinc and selenium, two other important immunity boosters.

Pumpkin seeds

Now you've got good reason to save those seeds when you're carving up pumpkins—a half cup contains about 6 milligrams of zinc, which is one of the most critical nutrients for overall immune function. Studies show that people who are zinc deficient (which is common with age) have a more difficult time fending off garden-variety infections.

Aim for: The current recommendation for zinc is 15 milligrams, though if you're prone to illness, you may want to aim for 30 milligrams daily. That's a lot of pumpkin seeds, so you may want to add some oysters or crab to your diet. Not a fan of shellfish? Dark-meat turkey is another good source, as is beef.

Helpful hint: You can quickly "roast" pumpkin seeds in your microwave. Put some olive oil in a microwave-safe baking dish and heat for 30 seconds. Then add the pumpkin seeds and cook on high for 7 to 8 minutes, turning every 2 minutes. Not into microwaving? You can also dry pumpkin seeds in the oven (15 minutes at 200°F/90°C).

Brazil nuts

These nuts are nature's number one source of the immunity-supporting antioxidant mineral selenium. When we're low on selenium, our white blood cells are slower to kill off microbes and tumor cells. In addition, because selenium protects cells from free radical damage, it's been suggested that a deficiency sets the stage for harmless viruses to mutate into more aggressive strains. And with a fatigued immune system, these more dangerous viruses can then mutate and reproduce out of control. Getting enough selenium rejuvenates immune cells so they're able to clobber the germs.

Aim for: Each Brazil nut contains 68 to 90 micrograms of selenium, so even one a day will do it because the recommended amount of selenium is relatively low—about 55 micrograms for men and women, though some experts believe 200 micrograms is more beneficial. If you tend to catch every cold going around, aim for the higher amount. You'll also find selenium in salmon, crab, and shrimp (between 34 and 40 micrograms in a 3-ounce (85 g) portion).

Yogurt with active cultures

About 70 percent of the immune system resides in your gut, so it stands to reason that a healthy gastrointestinal tract means a healthy immune system. The live cultures found in certain yogurts (be sure to check the label) work by populating your GI tract with friendly bacteria, like *Lactobacillus acidophilus,* to ward off the bad bugs. You can think of it as being like a neighborhood watch program in a small city. As in any city, good and bad elements coexist. But the more friendly bacteria you have, the less likely you are to be attacked by the nastier bugs.

Aim for: A cup a day.

Helpful hint: Opt for plain with no added sugar. Eating yogurt with sugar is counterproductive since sugar not only depresses immune function, it also attracts harmful microbes like yeast.

To get more beans in your diet, keep well-rinsed and ready-to-eat kidney or garbanzo beans in your refrigerator. Put them on the table at mealtime and add to salads and green vegetables, or just nibble on them throughout the meal.

Tea

It's believed that one reason the Japanese have lower rates of many diseases (including cancer) is that they drink so much green tea, a major storehouse of immunity-boosting compounds, including potent antioxidants like EGCG. Some research suggests that green tea is helpful for fending off the bugs that cause flu and diarrhea, whooping cough, pneumonia, and even cavities. Even black tea appears to have immunity-enhancing properties. A small study at Harvard Medical School that examined immune function in coffee drinkers compared to tea drinkers found that when blood taken from all the study participants was exposed to *E. coli* bacteria, the tea drinkers' immune cells responded about five times faster than the coffee drinkers'. Researchers believe it's the compound L-theanine in black tea that helps to rally immune function.

Aim for: 1 to 2 cups daily for general health. If you're sick, try to drink 3 to 4 cups.

FEATURED RECIPES

Ultimate Spiced Nuts *p. 288*
Sweet Potato Soup *p. 297*
Beef in Lettuce Wraps *p. 302*
Roasted Salmon with Sautéed Greens *p. 309*
Baked Chicken with Tomatoes *p. 311*
Beef and Broccoli Stew *p. 316*
Pumpkin Streusel Bread *p. 327*

Garlic

Garlic's a friend of the immune system, especially when eaten raw. For starters, it's an edible antibiotic, with strong antibacterial properties. It also fights viruses. And its sulfur compounds are surprisingly rich in antioxidants. Chop or crush your garlic, then let it stand for 10 to 15 minutes to fully release its healing potential.

Aim for: At least a clove a day.

A rainbow of fruits and vegetables

Brightly colored produce is a storehouse of antioxidants, substances our immune systems need in vast quantities when we're sick or under stress. Stress and sickness increase the body's production of the rogue, cell-attacking molecules known as free radicals. These molecules can damage the thymus gland, where many immune system cells are incubated. As the thymus goes, so goes the immune system. When the thymus is damaged, we become more susceptible to infections, which in turn produce more free radicals. Antioxidants help break this cycle.

Eating more fruit and vegetables is an easy way to naturally keep your body well supplied with antioxidants. But don't just go for the same old apples and oranges. Because antioxidants work best when they work together, the greater the variety of brightly colored fruits and vegetables you eat, the more types of antioxidants you consume—like the flavonoids found in red grapes and citrus fruits and the carotenoids that give carrots and sweet potatoes their bright orange color—and in turn the more effectively your immune system will function.

Aim for: 4 to 6 cups of fruits and vegetables a day.

Helpful hint: Think small, as in tiny berries. Blueberries top the USDA's list of antioxidant-packed fruits. Blackberries, strawberries, and raspberries also rate high.

NUTRITIONAL SUPPLEMENTS

Probiotics. In addition to eating yogurt with live cultures, you may want to take some probiotics—active cultures in supplement form—that enhance immune function by improving digestion and nutrient absorption and preventing an overgrowth of harmful bacteria and yeast in your gut. Because quality counts, look for refrigerated formulas that contain *Lactobacillus acidophilus* and *bifidobacterium*. And check the expiration date on the bottle. For the supplement to be effective, the organisms need to be alive when you take them. **DOSAGE:** 1 to 6 billion organisms daily. If you've recently taken antibiotics, you'll want more because antibiotics wipe out a good portion of your friendly bacteria. To repopulate your GI tract, take 30 billion organisms a day for two weeks, then scale back to 10 billion a day for six months. If you experience any gastric upset, scale back further.

Garlic. If garlic just burns your belly, supplements may be a good option, particularly around cold and flu season. A British study of 146 people found that volunteers who took garlic supplements for 12 weeks during cold season had fewer than half the number of colds compared to people in the placebo group. And when they got sick, they recovered four days faster. *Note:* If you take a blood thinner like warfarin (Coumadin), check with your doctor first because garlic can increase the drug's anti-clotting effects. **DOSAGE:** 300 milligrams two or three times daily is generally considered safe.

Zinc. Zinc is essential for the development and activation of T cells, white blood cells that help fight infection. Because you may not get all the zinc you need from your diet, you may want to get more from supplements in the form of pills or lozenges. When you feel a cold coming on, suck on zinc lozenges per the package directions. Some studies suggest that getting zinc right up against your mucous membranes cuts the duration of a cold by two to three days. And according to one study, taking a zinc lozenge every day throughout cold season may lower your risk of getting sick by 25 percent.

Should You Go Organic?

Recently, when Swedish researchers analyzed extracts from both organic and conventionally grown strawberries, not only did the organic strawberries contain more antioxidants, but when the researchers tested both extracts on colon and breast cancer cells, the organic extracts encouraged more cancer cells to destroy themselves. Organic produce generally contains higher levels of calcium, iron, magnesium, and chromium and about 30 percent more antioxidants than conventionally grown fruits and vegetables. Of course, organic foods are usually more expensive. When you can't buy organic, look for the freshest seasonal produce. The main point is to eat more fruits and vegetables, regardless of whether they're organic.

Indian cuisine is particularly rich in ingredients that bolster the immune system. Consider regular visits to an Indian restaurant, and order meals rich with lentils, chicken, dark green vegetables, and yogurt-based sauces.

Be sure to eat something before you pop a zinc lozenge; taking zinc on an empty stomach can cause nausea. **DOSAGE:** The recommended intake for zinc is 11 milligrams a day for men and 8 for women, although some practitioners recommend taking supplements of up to 25 milligrams a day. Zinc lozenges typically contain about 23 milligrams apiece. Note that too much zinc can actually depress immune function over time; don't take more than 40 milligrams a day, the upper safe limit.

B vitamins, including folic acid. B vitamins are involved with the production of our cellular DNA as well as many of the components of the immune system, such as antibodies and white blood cells. When we don't get enough B vitamins, we don't make enough of these infection fighters, and that leaves us vulnerable to illness. Stress depletes the B vitamins, which may help explain why we tend to get sick when we're under a lot of stress. **DOSAGE:** The B vitamins work together, and you want them all in balance, so choose a quality B-complex supplement and follow the label instructions for dosage.

Vitamins, A, C, and E. All of the nutrients in this vitamin "cocktail" work together to keep the immune system going strong and keep the number of immune cells high. Vitamins A and C help fortify the body's physical barriers, building collagen and strengthening the mucous membranes so germs are less able to slip through. They also rally the immune troops to do battle against germs that do make it past the barricades. Vitamin A helps C work, and it has significant antiviral activity. Vitamin C helps ensure that the body has enough infection-fighting T cells, and E partners with C to protect immune cells from free radical damage. It's also thought to enhance T-cell activity and assist in the production of antibodies. Vitamin E is considered an "immune-specific" nutrient, according to the Micronutrient Information Center at Oregon State University. That's because it protects and increases the activity of immune cells in the body. **DOSAGE:** *Vitamin E:* 15 milligrams daily. *Vitamin A:* Recommended intakes for vitamin A are complicated to understand because they are based on "retinol activity equivalents" (RAE), which account for the differences in activity between retinol (pre-formed vitamin A) and carotenoids (substances that convert to vitamin A in the body.) Since July 2018, dietary supplements will list vitamin A content in micrograms of these RAE's. Best bet? Look for supplements that provide close to 100 percent of the Daily Value for vitamin A from retinol as well as beta-carotene. *Vitamin C:* 400 milligrams a day.

CAUTION

Refined sugar and starches. Sugary and starchy foods (which convert easily into sugar in the body) deliver a double whammy to the immune system. For starters, eating sugar is like giving Valium to your white blood cells, knocking them out so they're less able to hunt down and destroy germs and cancer cells. In a study at Loma Linda University in California, when volunteers consumed about 100 grams of sugar (about the amount in two cans of soda), their white blood cell activity dropped by 50 percent and stayed low for up to 5 hours.

For fungi and cancer cells, sugar is like a champagne and caviar banquet—they just can't get enough. Sugar also encourages an over-growth of yeast, associated with chronic yeast infections and, according to some nutritionists, digestive problems like "leaky gut syndrome," which they believe burden the immune system. Some scientists are even singling out sugar as a cancer promoter.

Saturated fats and trans fat. Eating less of these fats—think marbled red meat and fried chicken—means better immune function. High levels of cholesterol and other blood fats, a common result of eating too many saturated and trans fats, contribute to inflammation in the body and may inhibit immune functions, including the ability of white blood cells to divide, move to areas of infection, and destroy organisms. In a small study done at Tufts University, when 18 men with high cholesterol switched from a diet in which 38 percent of the calories came from fat to a diet that included 28 percent fat, their immune function related to T-cell activity improved by up to 29 percent. Keep in mind that "good" fats like those in salmon, olive oil, avocados, and flaxseed are not thought to hamper immune function and may even improve it.

Alcohol. Whether alcohol is "off the menu" really depends on your state of health, along with how much and what you're drinking. While numerous studies show that light drinking has cardiovascular benefits, other research indicates that alcohol temporarily "intoxicates" your immune system, reducing the ability of all its cells to fight invading germs. This probably isn't a problem for light drinkers, but frequent imbibers take heed: Heavy drinkers are much more vulnerable to infections from bacteria (like pneumonia and tuberculosis) and viruses (such as the flu virus), certain cancers, and infections related to traumatic injuries. In fact, people who experience such injuries while drunk are six times more likely to die from them than nondrinkers with comparable injuries.

Still, all alcohol isn't equal. While hard liquor suppresses immune function, red wine, in moderation, doesn't, perhaps because of its antioxidants.

INFERTILITY

Creating another human being has something in common with growing a prize-winning garden: You need all the right conditions and good timing to boot. As with improving the soil in your backyard, you can help make the conditions in your body ripe for conception with the help of key food nutrients.

The reproductive system is awfully sensitive. In women, shifts in hormones, an abnormality in the reproductive organs, infection, disease, and even stress can lead to infertility. In men, the most common causes are low sperm count and slow "swimmers." Although food can't fix all fertility challenges, it can help improve your odds of fruitfulness.

YOUR FOOD PRESCRIPTION

Beans, spinach,
and other foods high in folate

Women are encouraged to take folic acid supplements when they're trying to conceive because doing so helps prevent certain birth defects. But men need folic acid, too. University of California researchers found that low levels of the B vitamin may affect sperm count and density (the number of sperm per milliliter of semen). Eating foods rich in folate (the natural form) can help meet these needs.

Aim for: 600 micrograms of folate per day, an amount found in 1 1/4 cups of fortified cereal or 1 cup of cooked lentils plus 1 cup of cooked spinach.

Helpful hint: Green vegetables like spinach and cabbage can lose 40 percent of their folate during cooking, so when you can, enjoy green vegetables raw.

FEATURED RECIPES

Broccoli Salad *p. 291*
Spinach Salad with Chickpeas *p. 293*
Shrimp and Grapefruit Salad *p. 294*
Beef in Lettuce Wraps *p. 302*
Mac 'n Cheese Primavera *p. 304*
Roasted Salmon with Sautéed Greens *p. 309*

Fatty fish, flaxseed, walnuts,
and other foods high in omega-3 fatty acids

The body uses omega-3 fatty acids to produce hormones called eicosanoids, which increase blood flow to the uterus, thus boosting the chances of pregnancy and facilitating fetal development. Omega-3s can also lower the risk of premature birth and low birth weight.

Omega-3s are important for potential dads as well. A recent study found fertile men had higher levels of omega-3s in their sperm than infertile men.

Aim for: 1,000 milligrams a day, the amount in a serving of salmon, 1/4 cup of walnuts, or 1 tablespoon of ground flaxseed.

Helpful hint: Women who are trying to conceive or are pregnant should not eat shark, swordfish, king mackerel, or tilefish because of their high mercury content.

Lean red meat, oysters, crab,
and other foods high in zinc

Low zinc levels translate into lowered sperm counts, less sperm movement toward the cervical goal, less semen, and even infertility. A zinc deficiency can affect a woman's fertility by lengthening her menstrual cycle, which means less frequent ovulation.

Aim for: 11 milligrams a day for men and pregnant women, the amount in 3 ounces (85 g) of lean beef plus 1 cup of fortified breakfast cereal. Do not exceed 40 milligrams a day, which is the established upper tolerable dose.

Milk, cheese, yogurt, *and other foods high in calcium and vitamin D*

At the University of Wisconsin, treatment with calcium and vitamin D restored fertility—at least in male rats. Other research shows that calcium levels increase in sperm during the last seconds before fertilization, providing the burst of energy needed to penetrate the egg. And for women, a Columbia University study found that in those with polycystic ovary syndrome, which interferes with ovulation, calcium and vitamin D helped restore normal menstruation.

Aim for: *Calcium:* 1,000 milligrams for men and 1,300 milligrams for women, the equivalent of three to four glasses of milk. *Vitamin D:* 1,000 IU daily, about the amount in 4 ounces (113 g) of salmon plus 3 cups of milk, and 1 cup of orange juice fortified with vitamin D.

Oranges, peppers, broccoli, *and other foods high in vitamin C*

Several studies have reported that low levels of vitamin C increase a woman's risk for miscarriage. In men, low levels of C can reduce the ability of sperm to do their job. Improving vitamin C intake to normal levels improved these conditions.

Aim for: 400 milligrams a day by boosting your intake of vitamin C–rich foods such as red bell pepper (190 milligrams per cup), orange juice (186 milligrams per cup), and broccoli (102 milligrams per cup).

NUTRITIONAL SUPPLEMENTS

Vitamin C. Daily supplementation may help boost fertility. **DOSAGE:** 400 milligrams a day.

Folic acid. Couples should begin taking folic acid supplements as soon as they decide to conceive. **DOSAGE:** 600 micrograms a day for women and men.

Calcium and vitamin D. Don't take calcium supplements derived from oyster shells or bonemeal. They may contain lead, which can harm an unborn child. **DOSAGE:** *Calcium:* 1,300 milligrams daily for women; men shouldn't take supplements because they may increase the risk of prostate cancer. *Vitamin D:* 1,000 IU daily for men and women.

Omega-3 fatty acids. These come in fish-oil capsules and in liquids such as flaxseed oil. Buy a brand with vitamin E, which helps keep the oil from becoming rancid. **DOSAGE:** 1 gram per day.

Zinc. High doses of zinc supplements can result in a copper deficiency. **DOSAGE:** Don't take more than 40 milligrams per day—the upper limit set by the National Academy of Sciences—without consulting your physician.

CAUTION

Coffee, cola, and other foods with caffeine. Some studies, though not others, suggest that caffeine affects fertility and may contribute to miscarriage. The theory is that it may affect ovulation by altering hormone levels. Moderate intakes of caffeine do not seem to pose a problem; however, most experts, including the American College of Obstetricians and Gynecologists (ACOG), recommend that women who are pregnant or planning to become pregnant should limit caffeine consumption to less than 200 milligrams a day—about the amount in 2 cups of coffee.

For men, the story's different. According to findings by Brazilian scientists, caffeine appears to make sperm nimbler.

INFLAMMATORY BOWEL DISEASE

If you have inflammatory bowel disease (IBD), the current wisdom on how to approach it can flip your perception of what constitutes a healthy diet: Don't overdo the fiber, hold back on the spices, and think twice before you eat fruit and vegetables. Nevertheless, research has revealed that such a diet may help alleviate some of the pain associated with IBD.

Characterized by persistent inflammation of the intestinal tract, IBD can be debilitating. Symptoms, including abdominal pain, diarrhea, appetite loss, and fatigue, can linger for weeks to years and disappear for periods of time. The two different conditions that fall under the category of IBD, Crohn's disease and ulcerative colitis, affect the GI tract in different ways. With Crohn's disease, inflammation in all layers of the intestinal wall prevents the small intestine from properly absorbing nutrients and disturbs the fine balance of water needed to usher foods along the intestine. That can lead to relentless diarrhea. Add appetite loss to the equation, and vitamin and mineral deficiencies become a real problem. With ulcerative colitis, the inner lining of the large intestine becomes inflamed, preventing the normal absorption of water from the colon, the last 5 feet (1.5 m) of the intestine. This causes diarrhea and extreme discomfort.

More than half of people who develop IBD eventually have surgery to remove part of their intestine or correct intestinal abnormalities. That can leave the digestive tract less robust and more sensitive to swings in dietary and other irritants. Food won't prevent or cure IBD, but the right diet may diminish symptoms. The strategy is to focus on foods that reduce inflammation, to reestablish healthy bacteria in the gut, and to pamper your intestinal tract. That means keeping a food diary to determine which foods trigger flare-ups and which seem to appease the sleeping giant. Work with your doctor to determine whether you have sensitivities to specific foods and establish whether you need supplements to replenish some of the nutrients lost during bouts of IBD.

FEATURED RECIPES

Salsa Tuna Salad Sandwiches *p. 300*
Tuna Kebabs *p. 306*
Tomato-Roasted Mackerel *p. 308*
Roasted Salmon with Sautéed Greens *p. 309*

Small, frequent meals rich in calories

Six small meals a day are often more easily digested than the traditional three and make it easier to get enough calories to maintain weight. People with IBD often lose significant weight, making it difficult for them to get sufficient nutrients. This is particularly true for people who have narrowed areas of the intestine as a result of IBD.

Aim for: Choose calorie-rich, nutrient-dense foods like whole grains, legumes, and nuts when your gut feels calm. During flare-ups, avoid the foods listed in Caution (see page 203) and focus on those that don't worsen your problem.

Potatoes, white rice, refined pasta, *and other low-fiber foods*

During flare-ups of IBD, the digestive tract is often inflamed and sensitive to irritation. Smooth, bland foods tend to be easier on the gut during this time. Because these foods often lack essential nutrients that we need for robust health, it's best to consult your doctor or a registered dietitian and to take a multivitamin to ensure that you're getting the nutrients you need.

Plantain

This green banana, common in South America, may have a soothing effect on the lining of the intestine. A study from England showed that soluble fiber from plantain creates an environment that resists inflammatory bacteria. If more studies follow suit, the plantain may find a regular place on the global menu of people with IBD.

Aim for: No one knows how much plantain may be the ticket to a healthy intestine, but boiled green plantain or sautéed yellow plantain is a lovely addition to any evening meal and may help soothe some of the irritation that comes with IBD.

Olive oil

Olive oil is rich in antioxidants called flavonoids, which protect the body's cells from daily wear and tear. Flavonoids may help reduce inflammation by neutralizing free radicals that contribute to it. One recent study showed that a combination of olive oil and fish oil reduced inflammation in the colons of rats with IBD.

Buy extra-virgin olive oil, which has the most flavonoids. For the highest quality and the most nutrient-dense oils, seek out estate oils that are produced in one region. Avoid "light" and "extra light" olive oil, which is often a mixture of less nutritious, refined olive oil and sometimes other types of lower-quality oil.

Aim for: Try to replace most of the oils in your diet with extra-virgin olive oil.

Helpful hint: Olive and canola oils are your best source of fats, but you don't necessarily need to cut out butter entirely. It's a source of butyric acid, needed to maintain a healthy mucosal lining in the gut.

Yogurt with active cultures *and other fermented milk products*

Although the cause of IBD remains a mystery, scientists are now exploring whether an overgrowth of bacteria in the intestine may contribute to the disease. Probiotics are beneficial bacteria found in fermented milk products like yogurt, buttermilk, and kefir. Getting more of them helps keep the "bad guy" bacteria in your gut in check.

Aim for: People with IBD respond differently to different diets, so there's no blanket recommendation here. You might start by having a daily half cup of yogurt or fermented milk with live, active cultures (look on the label for *lactobacillus, bifidus, Streptococcus thermophilus,* and *acidophilus,* among other active cultures) and gradually increase the amount you eat, up to 1 1/2 cups a day. Keeping a food and symptom diary during this trial period should help you establish the optimal amount for you.

Salmon, mackerel, walnuts,
and other sources of omega-3 fatty acids

With inflammation at the root of the problems caused by IBD, it makes sense to seek out foods rich in omega-3 fatty acids, which battle inflammation. Salmon and other fatty fish are the very best sources. In one study, patients with Crohn's disease who ate 3.5 ounces (100 g) or more of fish per day for two years lowered their chances of relapse from 58 percent to 20 percent. Ground flaxseed, flaxseed oil, and walnuts also contain essential fatty acids, but they aren't converted efficiently by the body to the kinds of omega-3s that fight inflammation (the kinds in fish). Still, if you don't eat fish, they're certainly better than nothing.

Aim for: Three fish meals per week.

Water *and other fluids*

The risk of dehydration is ever present with IBD because of chronic diarrhea. Kidney problems can also result when the amount of fluids entering the body doesn't keep up with the amount leaving it. Even when you don't have symptoms, it's smart to prioritize water.

Aim for: At least eight 8-ounce glasses (2 l total) of water or other fluids every day. Some acidic juices like pineapple or tomato may irritate your digestive tract, so stick to clear fluids whenever possible and avoid carbonated beverages, which can contribute to bloating.

NUTRITIONAL SUPPLEMENTS

A multivitamin/mineral. One of the more serious consequences of IBD is poor nutrient absorption. In fact, health-threatening deficiencies can happen when IBD is not monitored closely. **DOSAGE:** Check with your physician or dietitian to determine whether you need individual supplements or simply a high-quality multivitamin/mineral.

Vitamin B_{12}. This vitamin is absorbed in the lower part of the small intestine, an area that is sometimes surgically removed in severe cases of IBD. If you have had parts of your intestine removed, make sure that your doctor checks for vitamin B_{12} deficiency. **DOSAGE:** If you're B_{12} deficient, your physician can determine whether you would respond better to oral supplementation or monthly injections of B_{12} to replace this vital nutrient.

Vitamin D. Healthy bones are dependent in part on a healthy dose of vitamin D, the nutrient that aids in calcium absorption. But people with IBD may not absorb vitamin D well because of inflammation in the small intestine. Without enough D, the bones can soften and become vulnerable to fracture, a condition called osteomalacia. Research has shown that supplementation can help prevent this condition in people with IBD. **DOSAGE:** Check with your physician for the right dosage. Most people need at least 800 IU of vitamin D per day.

Get in the habit of making fruit smoothies at home—this blender drink is almost perfect for your health and digestion. Put a cup of plain yogurt, a banana, a fistful of berries, a teaspoon of honey, and a few ice cubes into your blender and process until smooth. It's that easy!

Vitamin K. Researchers are just starting to look at the possibility of vitamin K deficiencies in people with IBD. Because this vitamin is crucial to bone health, ask your physician to test your K levels. Vitamin K is found in leafy greens like spinach, lettuce, and watercress as well as soybean oil. **DOSAGE:** A multivitamin usually provides enough vitamin K, but check with your doctor.

Iron. Sometimes IBD causes bleeding in the intestinal walls, and this blood loss can lead to iron-deficiency anemia, a condition that causes fatigue and weakness. **DOSAGE:** Let your doctor decide whether you need to take supplemental iron and in what dose.

Omega-3 fatty acids. These anti-inflammatory "fish fats" may help people with Crohn's disease and ulcerative colitis. An Italian study recently found that when adults with IBD took supplements that included 400 milligrams of eicosapentaenoic acid (EPA) and 200 milligrams of docosahexaenoic acid (DHA)—the two main components of omega-3s—their relapse rates were lowered by 33 percent. **DOSAGE:** A combination of 400 milligrams of EPA and 200 milligrams of DHA daily. Be sure the capsules you choose are enteric coated so they won't break down until they reach the small intestine, where they can do their anti-inflammatory work.

Probiotics. If an overgrowth of "bad" bacteria may be to blame for IBD, increasing "good" bacteria with probiotic supplements may help relieve symptoms, especially if you're under stress. A study in Norway showed that rats fed a diet supplemented with probiotics were much less likely than those on a normal diet to develop harmful bacteria in their digestive tracts during stressful situations. **DOSAGE:** 10 billion colony-forming units (CFU) of probiotics once or twice daily.

CAUTION

High-fiber foods. Bran, the outer shell of many grains, can feel like sandpaper to an intestine affected by IBD, so eat bran cereals and foods made with whole-grain flour with caution. Other high-fiber foods, such as fresh fruits and vegetables, can cause already watery stools to take on even more water, producing more diarrhea. During bouts of IBD, eliminate whole grains and most produce and steer clear of nuts, seeds, and corn, which all can cause cramping in a narrowed bowel.

When a bout of IBD has receded, you can try to slowly reintroduce these foods to see whether your body will tolerate them. Eating fiber-rich foods when you're feeling okay may even be beneficial to a bowel prone to IBD because it can encourage production of butyrate, a fatty acid that helps keep inflammation under control and the intestinal lining healthy.

Fatty meats and fried foods. The saturated fats in burgers and the like can increase production of hormone-like compounds called prostaglandins that contribute to inflammation. Also, when fat is poorly absorbed, it can cause gas and diarrhea. Instead of doughnuts and french fries, try to eat foods with plenty of flavor that doesn't rely on fat.

Milk and other dairy foods. Many people diagnosed with IBD are lactose intolerant, which means they have trouble digesting lactose, a sugar found in milk and milk products. If your symptoms tend to flare up after eating dairy, try avoiding it for several weeks. A gastroenterologist can perform a test to see if you're lactose intolerant.

Alcohol and caffeine. Both can irritate an inflamed gut, and they act as diuretics, the last thing you need when you're prone to diarrhea.

INSOMNIA

If you find yourself walking around in a fog, having abandoned the dream of a decent night's sleep, you might consider padding on over to the kitchen. Grandma prescribed a glass of warm milk before bed, and modern science says she may have been onto something. Research has also discovered other "sleep medicines" hiding in your kitchen. Cheese, anyone?

The foods that appear the most effective in battling insomnia help boost chemicals that cause the body to relax, making for easier, more restful sleep. Combined with plenty of exercise and some stress reduction, they just may be the ticket to sweet dreams.

YOUR FOOD PRESCRIPTION

Warm milk with honey;

turkey; cheese; peanuts; and bananas

You've probably heard the jokes about the Thanksgiving turkey putting people to sleep, but this folk wisdom has a leg—make that two legs—to stand on. Turkey and the other foods listed above are rich in tryptophan, an amino acid that the body uses to produce serotonin, a kind of chemical lullaby, if you will. Serotonin slows nerve activity, calming the brain and spreading a "feel-good" message throughout your body. When darkness enters the picture, the brain converts serotonin to yet another hormone, melatonin, which regulates sleep.

In one recent Canadian study, when chronic insomniacs ate food bars containing 250 milligrams of tryptophan (the amount in two slices of provolone cheese, for example) plus a dose of carbohydrate, the time they spent awake during the night was decreased by 50 percent.

The reason we recommend honey with your warm milk—and the reason the study food bar included carbohydrate—is that a fast-digesting carbohydrate like honey or mashed potatoes stimulates the release of insulin, which in turn allows more tryptophan to enter the brain.

Aim for: Before going to bed, try a glass of warm milk with honey (heat can enhance the tryptophan effect of foods), a slice of turkey on a piece of whole-grain bread, a banana, a handful of nuts, some leftover baked beans, or a slice or two of cheese.

Whole grains

Oatmeal, whole-grain cereals and breads, and other complex carbohydrates increase production of serotonin.

Aim for: Make three of your daily carbohydrate servings whole grains (one serving is a small bowl of whole-grain cereal, a slice of whole-grain bread, or a half cup of brown rice or barley, for instance). Some experts recommend a bedtime snack of a complex carbohydrate to help prevent nighttime low blood sugar, which in some people may contribute to poor sleep.

FEATURED RECIPES

Edamame Hummus with Pita Crisps *p. 288*
Ultimate Spiced Nuts *p. 288*
Spinach Salad with Chickpeas *p. 293*
Lentil-Tomato Soup *p. 299*
Beef in Lettuce Wraps *p. 302*
Turkey Cutlets with Grapefruit Salsa *p. 313*
Banana-Peanut Bread *p. 326*

Chamomile tea

Sometimes all it takes to fall asleep is going to bed with the confidence that you *will* fall asleep. The scientific evidence on chamomile tea for insomnia is thin, but many people find it relaxing, and if you think a nice warm cup of this tea before bed will help you drift off, it probably will.

Aim for: A cup at bedtime.

Red meat, shellfish, tofu, lentils, *and other iron-rich foods*

If restless legs keep you awake, it's possible that you have a form of anemia caused by iron deficiency. Consult a physician to find out if you do. The doctor may prescribe supplements or a diet rich in iron to help correct the problem. Choose lean red meat for the least saturated fat, and eat it for lunch rather than dinner because its protein can counteract sleep-inducing serotonin.

Aim for: Women up to age 50 need about 18 milligrams of iron per day. Women 51 and older and adult men need 8 milligrams. A 3-ounce (85 g) portion of sirloin packs about 3 milligrams; a half dozen oysters, 14 milligrams; and 1 cup of lentils, 7 milligrams.

Helpful hint: To get more iron from plant foods, which contain the less absorbable nonheme type, eat them along with a food rich in heme iron (like meat) or in vitamin C, which also helps you soak up nonheme iron.

NUTRITIONAL SUPPLEMENTS

A multivitamin/mineral for iron and B vitamins. These nutrients can help you get a good night's sleep, especially if you're deficient in them. A deficiency of iron or the B vitamin folate may cause restless legs syndrome. Several of the B vitamins are important for brain function and help regulate both mood and sleep. For example, B_6 and niacin are directly involved in serotonin production.

Don't take more than the amount of iron in a multivitamin except under a doctor's supervision; too much can be harmful. If your multivitamin makes you feel energized, take it in the earlier part of the day. **DOSAGE:** One a day.

Magnesium. This mineral is involved in the production of sleep-inducing serotonin, and a magnesium deficiency may also cause restless legs syndrome. The glycinate and malate forms of magnesium are less likely than citrate and hydroxide forms to cause diarrhea. **DOSAGE:** 100 to 300 milligrams before bed.

OFF THE MENU

Alcohol. Even though alcohol is a sedative, you may wake up after a couple of hours, when most of the alcohol has been metabolized—that is, after the sedative effect wears off. Alcohol can also make snoring and sleep apnea worse by relaxing muscles in the airways.

Caffeine. Caffeine's the last thing you want in your system at night. If you're really sensitive to it, you should give it up altogether: One study showed that as little as 200 milligrams—the amount in 2 cups of coffee—in the morning was enough to cause sleep problems at night. Tea, cola, and chocolate also contain caffeine.

High-fat dinners. These can trigger indigestion and heartburn, which are difficult to sleep through.

A Fishy Solution?

Fish doesn't just help your heart; its omega-3 fatty acids (found in high concentrations in the normal brain) may also improve your mood by increasing levels of the feel-good hormone serotonin. Less depression often equals better sleep. Studies of omega-3s for insomnia have yielded mixed results, but there's no harm in eating more salmon as well as flaxseed and walnuts to see if it helps.

INSULIN RESISTANCE

It's great to be resistant to viruses, bacteria, and advertising—but not to insulin. You may never have heard of insulin resistance, but it's practically an epidemic in the United States—it's estimated that 25 percent of adults have it—thanks in large part to our aversion to exercise and our undying devotion to simple carbohydrates and processed, sugary foods. (Genes also play a role.) Insulin resistance puts you on the path to weight gain and diabetes and is now thought to contribute to heart disease, obesity, and even Alzheimer's disease.

Every time you eat your fill of french fries, scones, or sugary cereal—foods that spike your blood sugar—your body has to pump out insulin to get the sugar, or glucose, out of the bloodstream and into cells, where it can be used as fuel. Over time, repeated surges of insulin can tire out your cells' insulin receptors so they don't work as well and insulin can't be used as efficiently. The result? More and more insulin is needed to do the same job. That's insulin resistance. It's not that different from what happens when your spouse's hearing starts to go: You have to shout louder and louder to get him to change the channel (unless, of course, your beloved is simply ignoring you).

Extra insulin can raise blood pressure, cause problems with cholesterol levels, and even make it easier for certain cancers to grow. It also paves the way for weight gain. As your insulin resistance gets worse—which it will if you continue to follow the same diet—you may also develop high blood sugar, which carries its own risks.

Mild and moderate insulin resistance can be detected through a blood test that shows high levels of insulin. If you have severe insulin resistance, you may notice dark patches of skin on your neck, elbows, knees, or knuckles. You're more likely to be insulin resistant if others in your family have diabetes; if you have low levels of HDL ("good") cholesterol, high triglycerides, or high blood pressure; or if you've had diabetes during a pregnancy. African Americans and Hispanics are more at risk and so are overweight people, so shedding extra pounds is key if your pants are snug and your belt no longer goes the distance. Exercise also makes cells more "insulin-friendly," and if you have insulin resistance, you're probably not active enough. But there's no ignoring the fact that what you eat takes center stage in the development—and reversal—of this condition.

Switching to slow-digesting, high-fiber foods is the major goal; this helps keep blood sugar low so you need less insulin to bring it down. And weaning yourself from saturated fats (think marbled steak) and trans fat (think packaged snack foods and baked goods) in favor of unsaturated fats like those in fish, nuts, and olive oil can even crank up your cells' sensitivity to insulin.

Whole grains, beans, *and other complex carbohydrates high in fiber*

When's the last time you had whole-wheat pasta, barley, or beans on your plate? These are the types of foods that digest nice and slowly, keeping blood sugar spikes in check. But most of us eat perilously few of them. The same goes for legumes: Chickpeas, soybeans, and lentils are sadly underrepresented in our dishes. Fortunately, many of us have at least gotten the message as far as whole-grain cereals are concerned and are choosing higher-fiber brands. That's good. Data collected on almost 3,000 people in the Framingham Offspring Study shows that people who ate the most cereal fiber from whole grains were much less likely to have insulin resistance than those who ate the least.

Start by making sure your morning cereal contains at least 5 grams of fiber per serving. Next, make sandwiches with whole-grain bread (check that the first ingredient on the label includes the word *whole).* Then look to add beans to your diet. A can of black bean or lentil soup makes a terrific and extremely easy lunch, and it's simple enough to throw beans or chickpeas into salads.

Aim for: 25 to 35 grams of fiber per day. A cup of cooked lentils has 16 grams, as does a cup of cooked oatmeal.

Helpful hint: If you like oatmeal, buy the real stuff, not flavored instant oatmeal, which almost always contains added sugar.

Olives, olive oil, nuts, and avocados

All this time, you've probably thought guacamole was just party food, but when it comes to foods like avocados and nuts, party on (in moderation, of course). These foods are loaded with monounsaturated fats—fats that are actually good for you as long as you don't overdo them. (By the way, fats don't raise blood sugar; in fact, they help steady it.)

Unlike saturated fat, which raises the risk of insulin resistance, unsaturated fat can actually improve insulin sensitivity, as a Finnish study suggests. The researchers placed 31 people with impaired glucose tolerance (elevated blood sugar levels that accompany insulin resistance) on a diet high in saturated fat for three weeks. The participants were then switched to diets emphasizing monounsaturated or polyunsaturated fats—the kind in plant oils like canola oil. Those whose diet emphasized monounsaturated fats had the most improvement in blood glucose levels and insulin sensitivity.

Trying to lose weight? Don't shun fat entirely. A little bit of fat makes meals more pleasing and even helps you stay full longer. Just be sure to choose the "good" fats. Fortunately, veggies taste fantastic sautéed in olive oil, and salads are all the more appealing when topped with good stuff like nuts and seeds and olive oil–based salad dressings.

Aim for: Up to 1 tablespoon of olive oil–based salad dressing drizzled on a salad at lunch and vegetables at dinner, 1 ounce (28 g) of nuts, and 1/3 cup of guacamole or a few slices of avocado every day.

Helpful hint: Instead of cheese in your sandwich, try a slice or two of avocado. Squeeze the juice from a lemon wedge over avocado slices to keep them from browning and to boost vitamin C, a powerful antioxidant, as well.

FEATURED RECIPES

Spinach Salad with Chickpeas *p. 293*
Citrus Chicken Salad *p. 294*
Salsa Tuna Salad Sandwiches *p. 300*
Three-Bean Chili *p. 306*
Tuna Kebabs *p. 306*
Turkey Ragu with Spaghetti *p. 314*
Springtime Quinoa *p. 322*
Blueberry-Oat Scones *p. 324*
Chocolate Fondue *p. 330*

Dark chocolate, green tea,
and other foods high in flavonoids

Love dark chocolate? Here's your chance to indulge once in a while. Two recent Italian studies showed that people who ate a 3.5-ounce (100 g) bar of dark chocolate a day significantly lowered their insulin resistance compared to those who ate white chocolate. Researchers believe that the protection may come from the high levels of flavonoids in dark chocolate (actually, in the cocoa used to make it), which have both antioxidant and anti-inflammatory properties. Dark chocolate is also high in chromium, which helps increase insulin sensitivity. But the news isn't license to gorge on chocolate. Flavonoids are also found in green tea, wine, blueberries, apples with the skin, onions, cabbage, brussels sprouts, spinach, and asparagus.

Aim for: 1.5 ounces (42 g) of dark chocolate occasionally (buy a brand that contains 60 percent cocoa if you can find it), several cups of green tea a day, and several daily servings of citrus fruits and berries.

Helpful hint: Milk chocolate doesn't contain nearly as many flavonoids as dark chocolate and has more fat and calories, so make sure you satisfy your sweet tooth with the dark stuff.

Spinach, beans, fish,
and other foods high in magnesium

Beans may not be glamorous, but for people with insulin resistance, they're beauties where it counts. Studies show that low magnesium is linked with insulin resistance. People on diets rich in magnesium are also at much lower risk of type 2 diabetes than those who shun beans and leafy greens.

Aim for: Studies have shown doses of 300 to 400 milligrams of magnesium per day to be helpful in controlling blood sugar in people who have diabetes. A quarter cup of pumpkin seeds has 185 milligrams, and a cup of cooked spinach has 157 milligrams.

Helpful hint: Since some magnesium is lost in cooking, head for the salad bar.

NUTRITIONAL SUPPLEMENTS

Chromium. Chromium helps enhance the effects of insulin in the body. Yet recent studies have failed to show that chromium supplements can improve insulin sensitivity if a person does not have a deficiency of this nutrient. That said, it's difficult to measure whether you are deficient or not. **DOSAGE:** An adequate intake for adults 19 to 50 is 25 micrograms for women and 35 micrograms for men. (A cup of broccoli contains 22 micrograms.) Some studies have used supplemental doses as high as 1,000 micrograms. The Institute of Medicine has not set an upper limit for chromium but people with liver or kidney disease should not take high doses.

Magnesium. Supplements are recommended only for people with low blood levels of magnesium in their blood, as measured by a blood test. Chelated supplements like magnesium citrate are better absorbed than nonchelated forms like magnesium oxide. (*Chelated* means the magnesium is connected to another molecule, often an amino acid.) **DOSAGE:** Studies have shown magnesium doses of 300 to 400 milligrams per day to be helpful in controlling blood glucose in people with diabetes. This is about the same as the recommended amount of 400 to 420 milligrams daily for men and 310 to 320 milligrams for women.

CAUTION

Sugar and refined grains. White's fine for the tennis court but not for the majority of your food. Foods made from white flour (think most baked goods and white bread), sugary foods, most rice cereals, and other such "white foods" lack the fiber of whole grains and tend to be digested quickly, spiking blood sugar and in turn bumping up insulin production. Diets high in these foods also tend to be low in nutrients and full of calories, making it easy to pile on weight, which boosts the risk of insulin resistance.

Go "whole" by switching to whole-grain breads and cereals and eating whole fruit instead of drinking fruit juice. Instead of sugary soft drinks, try club soda with a slice of lime and imagine you're on a beach in the Bahamas. Processed and refined carbohydrates also figure heavily in many packaged snack foods, so be on your guard.

Fatty meat, full-fat dairy foods, and foods made with trans fat. It's time to seal the cookie jar (unless you bake your own treats). You may as well pack up the baloney and salami, too. The trans fat in many baked goods and the saturated fats in meats and cheese boost the risk of heart disease—already high for people with insulin resistance—and diabetes. They may also contribute directly to insulin resistance, and they may impair your body's ability to make insulin. Saturated fats are stored in cells as damaging triglycerides. When they accumulate in cells that produce insulin, they can actually kill those cells.

A Swedish study has also shown that decreasing saturated fat by replacing it with plant fats like olive oil increases insulin sensitivity as long as fat calories aren't more than 37 percent of the diet.

Fast food. In a 15-year University of Minnesota study of more than 3,000 young adults, researchers found that those who ate fast food more than twice a week gained an average of 10 pounds (4.5 g) and had a 104 percent increase in insulin resistance. Fast foods tend to be packed with hydrogenated oils and refined starches (think french fries and white hamburger buns) or sugar (think soda) that raise blood sugar. What's more, the serving sizes tend to be all too "super." The next time you feel the urge to zip through the drive-through, slam on the brakes—a healthy calorie expenditure.

Revealing Waistlines

Did you have trouble buttoning your skirt today? That could be a sign of insulin resistance. According to a survey commissioned by the National Women's Health Resource Center, 75 percent of women participants who had a family history of diabetes or heart disease reported having a burgeoning waistline, fatigue, and cravings for carbohydrates. The most common trait among the women was fat around the middle. If a woman's waist is at least 35 inches (89 cm), or a man's 40 inches (102 cm), it's time for a visit to the doctor, more exercise, and a healthier diet focused on whole grains, fruits and vegetables, and fish.

IRRITABLE BOWEL SYNDROME

If you have irritable bowel syndrome (IBS), you may start to feel that food is your enemy, since you never know how it's going to affect your sensitive digestive system. But don't despair! A diet tailored to your body's own quirks can make food your friend again.

In normal digestion, when you eat a meal, your esophagus, stomach, and intestine react with gentle contractions that move the food along the digestive tract. IBS changes that process, causing the contractions to sometimes speed up, sometimes slow down, and often increase in strength. The gut becomes irritated and vulnerable to any combination of the following symptoms: bloating, abdominal pain, diarrhea, constipation, or a seesawing occurrence of the latter two.

Experts used to think that IBS occurred only in the colon, the last 5 feet (1.5 m) of the intestine. We now know that IBS occurs throughout the entire digestive tract, starting in the mouth, and affects digestion, metabolism, and the excretion of waste. To make matters worse, stress often kick-starts and aggravates the symptoms, creating a vicious cycle because simply having IBS is stressful.

Because each person's case of IBS is different, the key to relieving discomfort is to keep a food and symptom diary. That diligence will pay off in helping you identify which foods to avoid and which appear to help.

If you haven't done so already, be sure to see your doctor to make sure you really have IBS. Many IBS symptoms can be warning signs of more serious diseases.

Keep a large container of plain yogurt in the refrigerator for quick, gut-healthy breakfasts and snacks. Make instant parfaits with granola and berries; use as the base for a quick smoothie; or merely mix in a spoonful of fruit spread.

Whole grains, legumes, nuts,
and other foods high in fiber

Filling your plate with these foods, as well as fruits and vegetables, is the best way to bulk up stool and keep the colon in tip-top shape for absorbing nutrients. Some types of fiber act like a snowball, gathering waste as it "rolls" through the digestive tract, then exiting the body in stool. Others act as Mother Nature's scrub brush, helping to clean off the sides of the digestive tract so nutrients can pass through intestinal walls easily. All fiber can help diminish IBS symptoms, from gas and bloating to constipation and, ironically, even diarrhea—at least in some people.

Fiber doesn't work for everyone with IBS; in some people, it can make symptoms like gas and bloating worse. So start by increasing your fiber intake very slowly. Add an extra serving of fruit or vegetables one week (starting with cooked rather than raw); eat a serving of whole grain like wild rice, quinoa, or barley the next; and by the end of the month, switch from white pasta to a whole-grain version. Try eating more beans as well: Lentils and other small beans are often more easily digested, especially when prepared with herbs and spices that help to combat gas, such as coriander and caraway. Keep a close watch on your symptoms with your food diary, and if fiber really does make your symptoms worse, cut back again.

Don't increase your fiber intake without also increasing the amount of fluids you drink. Without enough fluids, fiber hardens and shrinks in the stool, leading to constipation.

Aim for: General guidelines call for a minimum of 25 grams of fiber a day (more is better). You can get there by eating 2 cups of fruit, 2 1/2 cups of vegetables, and three servings of whole grains. For snacks, have an apple instead of pretzels; for breakfast, have whole oatmeal instead of white toast; for dinner, add fresh or frozen vegetables to your pasta sauce or soup. Spread fiber throughout the day for the best effect.

Fermented foods

The human digestive system is full of bacteria, some of it beneficial—helping to break down undigested foods—and some of it potentially harmful. A poor diet, antibiotics, and stress can all disrupt the ratio of "good" to "bad" bugs, leaving the gut susceptible to gas, bloating, and pain. Some studies have shown that yogurt and fermented milk products like kefir, which contain live, active cultures of friendly bacteria, can help reduce the symptoms of IBS. Milk sugars in kefir and yogurt help the bacteria survive the acids in your digestive system. If you're lactose intolerant, you may want to use a probiotic supplement, too (see Nutritional Supplements on page 214).

Other fermented foods such as sauerkraut and vinegar are currently being studied for their potential in treating digestive problems such as IBS. These foods contain acetate, a short-chain fatty acid that—along with its siblings butyrate and proprionate—shows promise for its role in maintaining a healthy gut, mainly by reducing inflammation.

Aim for: There's no magic target, since everyone with IBS responds differently. Start with a daily half cup of yogurt or fermented milk with live, active cultures, or try a tablespoon of apple cider vinegar in a glass of warm water. Use your food and symptom diary to help you determine if it's making things better.

FEATURED RECIPES

Tropical Fruit Salad *p. 286*
Ginger Butternut Squash Soup *p. 298*
Lentil-Tomato Soup *p. 299*
Roasted Salmon with Sautéed Greens *p. 309*
Springtime Quinoa *p. 322*
Raspberry-Almond Muffins *p. 324*
Pear Crisp *p. 332*

Low FODMAP diet

Some people with IBS find it hard to digest certain types of sugars such as fructose (found in honey, apples, and high-fructose corn syrups) and lactose (found in milk and other dairy products). Researchers at Monash University in Australia developed a diet called the low FODMAP diet, which limits these carbohydrates and others. If you're wondering, FODMAP stands for fermentable, oligosaccharides, disaccharides, monosaccharides, and polyols.

Unfortunately, this diet limits many healthful foods, including several types of fruits, vegetables, dairy products, and some whole grains such as whole wheat. Your doctor may suggest you try the low-FODMAP diet for a few weeks to see if your symptoms improve. If they do, you may be instructed to slowly add FODMAP foods back into your diet. Then you will know which ones you tolerate and which ones you don't.

Caraway seed, fennel seed, cardamom, and coriander

Used since ancient times as digestive aids, these spices are known to be carminative, or helpful to digestion. Caraway and fennel seeds help keep gas and bloating under control, while cardamom and coriander also help calm intestinal spasms that can lead to diarrhea.

Aim for: Heat the spices in a dry pan for a minute to release the flavor and then add to stews, soups, dips, and other recipes for a boost in digestion.

NUTRITIONAL SUPPLEMENTS
Enteric-coated peppermint-oil capsules.
Studies on using peppermint oil for IBS are numerous. It appears to help by relaxing smooth muscles in the digestive tract, relieving gas, and by possibly putting the brakes on the growth of bacteria in the small intestine. A study from Taiwan involving 110 people with IBS found that peppermint oil reduced stomach pain by 79 percent and bloating by 83 percent. **DOSAGE:** In the Taiwan study, volunteers took one capsule three or four times daily, 15 to 30 minutes before meals.

Probiotics. These beneficial bacteria can help get a disrupted digestive system back on track. In one study, women with IBS who took *Bifidobacterium infantis* for four weeks experienced 20 percent less bloating and pain than those taking placebos. **DOSAGE:** Take up to 10 billion live organisms, preferably *bifidus* or *lactobacillus,* once or twice daily.

CAUTION
Milk and dairy products. Many people with IBS can't tolerate lactose, a sugar found in milk. Instead of digesting the lactose, bacteria in the gut produce gas, bloating, and nausea. Yogurt may be an exception to the rule because

We often blame foods for our digestive woes, but sometimes, it's what we drink that is at fault. Coffee, soda, alcohol, milk, and even orange juice can irritate a sensitive digestive tract. The best plan: Stick to water or herbal tea.

the active bacteria in yogurt convert lactose to lactic acid (which gives yogurt its tart flavor). Avoid sugar-free yogurt (the sugar alcohols used as sugar substitutes can increase gas and bloating) and frozen yogurt that's been whipped (the air increases bloating). If you eliminate all dairy foods, make sure you get enough calcium from other calcium-rich foods or a supplement.

Raw tomatoes, citrus juices, and spicy condiments. All of these can irritate the GI tract, but not everyone reacts negatively, so keep a close eye on your body's reaction through your food journal. If you like spicy foods and are reluctant to give them up, try turning down the heat a bit. Some spices, like ginger and chile peppers, are antibacterial, so if they don't bother you, they could offer benefits. Cook with spices because heating them releases their healing potential.

Coffee. Coffee, even decaf, contains an enzyme that irritates the digestive tract, and irritants mean trouble to anyone with IBS. If you depend on coffee to get your bowels moving in the morning, as an alternative, consider using supplemental magnesium citrate (see "Nighttime Calming Remedy" on this page) at night. A cup of hot or warm water with a good squirt of lemon juice can also help start things moving.

Alcohol. Beer, wine, and spirits can all irritate the gut, making digestion painful and unpredictable. Avoid alcohol during bouts of IBS and drink only moderate amounts at other times.

Carbonated beverages. Any food that increases the amount of air in the gut will be a problem for someone suffering from bloating and gas. Opt for nonfizzy varieties of mineral water and other beverages.

Diet candy and sugar-free chewing gum. Sorbitol and mannitol—sugar alcohol used to sweeten sugar-free chewing gum and other low-sugar products—are a no-no on the low-FODMAP diet. They may also trigger diarrhea and stomach pain in people with IBS.

Nighttime Calming Remedy

The normal digestive process requires ongoing muscle contraction and relaxation in the gut. When we're under stress, or when we drink caffeinated drinks or use nicotine, contractions in the bowels tend to increase, throwing things off-balance and messing up the excretion process. Magnesium citrate, a muscle relaxant, can restore that balance and reduce symptoms of IBS, such as constipation, cramping, and bloating. Magnesium citrate also acts as a natural laxative; it works by drawing water into the intestine to help move waste along. Mix a 200- to 800-milligram dose of the powder in water, according to the directions on the label, and drink it warm like a tea before bed.

KIDNEY STONES

Like a little bullet that dams up your urinary tract, a kidney stone can stop you in your tracks and leave you writhing in agony. Stones can exist silently for years, but when a stone starts to move through one of the narrow tubes from the kidneys, the pain is so intense that women who've had attacks say it's worse than the pain of labor. Unfortunately, once you've had a kidney stone, the chances are high that you'll have another.

Luckily, turning on the kitchen tap and filling up with nature's most bountiful beverage may be the simple ticket to stone prevention. Certain foods can also help by correcting the balance of salts and minerals in urine and by breaking up crystals before they wreak havoc.

YOUR FOOD PRESCRIPTION

Water

On any given day, the kidneys filter about 45 gallons (180 l) of blood to remove salts, water, and waste products that form when the body processes food and liquids. All of this refuse passes as urine through tubes called ureters into the bladder. From the bladder, it flows through a slightly wider tube, the urethra, to exit the body when you urinate. When salts and waste overwhelm the liquid needed to flush them through the system, the waste materials clump together to form stones that can range from the size of a sugar crystal to the size of an apricot.

The more fluid you drink, the more quickly waste passes through your urinary tract, and the less likely you are to get kidney stones.

Aim for: At least 12 cups of fluid spaced throughout the day. If the weather is hot or you're exercising and sweating, you should drink even more.

Lemon water

A natural acid in lemons called citrate helps to break down waste in the kidneys and prevent stones from forming. In one study, when people drank 4 ounces (118 ml) of lemon juice combined with water, the amount of citrate released in the urine doubled.

Aim for: Squeeze fresh lemon juice into the water you drink over the course of the day. Aim for a total of about 1/2 cup of juice.

Low-fat milk, cheese,
and other calcium-rich foods

For years, researchers thought that calcium in the diet contributed to the most common type of kidney stones, those made of calcium oxalate. People prone to these stones were consequently told to cut back on milk, cheese, and other dairy products. But the Nurses Health Study, which has been analyzing the diets of thousands of women for decades, has found

FEATURED RECIPES

Open-Faced Sardine Sandwiches *p. 300*
Mac 'n Cheese Primavera *p. 304*

that the more calcium-rich foods a woman eats, the lower her risk of developing kidney stones. As a result, physicians now advise patients to eat plenty of dairy foods.

It appears that when calcium binds with salts called oxalates in the gastrointestinal tract, the oxalates never enter the bloodstream to reach the kidneys. People prone to kidney stones who take calcium supplements to improve bone strength should be careful to take them with food so the calcium can bind with the oxalates, effectively ushering them away from the kidneys.

Aim for: 1,000 milligrams of dietary calcium per day (1,200 milligrams for people over 50). Get it by drinking 3 cups of milk or having a combination of cheese, yogurt, milk, and other calcium sources like sardines.

CAUTION

Spinach, rhubarb, chocolate, and other foods high in oxalates. This odd trio, along with a number of other foods, contains oxalates, components of calcium oxalate kidney stones. If you have this type of stones, your physician may advise you to limit foods high in oxalates. These include the foods above as well as almonds, beets, figs, Swiss chard, and wheat bran.

Caffeinated coffee, black tea, and cola. Caffeine can cause problems for people prone to stones. It appears to increase the amount of calcium released in urine, increasing the likelihood that calcium will bind with oxalates to form kidney stones. Limit beverages with caffeine to 2 or fewer cups per day. Because

black tea also contains oxalates, you may want to limit this as well.

Salt. People who eat a lot of salt tend to excrete more calcium in their urine than they would on a low-salt diet. Again, the more calcium that passes through the kidneys, the higher the likelihood that it will bind with oxalates to form kidney stones.

Try to limit your salt intake to 2,300 milligrams a day, about a teaspoon. The best way to cut back is to watch the canned, packaged, and processed foods you eat. Some brands of canned soup, for example, pack more than 1,000 milligrams of sodium into just 1 cup. Even condiments such as ketchup and salad dressing can be loaded with sodium. Check labels; a low-salt food contains not more than 140 milligrams of sodium per serving. And of course, cut back on using the saltshaker, too.

Meat, fish, and poultry. Some people with kidney stones have excessive acid in their urine (called uric acid) that can contribute to kidney stones. Don't confuse this with other types of acid, like citrate, that can benefit you by preventing the formation of stones in urine. If you are prone to this type of stones, your physician may suggest that you limit meat, fish, and poultry because these foods are high in purines, substances that can break down into uric acid in the body.

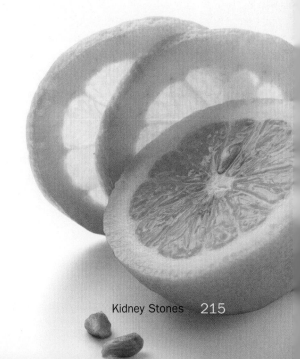

There are countless ways to get lemons into your diet, all of them delicious. Add lemon juice when you are cooking rice; squeeze on fresh vegetables; add to poaching liquids; roast a chicken with a pierced lemon in the cavity.

LEG CRAMPS

Here's a new reason to drink orange juice and eat bananas: Their potassium can help ease muscle cramps.

If you've ever had a charley horse—a sharp tightening of a muscle in the calf, foot, or other part of the leg—you know how painful it can be. Because these cramps often occur at night, they interrupt sleep. And they're more common with age.

A few smart tweaks to your diet can help. Some of the key nutrients that muscles depend on are electrolytes, minerals that work in tandem to balance the acidity and alkalinity of the body's fluids, so plan to get more calcium, potassium, and magnesium from your food. Some of the advice below should also help relieve restless legs syndrome (RLS), which causes uncomfortable sensations in the legs that are relieved only by moving.

YOUR FOOD PRESCRIPTION

Foods rich in calcium, potassium, and magnesium

In the right balance, these three minerals help muscles contract and relax. Having a steady supply of them helps prevent leg cramps that stem from an electrolyte imbalance. Pay special attention to magnesium; without enough, muscles can't relax after contracting—and many of us don't get enough. If you're taking a beta blocker to lower your blood pressure, check with your doctor to find out if it's the kind that depletes potassium from your system. Certain diuretics also deplete potassium and magnesium.

CALCIUM

Aim for: Three to four servings of low-fat dairy or other calcium-rich foods, like kale and other leafy dark greens, canned salmon with bones, and fortified orange juice.

POTASSIUM

Aim for: Frequent daily servings of avocados, asparagus, apricots, lentils, beans, yogurt, tomatoes or tomato juice, cantaloupe, and bananas.

MAGNESIUM

Aim for: Plenty of legumes, seafood, nuts, whole grains, leafy green vegetables—and a small amount of chocolate!

Water *and other fluids*

When an athlete gets muscle cramps during a workout, it's often due to dehydration. Most of us don't work out that hard, but fluids are still critical for keeping muscle cells hydrated (allowing muscles to contract and relax smoothly) and for getting electrolytes into cells, where they can be used for energy (otherwise, these key minerals could be lost through sweating).

If your cramps tend to come during or immediately following exercise, talk with your doctor. They could be a sign of atherosclerosis, or hardening of the arteries, which lets less oxygen reach muscles.

Aim for: At least eight 8-ounce glasses (2 l total) of water daily. If you exercise intensely, drink small amounts of fluid (3 to 5 ounces/88 to 147 ml) every 20 minutes during workouts.

Helpful hint: Athletes who exercise strenuously for 90 minutes or more may need to reestablish their electrolyte balance with a sports drink like Gatorade.

Tonic water

Quinine, a drug made from the bark of the cinchona tree, is prescribed by doctors in measured doses for some patients with leg cramps. It exists in small amounts in tonic water, providing it with that distinctive bitter flavor. The use of prescriptive quinine is controversial because too much can cause dizziness and dangerous blood problems, but tonic water is perfectly safe in moderate amounts.

Aim for: 8 to 16 ounces (227 to 473 ml) before bed.

Helpful hint: Brush your teeth after drinking tonic water at night. Like many other carbonated beverages, it often contains citric acids and sugars that can contribute to tooth decay.

NUTRITIONAL SUPPLEMENTS

B-complex vitamins. In one Taiwanese study, elderly patients with severe nighttime leg cramps found significant relief when they took vitamin B–complex pills for three months. Vitamin B_{12} is particularly important to the transmission of nerve impulses. **DOSAGE:** B-complex supplements vary in content, but the one used in the study contained 50 milligrams of B_1 (thiamin), 5 milligrams of B_2 (riboflavin), 30 milligrams of B_6, and 250 micrograms of B_{12}.

Folic acid. Some people's leg cramps may be due in part to a deficiency of folate. Women who take prenatal multivitamins (which include folic acid, the supplement form of folate) have a lower incidence of RLS, and in one study, pregnant women with the condition experienced relief after being treated with folic acid.

Check with your doctor before taking folic acid supplements, since they may mask a vitamin B_{12} deficiency. **DOSAGE:** 400 to 800 micrograms per day.

Vitamin E. Several studies have found that E can help alleviate leg cramps. The effective dose may vary from person to person. **DOSAGE:** 30 IU, the amount typically found in a multivitamin. Dosages over 1,200 IU can cause side effects like blurred vision, dizziness, and headaches.

Iron. Iron-deficiency anemia can cause muscle cramps, so check with your doctor to see if you may be anemic. Women and elderly people are particularly prone to this condition. Too little iron can also cause restless legs syndrome. **DOSAGE:** For women up to age 50, 18 milligrams a day, the amount in many multivitamins formulated for women. Men should avoid iron supplements unless a physician prescribes them for diagnosed anemia. Too much supplemental iron can cause constipation, so eat plenty of fiber and drink at least 8 cups of water a day to help avoid it.

Magnesium. There is some evidence that magnesium supplements can help pregnant women with leg cramps; if you're pregnant, check with your doctor before taking supplements. But almost everyone can do with more magnesium than they get in their diets. An extra 400 milligrams per day, taken with food, may help and certainly does no harm. The glycinate and malate forms of magnesium are less likely than citrate and hydroxide forms to cause diarrhea. **DOSAGE:** Typically, 100 to 400 milligrams per day will correct a deficiency.

CAUTION

Caffeine. Caffeine is a diuretic, flushing the body of fluids that the muscles need to function smoothly. It also constricts blood vessels, decreasing circulation to muscles, and interferes with the body's absorption of magnesium. If you have restless legs syndrome, definitely avoid caffeine. It increases levels of the brain chemical dopamine, and overproduction of dopamine is thought to be a cause of RLS.

FEATURED RECIPES

Tuna and White Bean Salad p. 295
Lentil-Tomato Soup p. 299
Salmon Cake Sandwiches p. 302
Thai Roasted Shrimp p. 310
Banana-Peanut Bread p. 326

LUNG CANCER

First things first: If you smoke, stop. Tobacco use is responsible for 87 percent of lung cancer deaths. Of course, even nonsmokers get lung cancer (and being around secondhand smoke can increase your risk by up to 30 percent).

What can you do to protect yourself, besides run screaming from cigarettes? Eat more fruits and vegetables. Swedish scientists recently found that people—smokers and nonsmokers alike—who eat a lot of vegetables have half the lung cancer risk compared to non–veggie eaters. That's because vegetables contain a grab bag of cancer-protective compounds, like the carotenoids in dark green and deep yellow, orange, and red produce. So while it's certainly not license to puff away, eating some extra broccoli, papaya, or red peppers may help you breathe a little easier.

YOUR FOOD PRESCRIPTION

Cruciferous vegetables

If carcinogens are like a heavy metal band that's prone to trashing hotel rooms, think of cruciferous vegetables as a crack security squad that hustles them out before they do harm. What makes vegetables like cauliflower, brussels sprouts, and especially broccoli such great bodyguards is their sulforaphane, considered one of the most potent cancer fighters found in food.

Cruciferous vegetables also contain a substance called indole-3-carbinol, which works like a cleanup crew, repairing damage that carcinogens do to cells before they can turn cancerous. No wonder some research suggests that eating more broccoli and brussels sprouts may lower the risk of lung cancer by as much as 40 percent.

FEATURED RECIPES

Tropical Fruit Salad *p. 286*
Edamame Hummus with Pita Crisps *p. 288*
Broccoli Salad *p. 291*
Citrus Chicken Salad *p. 294*
Open-Faced Sardine Sandwiches *p. 300*
Tomato-Roasted Mackerel *p. 308*
Roasted Salmon with Sautéed Greens *p. 309*
Brussels Sprouts with Caramelized Onions *p. 319*

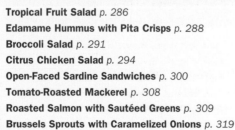

Aim for: At least four 1/2-cup servings weekly.

Helpful hint: Steaming broccoli for 3 to 4 minutes, until it's crisp-tender, makes more of its sulforaphane available.

Oranges, papayas, peaches, red bell peppers, and carrots

Notice something these foods have in common? The colors orange and red, of course. Those colors come from a type of carotenoid (an orange antioxidant pigment) called beta-cryptoxanthin that specifically seems to safeguard smokers.

According to the World Cancer Research Fund and the American Institute of Cancer Research, the evidence is consistent yet still limited that the consumption of foods containing carotenoids reduces the risk for lung cancer. Skip the beta-carotene supplements, however. High doses are a convincing cause of lung cancer if you have ever been a smoker, says this same report.

Aim for: Include red-orange fruits and vegetables among your daily 4 to 6 cups.

Soy foods

Some very early research suggests that as in breast cancer, estrogen may encourage the growth of lung tumors, and researchers suspect that blunting estrogen's effects may help slow or even stop lung cancer's development.

Here's how it's thought to work: Lung cancer cells have estrogen receptors; you can think of them as parking spots reserved for estrogen. But soy's estrogen-like compounds (phytoestrogens called isoflavones) may block those spots so "real" estrogen can't park there. The research is still limited but in one study of more than 3,400 people conducted at MD Anderson Cancer Center in Houston, volunteers who ate more foods high in isoflavones (soy, as well as broccoli, spinach, and carrots, which contain isoflavones called lignans) had about a 46 percent lower risk of lung cancer.

Aim for: Research suggests that one to three servings a day of soy foods like tofu, soy milk, and edamame are enough to alter estrogen activity. More isn't better when it comes to phytoestrogens, so stick with soy foods rather than isoflavone supplements.

Salmon, sardines, mackerel, *and other foods high in omega-3 fatty acids*

Some research suggests the combination of cigarette smoke and animal fats promotes lung cancer. Substituting fish high in omega-3 fatty acids for meats appears to minimize the effect.

According to a Belgian study that examined fish consumption in 36 countries over 30 years, eating more fatty fish appeared to reduce lung cancer mortality. For instance, Hungary and Iceland both have high smoking rates, and animal fats are a big part of the diet. But fish consumption is higher in Iceland, which may explain why lung cancer deaths among men are more than three times lower there than in Hungary.

Aim for: Two to three servings a week.

Spinach, kale, beans, *and other foods rich in folate*

If you smoke (or recently quit), load up on folate, a B vitamin that safeguards cells from tobacco carcinogens. Another study done at the

MD Anderson Cancer Center found that former smokers who had enough folate in their diets lowered their risk of lung cancer by 40 percent. Smoking drains folate from the body, as does alcohol consumption.

Aim for: 400 micrograms of folate each day. You may be getting that much if you take a multivitamin. But you can also get it from food if you eat at least three servings of whole grains each day, along with four to six servings of fruit and vegetables. At least one of those vegetable servings should be leafy dark greens or legumes. The safe upper limit for folate is 1,000 micrograms from food and supplements.

Helpful hint: Spinach packs a double anticancer punch—it's a great source of folate as well as other cancer fighters like carotenoids and phytoestrogens.

NUTRITIONAL SUPPLEMENTS

Vitamin C. If someone in your family smokes, or you frequent smoky places, take some vitamin C "insurance." A study at the University of California, Berkeley, found that for nonsmokers, C supplements reduced free radical damage caused by secondhand smoke by about 11 percent. (Free radicals can alter cell DNA, which over time can cause cells to turn cancerous.) In addition, C helps vitamin E protect the lungs from cigarette damage. While smoking quickly depletes E, according to a study done at Oregon State University, taking extra C maintains E at levels typically found in nonsmokers. **DOSAGE:** 500 to 1,000 milligrams daily if you are frequently exposed to smoke.

CAUTION

Red and processed meat. Several population studies suggest a link between meat (particularly if it's grilled or fried) and lung cancer. The evidence that links red and processed meat to lung cancer is still limited but consistent, says the American Institute for Cancer Research. These experts recommend limiting red meat to no more than 18 ounces (510 g) a week and avoiding processed meat if possible.

LUPUS

Lupus remains one of medicine's biggest mysteries. Researchers still don't fully understand exactly what triggers this autoimmune disease, but it's thought to develop when certain types of genes that may predispose someone to lupus interact with environmental factors like common viruses. The immune system gets misdirected and produces antibodies that target the body's tissues and organs. As these antibodies, called auto-antibodies, build up in various organs, inflammation results. There are several types of lupus, the most common being systemic lupus erythematosus (SLE). It can be mild, causing fatigue, joint pain, or skin rashes, or severe, affecting major organs like the kidneys.

People with lupus are always instructed to eat a healthy diet low in fat and high in fresh vegetables. But is it possible that nutrition can do more to alleviate symptoms and perhaps even stymie the disease? Since many of the medications used to treat lupus work by reducing inflammation and calming an overactive immune system, it makes sense that eating foods and taking supplements that do likewise can help, too (in addition to—not in place of—medication). Although there is no "lupus diet" per se, some very preliminary studies in animals and humans suggest that nutrition may be useful for reducing the severity of flare-ups and encouraging remission.

YOUR FOOD PRESCRIPTION

Fish *and other foods high in omega-3 essential fatty acids*

There's some evidence that in cultures like Japan and the Eskimo communities in Greenland, where people consume a lot of omega-3 essential fatty acids from fish, seafood, and other sources, the rates of autoimmune disease are lower than in countries where intake of omega-3s is low. That doesn't necessarily mean that fish low-

ers the risk of lupus, but it's worth noting that there's already a fairly well established association between high fish consumption and lower rates of conditions like depression and heart disease, so the idea isn't very far-fetched.

There haven't been specific studies on eating fish to decrease lupus flare-ups, but research does suggest that taking supplements of the omega-3s EPA and DHA (found in fatty cold-water fish) reduces autoimmune disease–related inflammation and may slow the progression of disease (see Nutritional Supplements on the next page)—though it's hard to say whether this is due to the supplements or the natural ebb and flow of the disease. In a 24-week study of 60 people with SLE, researchers at Ulster University in Northern Ireland found that those taking 3 grams of an EPA supplement reported about a 23 percent decline in disease activity compared to those taking placebos. In a British study of 27 patients taking 20 grams daily of EPA for 34 weeks, about half the participants found it beneficial.

FEATURED RECIPES

Spinach Salad with Chickpeas *p. 293*
Tuna and White Bean Salad *p. 295*
Open-Faced Sardine Sandwiches *p. 300*
Tomato-Roasted Mackerel *p. 308*
Roasted Salmon with Sautéed Greens *p. 309*

Flaxseed is another source of omega-3s, particularly alpha-linolenic acid (ALA). In one very small, two-year study done in Canada, kidney function improved among eight participants who mixed 30 grams (about an ounce) of flaxseed into their daily cereal or juice.

Aim for: At least two servings of fish per week. To get the amounts of omega-3 fatty acids used in the studies, you'll need supplements.

Helpful hint: For a double anti-inflammatory whammy, choose fish like salmon, rainbow trout, and scallops. They all contain omega-3s as well as high levels of the antioxidant mineral selenium, which is also anti-inflammatory.

Green tea

Some population studies suggest that lupus incidence is lower in countries like China and Japan, where green tea is a diet staple. One explanation may be that green tea contains potent compounds called polyphenols that are both antioxidant and anti-inflammatory. It's possible that adding green tea to your diet or even applying it directly to the skin rashes that often accompany lupus may be helpful. When green tea polyphenols were mixed with skin and salivary gland cells in lab studies done at the Medical College of Georgia, researchers noted a significant decrease in the markers for SLE.

Aim for: Because the research is still so preliminary, more studies need to be done before any definitive recommendations can be made. But it couldn't hurt to start drinking a few cups of green tea a day.

NUTRITIONAL SUPPLEMENTS

Omega-3 fatty acids. Researchers are still divided over whether omega-3s are helpful for autoimmune diseases, particularly since more dramatic results are seen in animal studies than in human ones. But a small study done in India found that supplementing with EPA and DHA (which work better together than alone) appeared to induce remission in 10 patients with SLE. In other studies, when people with

Can a Vegetarian Diet Help?

The answer is "probably." Research suggests that vegetarian and low-fat vegan diets (no animal products at all) significantly reduce symptoms of other chronic inflammatory diseases like rheumatoid arthritis.

Vegetarian diets usually contain less protein than meat-centered diets. Since getting too much protein puts added strain on the kidneys, a switch may help if lupus is affecting your kidneys, as it does in about 60 percent of cases. If your doctor wants you to eat less protein, this may mean you'll need to cut back on fish, too (when it comes to kidney function, protein is protein), but it's possible to get anti-inflammatory omega-3 fats from plant sources like flaxseed or from supplements.

Another reason to avoid or cut back on animal fats: They contain arachidonic acid, which stimulates inflammation.

chronic inflammatory conditions took fish oil, they were able to reduce their use of non-steroidal anti-inflammatory medications. **DOSAGE:** 3 to 6 grams of high-quality fish oil daily only under your doctor's supervision. Fish oil should always be refrigerated. If you find that a fishy taste or smell is "repeating" on you, it's an indication that the oil is rancid and needs to be replaced.

Antioxidants, especially vitamin E, vitamin A, and selenium. Some research suggests that low levels of vitamins A and E, thought to be a risk factor for rheumatoid arthritis, may also be a risk factor for lupus. Animals deficient in vitamin A seem to have more severe lupus symptoms. A recent review of dietary strategies for the treatment of SLE found that a diet high in antioxidant nutrients can help suppress inflammation and protect against tissue damage. **DOSAGE:** Look for a multivitamin formula that contains close to 100 percent Daily Value for antioxidant vitamins A, C, and E, beta-carotene, and selenium.

Vitamin D. Recent studies show that a deficiency of vitamin D may predispose people to a variety of autoimmune diseases. Additionally, many people in the United States, particularly in the northern states, are deficient in D. Vitamin D deficiency clearly contributes to the widespread osteoporosis that's seen in women and even men, and especially in people treated with certain lupus medications, such as steroids. A recent prospective study of 18,000 women over 22 years found no evidence that vitamin D intake was protective against SLE. Other studies, however, have shown a decrease in inflammation in patients with SLE at doses as low as 200 IU per day. **DOSAGE:** 400 to 1,000 IU per day. Check with your doctor if higher doses are recommended.

CAUTION

Safflower, sunflower, and corn oils and most margarines. These are rich in omega-6 essential fats, but the type that some experts say we eat too much of. In the United States, most of us consume far too many omega-6s and too few anti-inflammatory omega-3s. This imbalance is believed by some experts to be a contributing factor in other chronic inflammatory conditions, like rheumatoid arthritis.

In a very small study of 11 lupus patients who reduced their dietary intake of omega-6s for a year, 8 participants experienced a reduction in their symptoms. A German study of 60 people with rheumatoid arthritis gives further credence to the idea: Among those who consumed an anti-inflammatory diet, the number of tender, swollen joints decreased by 14 percent compared to those eating a standard Western diet. When the participants on the anti-inflammatory diet then added fish-oil supplements for two months, their joint swelling and pain decreased even more.

Alfalfa. Alfalfa seeds and sprouts contain the amino acid L-canavanine, which appears to aggravate lupus symptoms.

Foods high in zinc. You never want to become zinc deficient, because this nutrient is critical to so many body functions. But it's also one of the most effective natural immune system boosters, so if you have lupus, you may not want to take extra. Stick to the recommended amount of 15 milligrams a day and steer clear of zinc-rich foods like oysters and Brazil nuts.

Echinacea. Because this herb stimulates immune function, people with lupus are advised not to take it because it may initiate flare-ups. Indeed, in European countries, echinacea labels state that it's contraindicated in people with autoimmune diseases.

DHEA: Another Solution?

Sex hormones play a role in immune function, and because estrogens are known to increase production of auto-antibodies, an imbalance in estrogen may be one reason that lupus primarily affects women. Although it's still very controversial, balancing estrogen with an androgen or male sex hormone, like the dietary supplement DHEA, may prove helpful, particularly because androgens reduce inflammation and suppress the immune system. Indeed, a California company is currently testing pharmaceutical-grade DHEA for lupus.

In a Taiwan study, 120 women with active SLE took either 200 milligrams of DHEA a day or a placebo for 24 weeks. The number of women with flare-ups was 16 percent lower in the DHEA group than in the placebo group. In other studies, participants who took DHEA were able to reduce their dosages of steroid medications.

Studies on DHEA typically used 200 milligrams a day. But there are some caveats with DHEA, so it should be used only under a doctor's supervision. DHEA boosts testosterone levels, resulting in increased acne, facial hair, and abnormal cholesterol and triglyceride profiles. Long-term use is associated with liver cancer in rats, and over time, it may even aggravate lupus symptoms. Also, because dietary supplements aren't regulated by the FDA, the amount of DHEA in over-the-counter preparations may vary from formulation to formulation and may even differ from what's stated on the label.

MACULAR DEGENERATION

When someone says "Feast your eyes on this," he's not usually pointing to a big salad or a plate of steamed spinach. But maybe he should be. Recent studies have shown that certain foods—especially fruits and vegetables—can protect our eyes from age-related macular degeneration (AMD).

AMD is the most common cause of severe, irreversible vision loss in people 50 and older. Its target is the macula, a tiny yellow area near the center of the retina that's highly specialized to allow you to see details and provide clear central (not peripheral) vision, the kind you need to read and drive.

Although experts aren't sure what causes AMD—they now believe that heredity plays a role in many cases—it's usually characterized by a loss of pigment in the retina as well as yellowish deposits called drusen. And there's strong evidence that nutrition plays a role in preventing it. In fact, parts of the macula are actually made of certain nutrients that we get from food. Loading up your plate with the right foods won't cure AMD, but it can slow its progress and also lower your risk of developing it in the first place.

YOUR FOOD PRESCRIPTION

Spinach, collard greens, kale,
and other green leafy vegetables

One of the very best things you can do to keep your vision sharp is to eat more greens. They're loaded with lutein and zeaxanthin (pronounced zee-uh-ZAN-thin), a pair of natural plant pigments often found together in foods. These antioxidant pigments are part of the carotenoid family (think beta-carotene), and they're the only carotenoids found in the eye. Studies have found that people with high levels of lutein and zeaxanthin have as much as three times less risk of AMD than those with lower levels.

That's not so surprising, since the macula's yellow pigment is made up of lutein and zeaxanthin. Researchers believe they act as a kind of super sunscreen, protecting the retina by absorbing a damaging part of sunlight called blue light. The two antioxidants also protect the retina's cells from damaging free radicals. Zeaxanthin, the main component of the macula, may also bulk up its pigment, which in turn appears to shore up the macula's sensitivity to visual signals.

Although greens—especially cooked ones—carry the largest share of lutein and zeaxanthin, the pair is also plentiful in brightly colored fruits and vegetables like orange bell peppers, corn, persimmons, and tangerines.

Aim for: 6 to 10 milligrams of lutein and zeaxanthin per day—a bit more than the amount in 1/2 cup of cooked spinach or kale.

Helpful hint: Sauté your greens in olive oil or add some oil-based dressing to your salad. Fat helps the body absorb lutein and zeaxanthin. Indulge in a spinach omelet as well. Although eggs don't have the wealth of the two antioxidants that greens do, they have enough fat to make sure you get what's there.

Fish *and other foods rich in omega-3 fatty acids*

Fish has been touted as a heart-healthy food, but researchers have also found that fish and other foods high in omega-3 fatty acids can lower the risk of AMD by as much as 30 percent.

The two main components of the omega-3s in fish, known as EPA and DHA, are essential for the development and function of the retina. The membranes of the photoreceptor cells—especially the rods—are also packed with DHA. It helps the membranes remain fluid, which in turn may help protein molecules in the rods respond to light. Omega-3s also help produce beneficial types of prostaglandins, hormone-like substances that affect many processes in the body, including blood flow and nerve transmission, both of which affect eye health.

Not a fish fan? Look to walnuts, flaxseed, flaxseed oil, and soybeans for alpha-linolenic acid (ALA), which the body converts (poorly, unfortunately) to DHA and EPA. ALA is essential because it can't be made by the body.

Aim for: 8 to 12 ounces (236 to 340 g) of fatty fish a week. Too busy to grill fish? Toss a quarter cup of walnuts into a salad or add a tablespoon of ground flaxseed to oatmeal to get your daily dose of omega-3s.

Helpful hint: To avoid contaminants in fish, avoid swordfish, which is generally high in mercury, and try to eat a variety of fish. Fill out your diet with more omega-3s by eating walnuts and flaxseed.

Carrots, red bell peppers, almonds, and sunflower seeds

In a major clinical trial, the National Eye Institute found that high doses of beta-carotene and vitamins C and E, coupled with zinc, stopped or slowed the progression of AMD by 25 percent over a five-year period. Although the effective doses were far higher than you can get from diet alone, heaping your plate with food dense in these nutrients makes sense, especially for people who already have AMD or are at increased risk for it (such as those with a family history of the disease and possibly people with light eye color).

You'll get plenty of beta-carotene from the leafy greens we've already recommended; other great food sources are carrots and sweet potatoes. Spinach also provides vitamin E, and almonds and sunflower seeds are even better sources. For vitamin C, turn to red bell peppers, orange juice, citrus fruits, and broccoli.

Scientists aren't certain why the antioxidants in these foods protect the eyes, but they have some clues. Beta-carotene converts to vitamin A in the body, and in the retina, that's converted to a rod protein essential for the perception of light.

Like beta-carotene, vitamins C and E are powerful antioxidants that protect cells—including those in the macula—from damaging free radicals. And the mix of these antioxidants is apparently more effective than the nutrients acting singly. For example, vitamin E requires vitamin C to do its job as an antioxidant.

Aim for: *Beta-carotene:* 15 milligrams daily, about the amount in a sweet potato with skin or a cup of cooked spinach. You'll get even more from a cup of carrot juice. *Vitamin E:* 400 IU (about 268 milligrams) daily. This amount is virtually impossible to get from foods, especially on a low-fat diet, so you'll need help from supplements. A quarter cup of sunflower seeds has about 8 milligrams, an ounce (28 g) of almonds has about 7, and a cup of cooked spinach has almost 4. *Vitamin C:* 500 milligrams daily, which you can get from a cup of orange juice plus a cup of chopped red bell pepper.

FEATURED RECIPES

Spinach Salad with Chickpeas *p. 293*
Sweet Potato Soup *p. 297*
Roasted Salmon with Sautéed Greens *p. 309*
Beef and Broccoli Stew *p. 316*
Creamed Spinach *p. 320*
Raspberry-Almond Muffins *p. 324*

Oysters, crab, beef, baked beans, *and other foods rich in zinc*

Zinc, an essential mineral found in meats (especially liver) and seafood (especially oysters), acts as vitamin A's partner, ensuring that it can be used by the body, including the retina. Scientists believe the retina's high levels of zinc help protect its membranes.

Aim for: 15 to 20 milligrams of zinc daily. A can of baked beans in tomato sauce contains about 14 milligrams; 3 ounces (118 g) of lamb or crab, about 6 milligrams; and 3 ounces (118 g) of ground beef, about 5 milligrams. If you like oysters, 3 ounces (118 g) will get you to 76 milligrams of zinc.

Helpful hint: A serving of fortified cereal contains all the zinc you need for the day.

NUTRITIONAL SUPPLEMENTS

Lutein and zeaxanthin. In a second clinical trial called AREDS2 (Age-Related Eye Disease Study 2), the National Eye Institute found that doses of 10 milligrams of lutein and 2 milligrams of zeaxanthin (carotenoid substances) reduced the risk for advanced AMD slightly more than formulas that contained beta-carotene. Supplements with this formulation are now available over the counter. (Look for AREDS2 on the label.)

Omega-3 fatty acids. Omega-3s come in soft-gel fish-oil capsules or in liquid form. Because omega-3s are sensitive to heat, light, and oxygen, store supplements in the refrigerator. Also, choose a supplement with vitamin E, which will help keep the omega-3s from becoming rancid.

Although previous studies found that the omega-3 fatty acids DHA and EPA helped promote eye health, taking supplements that contained 350 milligrams of DHA and 650 milligrams of EPA did not reduce the risk of advanced AMD in the AREDS2 clinical trial. **DOSAGE:** A safe dose of omega-3s is about 1,000 milligrams a day. Talk to your doctor if you are considering higher doses.

Vitamins C and E, and zinc. This combination of nutrients is thus far the only proven way to halt or slow the progression of AMD. In the AREDS2 trial, researchers found that a reduced—and safer—dose of zinc (25 milligrams instead of 80 milligrams in the original AREDS trial) was still as effective in reducing the risk for advanced macular degeneration. And the AREDS2 formula also eliminated beta-carotene due to the finding that beta-carotene supplements increased the risk for lung cancer in

Can steak be bad for your eyes? If it's fatty, the answer is yes. Animal fats boost free radical activity in your body, which can harm cells in your retinas.

smokers or former smokers. Substituting lutein and zeaxanthin (other types of carotenoids) for beta-carotene in the AREDS2 formula was effective in some participants, however. **DOSAGE:** *Vitamin C:* 500 milligrams daily. *Vitamin E:* 400 IU daily. *Zinc:* 25 milligrams of zinc oxide daily. *Lutein:* 10 milligrams daily. *Zeaxanthin:* 2 milligrams daily.

If you have macular degeneration, talk to your doctor to see if the AREDS2 formula may be helpful.

CAUTION

Fatty meats, butter, and other sources of saturated fat. Saturated fats boost free radical activity, undermining antioxidants' good work. Keep your meat choices as lean as possible and stick to small servings (3 to 6 ounces/85 to 170 g). Use only small amounts of butter (a teaspoon at a time) or use a soft tub margarine with no trans fat. Cheese is another source of saturated fat, so use it sparingly and buy low-fat or part-skim cheese whenever possible. Soft cheeses like goat cheese have slightly less fat per ounce (28 g) than hard types.

Alcohol. Too much alcohol also undermines the work of antioxidants. Alcohol forms two harmful compounds called acetaldehyde and malondialdehyde, which stoke up cellular damage by free radicals (and which make us feel so bad the day after one too many). It also depletes vitamin A, one of the antioxidants proven to slow AMD.

Corn, sunflower, and safflower oils. Many experts think that consuming more omega-6 fatty acids in these oils and the packaged foods made with them at the expense of omega-3s (fish, walnuts, and flaxseed) may contribute to inflammation. And recent studies show that, while an increased intake of omega-3s decreases the risk for macular degeneration, higher intakes of one type of omega-6 fatty acid increased the risk.

Squeezing More Nutrients from Your Food

Want to get more omega-3s from your flaxseed and more antioxidants from your spinach? Buy, store, and prepare them properly.

Nuts and flaxseed: Exposure to heat, light, and oxygen not only lowers the nutritive value of omega-3 fatty acids but also releases free radicals, the enemies of the retina (as well as other body tissues). Store nuts, ground flaxseed, and ground cloves (surprisingly high in omega-3s) in dark jars in the refrigerator or freezer. Buy whole flaxseed and grind it as needed; the seed's shell and the vitamin E within the seed protect the omega-3 oils from oxidation.

Walnut and flaxseed oils: Use these heat-sensitive oils for salads, not stir-fries.

Leafy greens: Leafy greens and other vegetables are highest in sight-saving nutrients right after they're picked. Buy the freshest greens you can and eat them within two days. The greener the leaves, the more packed they are with antioxidants, and leaves trump stems, so fill up on stemless outer leaves. Although cooking greens, especially in water, destroys a small percentage of some vitamins and minerals, such as vitamin C, steaming, microwaving, or stir-frying will minimize the loss. And cooking actually makes some nutrients like carotenoids more available.

Fruits: Once you cut them, dig in, because vitamin C is destroyed by the air exposure.

MEMORY LOSS

If we lose our keys, we think we're losing our marbles. But in fact, everyone experiences some "recall shortfalls" from time to time. It's a normal side effect of stress, distractions, multitasking, and yes, getting older. Serious memory lapses could be a sign of dementia (see the Alzheimer's Disease entry on page 94), but plain old forgetfulness isn't usually something to fret about. The fact is, the memory usually serves us well enough even when our joints and other body parts start to go. That said, brain cells do shrink over the years, and eventually our brains make fewer chemicals called neurotransmitters that carry messages from one nerve cell to the next. Attacks from free radicals, which roam the whole body, also take their toll on brain cells over time.

Want to remember why you walked into a room? Start by walking into your kitchen. There you'll find "brain foods" rich in protective nutrients, such as antioxidants that neutralize free radicals, B vitamins that help ensure sufficient quantities of neurotransmitters, and inflammation-dousing oils and even spices. If, after adding more of these foods to your daily diet, you still can't remember the name of your dentist to make an appointment … well, you've gone too long without a cleaning.

YOUR FOOD PRESCRIPTION

Fruits, vegetables, nuts,
and other foods rich in antioxidants

Brain cells called neurons are particularly vulnerable to oxidation by free radicals. These rogue molecules attack cells much like oxygen "attacks" a freshly cut apple, turning it brown and "aging" it prematurely. Antioxidants, found in abundance in most fruits and vegetables and in nuts and beans, neutralize free radicals. When you eat enough of these foods, your brain collects antioxidants, and this offers protection to various parts of the brain, including the hippocampus, a region that's key to forming and retaining memories. Antioxidants also help prevent atherosclerosis, or hardening of the arteries, which limits the flow of oxygen and nutrients to the brain.

You can get your fill of three particularly important antioxidants—vitamins C and E and the mineral selenium—by filling your plate with fruits, vegetables, and nuts.

Aim for: 4 to 6 cups of fruits and vegetables a day, plus a handful of nuts a few times a week.

Helpful hint: An ounce (28 g) of almonds offers 7 milligrams of vitamin E (you need 15 milligrams daily). One kiwifruit provides 75 milligrams of vitamin C, close to your daily requirement.

Spinach

Popeye had it right: Eating lots of spinach does make you stronger, at least mentally. Spinach-rich diets have proven particularly useful in helping patients recover motor skills like walking following a stroke or other neurological damage, and at least one enzyme in spinach has also proven effective in recovering memory in rats.

Aim for: Make spinach at least one of your daily servings of fruits and vegetables.

Helpful hint: Cook or serve spinach with a drizzle of olive oil. The fat helps the body absorb fat-soluble nutrients like vitamin E from the leafy greens.

Blueberries

When summer rolls around, there's nothing like fresh blueberries. But here's a reason to stock your freezer and eat them all year long: a better memory. The sweet blue globes are powerhouses of phytochemicals called anthocyanins—the compounds that give the berries their hue, act as strong antioxidants, and may, according to studies in aging lab animals, enhance memory. Rats did better on water maze tests after they were fed blueberry extracts over the course of eight weeks. According to the study authors, the blueberries improved age-related deficits in neuronal signaling, which translates to better message carrying between nerve cells.

Aim for: 1/2 cup a day.

Salmon, mackerel,
and other fish rich in omega-3 fatty acids

The brain contains tremendous amounts of fats, so it comes as no surprise that healthy fats in the diet benefit your "think tank." Brain cells are lined with omega-3 fatty acids that help reduce inflammation. These same fats help keep blood vessels elastic so oxygen and nutrients can flow upstairs unimpeded.

Although some research suggests that a diet rich in omega-3 fatty acids can protect the brain, a recent clinical trial with 4,000 older patients found that supplements of omega-3 fatty acids did not slow memory decline. Best to get your omega-3s in food, especially fish. Studies have shown that people who consume fish once or twice a week have slower declines in cognitive function.

Aim for: Two fish meals a week. Bake, poach, or broil fish instead of frying, or pan-fry it in a little olive oil.

Olive oil

Researchers have linked getting a relatively high proportion of calories from monounsaturated fats like those in olive oil with lower rates of cognitive decline. This is particularly true when these fats are consumed as part of the typical Mediterranean diet (rich in vegetables, whole grains, legumes, and fish). While low-fat diets are touted for many health conditions, the brain needs these "good" fats to function well.

Aim for: 1 to 2 tablespoons a day. Use olive oil and other monounsaturated oils like canola oil in place of butter and margarine.

Eggs

One of the few foods known to contain choline, the vitamin-like compound that cells need to function properly, eggs are particularly important in the diets of pregnant women while their babies' brains are developing. Studies have shown that rats whose mothers ate plenty of choline had stronger memories even into old age. Choline appears to be crucial to the development of the hippocampus, the memory center of the brain. Egg yolks also contain lots of vitamin B_{12}, which is known to help lower homocysteine. At high levels, this amino acid has been linked to cardiovascular disease that can lead to memory-impairing stroke. In fact, homocysteine is toxic to the brain and is linked to poor brain performance.

Aim for: One egg a few times a week. If you have high cholesterol, talk to your doctor about the number of eggs appropriate for your diet.

FEATURED RECIPES

Zucchini Frittata *p. 287*
Updated Waldorf Salad *p. 290*
Broccoli Salad *p. 291*
Open-Faced Sardine Sandwiches *p. 300*
Tomato-Roasted Mackerel *p. 308*
Roasted Salmon with Sautéed Greens *p. 309*
Curry-Seared Scallops *p. 310*
Blueberry-Oat Scones *p. 324*

Garlic

You probably think of your heart when you think about garlic and health, but your brain also benefits from these pungent cloves. Their sulfur compounds are potent antioxidants. Garlic also helps lower cholesterol and high blood pressure and reduce inflammation, three factors that increase the risk of heart disease and dementia.

Aim for: At least one clove a day, although more is better.

Helpful hint: When using garlic in recipes, chop it and let it stand for 10 to 15 minutes before cooking. The waiting period allows the garlic's active compounds to develop.

Cinnamon

Pop a stick of cinnamon chewing gum the next time you have to take an exam or recite a poem from memory. One study showed that when volunteers chewed cinnamon gum before being tested on various tasks, they performed better than those who chewed no gum or gum of other flavors (including peppermint). Researchers hope to someday use cinnamon to help the elderly improve brain function and performance. Cinnamon also has anti-inflammatory properties that may help keep your brain sharp when you add the spice to your meals.

Aim for: Sprinkle cinnamon on sliced fruit, hot breakfast cereal, lattes, and even soups and stews.

Apples

Could a daily apple in your lunch bag help sharpen your memory skills? It's possible, especially if you eat the skin, where most of the apple's quercetin is stored. In at least one study, this antioxidant proved more effective than vitamin C at protecting brain cells from oxidative damage.

Aim for: An apple a day, of course!

Wine, beer, and spirits

Although too much alcohol is bad for the brain, some studies have found that people, older people in particular, who have one to two drinks a day have a lower risk of memory loss than those who never drink. Other studies, however, show that even moderate alcohol consumption is not protective for the brain.

Aim for: If you choose to drink, up to one drink a day for women, two for men. One drink is either 4 ounces (118 ml) of wine, 1.5 ounces (44 ml) of hard liquor, or 12 ounces (355 ml) of beer.

Curry dishes
and other foods containing turmeric

The bright yellow spice called turmeric, used in traditional Indian curries and other dishes, gets its lovely hue from an antioxidant compound called curcumin. Animal studies have shown that curcumin helps prevent the formation of amyloid, the gummy protein buildup that can clog neural pathways in the brain. Curcumin also helps prevent oxidation and inflammation.

Aim for: 1 tablespoon of turmeric daily, about the amount found in two traditional curry dishes. You may also opt for up to 400 milligrams of curcumin in supplement form, but check with your doctor first.

Tea

Want to get your fill of antioxidants? Take up a tea habit. One animal study from England has shown that the antioxidants in both black and green teas can inhibit several of the enzymes that have been linked to the progression of Alzheimer's disease. Studies also suggest that tea may help prevent the protein buildup that slows communication between neurons, damming the brain's memory channels.

Aim for: Scientists need to do more studies before they'll suggest just how much tea is the right amount for protecting memory. In the meantime, a few cups a day can be healthful.

Oatmeal, high-fiber breakfast cereals, and whole grains

Where memory is concerned, the best breakfast cereal may be good old-fashioned oatmeal. In one recent study, when children ate oatmeal rather than cold cereal or no breakfast, their memory skills improved by 5 to 12 percent. In other research, the more whole grain the cereal, the more it appeared to improve memory. Scientists suspect that it may be the high fiber and protein content of oatmeal and whole-grain cereals that helps slow digestion, releasing glucose (blood sugar) more gradually into the bloodstream. The brain uses glucose as a source of energy, and a steady flow appears to help the brain retain information for tasks that require memory skills.

Aim for: One bowl of oatmeal or other cereal with at least 5 grams of fiber per serving. Top it with blueberries and toasted nuts for a real brain boost.

Helpful hint: Old-fashioned or steel-cut oats digest somewhat slower than instant oatmeal does. If you opt for instant, buy the plain (unsweetened) stuff and add your own flavorings, such as cinnamon.

Leafy greens, lentils, fish,
and other foods rich in B vitamins

Folate (also known as folic acid) and vitamins B_6 and B_{12} help lower levels of homocysteine, an amino acid in blood that has been linked to increased risk of dementia. High levels usually signify a deficiency of B vitamins. One study showed that people with high homocysteine levels and low folate levels had difficulty remembering words and details from a short story.

Aim for: A banana at breakfast; a spinach salad with chickpeas, bell pepper, and avocado at lunch; and a serving of fish at dinner should deliver the B vitamins you need for the day. Most breakfast cereals are also excellent sources of B vitamins, added by the manufacturers to replace the vitamins lost when grains are refined.

NUTRITIONAL SUPPLEMENTS

A multivitamin/mineral. The brain is so complex that its proper care and feeding remain a bit mysterious. For added insurance, take a daily multivitamin to make sure that your noggin gets all the nutrients it needs. **DOSAGE:** One a day.

Iron. Blood depends on iron to help deliver oxygen to the brain. People with iron-deficiency anemia can have significant memory loss. **DOSAGE:** Recommended daily amounts are 18 milligrams for women up to age 50 and 8 milligrams for women 50 and older and for men. You can usually get what you need from a multivitamin formulated for your age group or gender. If you suspect you have anemia, consult your doctor to confirm your suspicion and determine the amount of iron you need to correct the problem.

CAUTION

Fatty meats, butter, and other sources of saturated fat. Foods rich in saturated fat can trigger inflammation, not good for your heart or your brain.

White bread and flour, white rice, and sugary foods. These send blood sugar up and down in a hurry, but what the brain really needs is a steady supply.

MENOPAUSE

If you break into hot sweats more often than a diva changes clothes, look to your diet for help. By eating delicious vitamin E–rich foods like almonds and leafy greens or adding edamame (green soybeans) and flaxseed to your soups and salads, you may be able to turn down those "power surges" and reduce other symptoms of menopause, like insomnia, mood swings, or depression—and boost your overall health. And unlike hormone replacement therapy, these foods won't raise your risk of breast cancer or heart disease, and they may even lower it.

YOUR FOOD PRESCRIPTION

Soy foods, peas, flaxseed,
and other foods high in phytoestrogens

Soy is no cure-all for hot flashes and other menopause complaints, but for some women, it may help. Tofu, soy milk, edamame, and soy nuts all contain estrogen-like compounds called isoflavones. In the body, these act like weaker versions of estrogen, blocking the real stuff and, the theory goes, those annoying symptoms. Results on soy for hot flashes have been mixed, but some evidence suggests that foods high in phytoestrogens, like soy, beans, and peas, may reduce hot flashes by 9 to 40 percent.

One possible reason for the mixed study results is that only 30 to 40 percent of Americans can convert isoflavones into the active form, while 90 percent of Asians and all rats (often used in studies) can. Still, it's worth giving soy foods a try for a month to see if they make a difference.

You can also get around the conversion problem by enjoying fermented soy products like miso (a paste delicious in soups) and tempeh (the healthy person's french fry; brown it and add to stir-fries). The isoflavones in fermented soy are already converted.

Flaxseed's a great choice as well because it offers a triple package of fiber, heart-healthy omega-3 fatty acids, and chemicals called lignans that reduce the risk of breast cancer. And some studies show that it helps reduce hot flashes. The best way to use flaxseed is to grind 1 to 2 tablespoons a day in a coffee grinder used just for that purpose and enjoy it sprinkled on cereal and salads and in soups.

Aim for: There's no recommended amount for menopause, but try replacing some of your regular milk with soy milk (try it on your morning cereal) and some of the protein in your recipes with soy protein.

Almonds, sunflower seeds, wheat germ, leafy greens, olive oil, *and other foods high in vitamin E*

Limited research but lots of clinical evidence suggests that vitamin E may help prevent hot flashes. And a recent Tufts University study indicated that E helps prevent blood vessel blockage by keeping vessels dilated. This is important for menopausal women, whose risk of heart disease is two to three times higher than that of nonmenopausal women. Whole-grain cereals fortified with vitamin E are also excellent sources.

Aim for: There is no specific recommendation. Try starting your day with a bowl of whole-grain breakfast cereal sprinkled with wheat germ, and at dinner, toss a handful of sunflower seeds on top of a serving of spinach sautéed in olive oil.

Helpful hint: Because vitamin E requires vitamin C to remain active, toss your spinach salad with some slivered almonds, orange segments, or strawberries, and add some dried cranberries to nuts as a snack.

Chickpeas, fish, turkey,
and other foods high in vitamin B_6

If your spirits are lower than usual during menopause, consider serving yourself more fish, bananas, and other foods high in B_6. This vitamin spurs the production of hormones, including mood-boosting serotonin. It also helps prevent a buildup of homocysteine, an amino acid that ups the risk of heart disease. Some studies have also found that people with higher B_6 levels have better memory skills compared to people with lower levels.

Yams, often recommended for menopausal women, happen to be an excellent source of B_6. (They also contain compounds that resemble progesterone, another hormone that dips during menopause, but researchers have proven that our bodies can't use these compounds as they would progesterone.)

Aim for: Women need a minimum of 1.3 to 1.5 milligrams of vitamin B_6 daily, about the amount in a 4-ounce (113-g) serving of tuna or two bananas.

Helpful hint: You can sneak some B_6 into your meal by spicing things up; turmeric, cayenne, and ginger all contain small amounts.

Salmon, mackerel, flaxseed,
and other foods high in omega-3 fatty acids

Fish comes packed with omega-3 fatty acids that help reduce bone loss and lower risk of heart disease; menopausal women are at greater risk for both than are premenopausal women. Flaxseed also contains an omega-3 called alpha-linolenic acid (ALA), but our bodies can convert only 5 to 10 percent of that into the forms we need, which we get directly from fish.

Aim for: Two to three 4-ounce (113-g) servings of fish a week.

Salmon, sardines, meat, poultry,
and other foods high in vitamin B_{12}

B_{12} helps the body produce neurotransmitters, chemicals that transmit nerve signals and affect mood. In fact, low levels of B_{12} are associated with depression. B_{12} deficiency also leads to higher levels of homocysteine, which in turn raises the risk of heart disease and stroke.

Aim for: At least 2.4 micrograms daily, about the amount in 3 ounces (85 g) of light tuna. However, the amount needed to normalize homocysteine levels—about 500 micrograms

Create a twice-a-week fish-for-dinner habit. Simply cook fresh fillets on the stove or in the oven with olive oil, garlic, salt, and pepper, as you would a chicken breast. Then top with a simple sauce or, if you wish, just a tablespoon of salsa.

a day—would be tough to get from diet alone (see Nutritional Supplements, below).

Helpful hint: Most breakfast cereals are fortified with twice the recommended daily amount of B_{12}.

Beans and peas, leafy greens,
and other foods high in folate

Several studies have shown that folate (called folic acid in supplement form) fosters heart, bone, and cognitive health by lowering levels of homocysteine. Research has also linked low levels of folate to depression. In short, this B vitamin seems an ideal match for menopausal women.

Aim for: 400 micrograms of folate daily, the amount in a bowl of fortified cereal or in 1/2 cup of sautéed spinach, 1/2 cup of chickpeas, and an ear of corn.

Helpful hint: Cooking vegetables can reduce their folate content by up to 40 percent, so enjoy raw spinach salads when you're looking for a vegetarian folate boost.

Milk, cheese, salmon, greens,
and other foods high in calcium

With menopause comes a higher risk of osteoporosis, so if you're not already eating plenty of calcium-rich foods, it's high time to start. The calcium in foods can't help replace bone that's already lost, but studies have shown that it does rein in the loss. To protect your heart, choose low-fat versions of dairy foods and switch to fat-free milk.

Aim for: 1,000 to 1,200 milligrams of calcium daily, about what you'll get from a cup of yogurt, an ounce (28 g) or two of mozzarella cheese, and a cup of white beans.

Helpful hint: If you down a lot of sodas, you're losing calcium. Sodas contain phosphorus, another mineral that gives our bones density. But our bodies eliminate any extra phosphorus through urine—and calcium goes with it.

Fortified milk and cereals
and other foods high in vitamin D

The "sunshine vitamin" (which your body makes when exposed to sunlight) stimulates the absorption of calcium, especially important for menopausal women with thinning bones. Sockeye salmon is a particularly rich source of D because the fish eat a steady diet of plants that create lots of vitamin D from sunlight, as well as small sea creatures that eat those plants.

Aim for: 1,000 IU per day; 3 ounces (85 g) of salmon has 425 IU.

NUTRITIONAL SUPPLEMENTS
Vitamin E. Opinions are mixed whether supplemental vitamin E is beneficial—or even helpful—for hot flashes. Best bet: Get your vitamin E in a reliable daily multivitamin mineral supplement. You can also pop open a vitamin E soft-gel and apply the oil topically once a day for vaginal dryness. **DOSAGE:** Some doctors recommend 400 to 800 IU daily for hot flashes, which is much higher than the recommended 22.5 IU per day.

Vitamin B_6. Most people get the B_6 they need from their diets, although heavy drinkers and the elderly risk deficiency because of absorption difficulties. **DOSAGE:** 2 to 20 milligrams a day are typical doses for people who are deficient. Ask your doctor about the amount you should be taking, if any.

Omega-3 fatty acids. Omega-3s such as DHA and EPA come in soft-gel fish-oil capsules or in liquids such as flaxseed oil. Skip the flaxseed oil: It doesn't have the fiber or cancer-preventing lignans that whole flaxseed does, it's expensive, and it goes rancid. Because omega-3s are sensitive to heat, light, and oxygen, store the supplements in your refrigerator. Also, choose a supplement with vitamin E, which will help prevent rancidity. Taking the supplements with food or freezing them first can help reduce the burping often associated with fish oils. So can choosing a fish-oil supplement that contains citrus essence. **DOSAGE:** 1 gram a day of a combination of EPA and DHA is often recommended.

Vitamin B$_{12}$. As we age, it's harder to absorb B$_{12}$ from food. Because of that, the Institute of Medicine recommends that people over 50 take B$_{12}$ in supplement form. Therapeutic doses of 500 micrograms a day, along with vitamin B$_6$ and folic acid, have been shown to help decrease dangerous homocysteine levels in the blood, thus decreasing the risk for heart disease. **DOSAGE:** Look for a multivitamin formula that contains 100 percent of your Daily Value (DV) for vitamin E, or about 6 micrograms. Up to 500 micrograms a day is considered safe but check with your doctor first.

Calcium. Scientists are still researching the optimal amount of calcium necessary to slow bone loss. For now, the National Academy of Sciences recommends taking the amount below. Look for a supplement that also contains vitamin D. **DOSAGE:** 1,000 to 1,200 milligrams daily, divided into two doses.

Vitamin D. Those of us who live in sunny climates usually get vitamin D from sunlight or by eating vitamin D–rich foods. But people who live in less sunny northern climates or who take certain medications, such as laxatives and antacids, may need a supplement boost. Ask your doctor to check your D level, especially if you live in the north. As we get older, our bodies don't convert sunlight into D as well as they once did. **DOSAGE:** 1,000 IU daily.

CAUTION

Caffeine, alcohol, and spicy foods. All three may crank up the ol' hot flash burner. Alcohol lowers your body temperature as you drink, especially to excess, then raises it as the alcohol leaves your system.

Corn, sunflower, and safflower oils. These are rich in omega-6 fatty acids that in excess may overpower the benefits of omega-3 fatty acids in fish and other foods. In a study at Purdue University, researchers found that for menopausal women who had a low ratio of omega-6s to omega-3s, bone loss was minimized.

Should You Go Meatless?

More and more people are becoming vegetarians, and if menopausal symptoms plague you, perhaps you should consider jumping on that bandwagon. As we've noted, a diet full of the phytoestrogens in soy foods, beans, and flaxseed helps reduce hot flashes and lowers the risk of heart disease and osteoporosis. Studies have also shown that women who eat lots of fruits and vegetables have a 54 percent lower risk of stroke than women who do not. And research has shown that vegan diets (no animal products at all, including milk and eggs) help postmenopausal women lose weight and improve their sensitivity to insulin, which is important for preventing diabetes. But vegetarians who eat no meat or dairy products need to be certain they get enough vitamin B$_{12}$, calcium, and iron in their diets. Most breakfast cereals are fortified with adequate amounts of B$_{12}$ and iron, and soy milk and many brands of orange juice are fortified with calcium.

MENSTRUAL PROBLEMS

PMS, cramps, and bloating are the price women sometimes pay for being designed with the ability to produce children. After ovulation—about halfway through the monthly cycle—the hormone progesterone increases, preparing the lining of the uterus for a fertilized egg. But about seven days before a period starts, if no egg is implanted, levels of both progesterone and estrogen drop. For many women, those seven days can bring symptoms of premenstrual syndrome, or PMS, including irritability, depression, cramping, bloating, cravings, breast pain, and headaches. For other women, problems such as heavy bleeding and cramps start with menstruation.

Ibuprofen is a godsend for many, but other helpful "medicines" come in foods, not pills. Although food isn't a cure-all for menstrual problems, women whose diets are healthful and who cut out certain foods seem to do better than others. In part, that's because some foods help balance hormones, improve mood, and diminish water retention, all of which affect how we feel during menstruation.

YOUR FOOD PRESCRIPTION

Dairy products *and other foods high in calcium and vitamin D*

You've probably never thought to reach for milk for your PMS, but maybe you should. In a long-term study of more than 3,000 women, researchers found that the women who drank four servings of low-fat or fat-free milk a day (or the calcium and vitamin D equivalent in fortified orange juice, low-fat yogurt, and other low-fat dairy foods) had a 40 percent lower risk of developing PMS than the women who had only one serving of milk a week. Other studies have also shown calcium's ability to curb PMS symptoms.

Researchers aren't certain why calcium and vitamin D are such a winning pair, but one theory is that PMS may stem from—or at least reveal—a lack of calcium (PMS symptoms are similar to those of calcium deficiency). And researchers do know that in women with PMS, estrogen levels tend to be higher and calcium levels lower than in women without PMS.

Vitamin D helps the body absorb calcium, and it probably affects both the brain and estrogen in ways scientists don't yet understand.

Aim for: 1,000 to 1,200 milligrams of calcium and 400 IU of vitamin D daily, the equivalent of four glasses of fat-free or low-fat milk.

Helpful hint: Be sure to drink "skinny" milk. According to researchers, women who drink fat-free or low-fat milk have a lower risk of PMS than those who drink whole milk.

Spinach, soybeans, grains, *and other foods high in magnesium*

Munching on spinach salads and even baked goods made with whole-grain flour, buckwheat, or whole-grain cornmeal—all rich in magnesium—could help put a stop to the PMS blues. Although it's not clear how magnesium affects PMS, the nutrient is essential for dopamine production. This mood-boosting hormone also helps balance adrenal and kidney function, which in turn helps minimize fluid retention. And in a two-month British study, women who took just 200 milligrams of magnesium daily—about the equivalent of a quarter cup of almonds or two servings of spinach—had less weight gain, bloating, and breast tenderness during the second month of the study than women taking a placebo. Another study found that the ratio of magnesium to calcium was significantly lower in women with PMS than in women without it.

Aim for: The women in the British study took only 200 milligrams of magnesium daily, but the recommended amount is 320 milligrams. Half a halibut fillet contains 170 milligrams; a cup of whole-wheat flour, 166 milligrams; a cup of cooked spinach, 157 milligrams; and a cup of soybeans, 148 milligrams.

Helpful hint: Develop a yen for raw spinach. About one-third of spinach's magnesium is lost in cooking.

Nuts, seeds, wheat germ,
and other foods high in vitamin E

Eating foods like almonds and sunflower seeds is never a chore, and doing so may help relieve symptoms of PMS. In a small three-month study of 46 women with PMS, those who took a daily 400 IU dose of vitamin E—admittedly the equivalent of far more nuts than you'd want to eat in one day—saw their mental and physical symptoms of PMS abate.

Aim for: The women in the study took 400 IU daily, an amount that's nearly impossible to get from diet alone. One tablespoon of wheat germ oil has more than 20 milligrams, and an ounce (28 g) of almonds has more than 7. The recommended amount of vitamin E is 15 milligrams (about 23 IU).

Clams, oysters, beef, soybeans,
and other foods high in iron

If heavy bleeding is your monthly burden, try adding more iron to your diet; too little can cause heavier flow. Lean red meat and oysters are terrific sources. One note of caution: Eating too much red meat may increase the risk of endometriosis, a painful condition in which uterine tissue grows on organs outside the uterus, such as the ovaries or fallopian tubes. In an Italian study, women who ate meat every day had double the risk of endometriosis compared to women who ate less meat and more fruits and vegetables.

Aim for: For women, the recommended amount of iron is 18 milligrams per day, about what you'll get from a bowl of oatmeal and a cup of soybeans.

Helpful hint: Women who eat low-fat vegetarian diets have fewer premenstrual symptoms than those who eat meat. But if blood flow is heavy, they need iron. The solution: Eat iron-rich beans, tofu, and spinach.

Tofu, soy milk, flaxseed,
and other foods with phytoestrogens

If you snack on edamame (green soybeans) or add them to soups and salads, you may be serving up some menstrual relief. Soy and flaxseed contain phytoestrogens, plant chemicals that imitate estrogen, which may help balance hormones during menstruation. Study results are mixed, however. One Korean study found

For dinner, steam clams—it's easy! Pour some no-iodine salt and cornmeal in cold water and soak the clams for 30 minutes. Scrub the shells and rinse thoroughly. Then steam in a mix of water, white wine, garlic, and pepper until the clams open.

that soy lessened premenstrual symptoms, and in a small two-month British study of young women, soy protein significantly reduced breast tenderness and swelling compared to a placebo. Yet a Japanese study found soy had no effect.

Aim for: Try serving yourself some soy milk, edamame, or tofu a few times a week over the course of a month and see if it helps.

Complex carbohydrates
from whole grains, fruits, and vegetables

Many women crave sugary carbohydrates like chocolate and ice cream before and during their periods. But instead of having a sugar fix, eating meals plump with whole grains, fruits, and vegetables may double-cross PMS symptoms, including the cramping that often accompanies heavy bleeding.

Carbohydrates boost levels of the feel-good neurotransmitter serotonin, the same one targeted by certain antidepressants. In a study at the Massachusetts Institute of Technology, researchers found that women who ate large amounts of carbohydrates became less depressed, angry, and anxious and had more stable moods than women who ate fewer carbs. Complex, or high-fiber, carbohydrates are best because they're digested more slowly than carbs that come from sugar or refined grains, so they help keep blood sugar levels stable. When blood sugar drops too low, most of us get tired and grouchy, which can worsen PMS symptoms. Complex carbs also help prevent the constipation that's common in women with menstrual cramps.

Another benefit of whole grains: They contain the mineral manganese. In a USDA study, researchers found that when women had low levels of manganese (and calcium), they had much more severe premenstrual symptoms than they did when they supplemented their diets with both minerals. Researchers aren't sure why manganese may help, but it is involved in blood clotting, and women with low levels tend to bleed more heavily than women with normal levels. Manganese also helps the body maintain normal blood sugar levels. Top-notch sources include oat bran, whole-grain wheat flour, fortified cereals, and buckwheat flour.

Include lots of citrus fruits and berries in your choices as well. Citrus fruits contain vitamin C, and berries, grapes, and cherries offer antioxidants called flavonoids, both of which help reduce heavy bleeding. An Italian study showed that women who ate lots of fresh fruit and vegetables also cut their risk of endometriosis by 40 percent.

Aim for: Three servings of whole grains a day (that's 1/2 cup of cooked oatmeal or cooked wheatberries, one slice of whole-grain bread, and 1/2 cup of whole-wheat pasta), five to six servings of vegetables, and three to four servings of fruit.

NUTRITIONAL SUPPLEMENTS

Calcium and vitamin D. Most women could benefit from a daily calcium supplement, although it's unclear whether supplements affect PMS the same way foods high in calcium and vitamin D do. **DOSAGE:** *Calcium:* 1,000 to 1,200 milligrams daily, in two doses (it's best absorbed in 500- to 600-milligram amounts). *Vitamin D:* 400 IU daily.

Magnesium. Several studies have found that magnesium can improve PMS symptoms. A study in Britain, for instance, found that taking 200 milligrams of magnesium a day for two months reduced fluid retention and breast tenderness. Another study found that 360 milligrams three times a day, taken from day 15

FEATURED RECIPES
Buckwheat Pancakes with Fruit Sauce *p. 286*
Edamame Hummus with Pita Crisps *p. 288*
Ultimate Spiced Nuts *p. 288*
Spinach Salad with Chickpeas *p. 293*
Mac 'n Cheese Primavera *p. 304*
Roasted Salmon with Sautéed Greens *p. 309*
Chicken-Barley Bake *p. 312*
Beef and Broccoli Stew *p. 316*
Zesty Cornbread *p. 326*
Pumpkin Streusel Bread *p. 327*

to the start of a period, helped diminish mood swings. Magnesium chloride and magnesium lactate are the easiest forms to absorb. **DOSAGE:** The studies showed an effect in doses from 200 to 1,100 milligrams a day.

Vitamin B₆. Several studies have found that doses of 50 to 100 milligrams can help relieve breast pain and depression related to PMS. **DOSAGE:** 50 to 100 milligrams.

CAUTION

Salt. Salt causes the body to retain fluids, which only adds to bloating and breast pain.

Sugar and fat. Sugary foods like candy bars and cake make blood sugar spike and then drop, and that rollercoaster ride can affect your mood and energy level. If you want a sweet treat, try fresh or dried fruits (these are high in calories, so just a small handful will do) instead. Their fiber slows digestion, which results in slower fluctuations in blood sugar.

Saturated fat in fatty meats and full-fat cheese cranks up production of certain prostaglandins (hormone-like chemicals) in the uterus that stimulate the muscles and can cause cramps. (Of course, as we noted earlier, heavy bleeders need the iron from these very foods. If you're a heavy bleeder with cramps, choose lean cuts of meat or get iron from nonmeat sources like oysters, beans, and spinach.)

If you're eating a lot of sugar and fat, chances are good that you weigh more than you should, and your waistline could be contributing to your menstrual problems. A University of Michigan study found that women who carry extra pounds have double the chance of longer episodes of pain compared to thinner women.

Caffeine and alcohol. Caffeine is a stimulant, which can lead to anxiety and mood swings, not the effect you want during menstrual periods already awash with drama. Studies with alcohol have been mixed. If you drink, keep it moderate.

Sleuthing for Hidden Salt Sources

Salt is sneakier than a cat burglar, cropping up even in foods we think of as healthy, like canned vegetables and soup, as well as more obvious sources like pizza and salty snack foods. It's also in condiments such as ketchup and barbecue sauce. Thus, even if you banish salt from the table—a great way to start cutting back—you may be eating more sodium than you think. Check food labels before you buy. The recommended daily intake of sodium is 2,300 milligrams, which is the amount in 1 teaspoon of salt.

When You Don't Feel Like Eating

Cramps, bleeding, mood swings, and bloating aren't exactly clarion calls to dinner. But even if you don't feel like eating, you can still drink water, herbal tea, green tea, and fruit and vegetable juice. Oddly enough, drinking more fluids lessens bloating: The body releases fluid when you're well hydrated but holds on to it when you run low. And fruit and vegetable juices provide nutrients that can be helpful in reducing symptoms.

MIGRAINE

"That no one dies of migraine seems, to someone deep into an attack, an ambiguous blessing." So Joan Didion wrote in her essay collection, *The White Album*. What causes such distress that dying doesn't seem unreasonable? That's one of the more frustrating things about migraines—headache experts aren't quite sure.

The new thinking is that people who get migraines have extra-sensitive, hyper-reactive brains. Something sparks a region deep in the brain, dubbed the "migraine generator," and that unleashes a cascade of brain chemicals that inflame nerve endings, dilate blood vessels, and flood the brain with pain signals. So what's the "something" that triggers this reaction? That's even more frustrating. Almost *anything* can cause a migraine, including weather changes, strong odors, stress, loss of sleep, and certain foods and drinks. A good many migraines are also related to fluctuations in estrogen levels, which is no doubt why three times more women than men get migraines (often coinciding with their periods) and why the headaches tend to disappear during pregnancy and after menopause.

Avoiding the foods that often trigger migraines while making a point of eating those that help prevent them may reduce the number—and intensity—of headaches you get. And compared to dying, that sounds pretty good.

YOUR FOOD PRESCRIPTION

Fruits, vegetables, and legumes

This is good general advice, but it may be particularly helpful for women who get migraines with their periods—which may be due to a sudden drop in estrogen. The higher your overall estrogen level is to begin with, so the reasoning goes, the farther it can fall during the drop. The fiber in these foods helps by removing excess estrogen from the body along with waste, so it's not recycled back into your bloodstream.

In addition, fruits, vegetables, and legumes all contain plant estrogens that blunt the negative effects of the estrogen our bodies naturally make. Another major plus of these foods: They're low in fat. When you eat more fat, your body makes more estrogen.

Aim for: Getting the recommended 4 to 6 daily cups of fruit and vegetables is a great place to start.

Fatty fish

You know it as heart-healthy fare, but salmon and other fatty fish (like mackerel, trout, and herring) just may help reduce migraines, too. These fish are rich sources of the omega-3 fatty acids EPA and DHA. Some preliminary research on these anti-inflammatory compounds done at the University of Cincinnati showed that when they

FEATURED RECIPES

Buckwheat Pancakes with Fruit Sauce p. 286
Spinach Salad with Chickpeas p. 293
Tuna and White Bean Salad p. 295
Ginger Butternut Squash Soup p. 298
Lentil-Tomato Soup p. 299
Roasted Salmon with Sautéed Greens p. 309
Beef and Broccoli Stew p. 316
Brown Rice Risotto p. 321
Almond Rice p. 322
Zesty Cornbread p. 326

were taken in supplement form, they appeared to reduce the frequency and severity of migraines in some people over the course of six weeks.

Aim for: The University of Cincinnati study used capsules containing 300 milligrams of EPA and DHA and 700 milligrams of other oils. Four 4-ounce (113 g) servings of fatty fish a week would provide about the same amount of the beneficial fish oils used in the study.

Coffee

Although caffeine may trigger migraines in some people, when a migraine strikes, a few cups of coffee do help relieve the pain. Caffeine is so effective at helping to shrink swollen blood vessels in the brain, it's one of the key ingredients (together with acetaminophen and aspirin) in over-the-counter migraine medicines like Excedrin Migraine.

Aim for: A cup or two when a migraine hits.

Ginger

Research shows that this warming spice contains some potent compounds that are similar to the ones in nonsteroidal anti-inflammatory drugs. It may work against migraines by blocking inflammatory substances called prostaglandins. Ginger hasn't been rigorously tested for headache relief, but even if it doesn't stop your migraine, it should help relieve the nausea that often comes with it.

Aim for: There's no recommended dose for ginger, but you might start using powdered or fresh ginger liberally in cooking or ordering dishes flavored with ginger when dining out. And when a migraine strikes, drinking a glass of water with a few teaspoons of powdered ginger mixed in every few hours may help alleviate the pain. You can also suck on dried ginger candy.

Whole grains, beans, leafy dark green vegetables, *and other foods high in magnesium*

What do these foods have in common? They're all high in magnesium, which research shows is often deficient in people who get migraines. Low levels of magnesium are thought to make the brain extra sensitive to migraine triggers.

Aim for: The recommended daily amount for magnesium is 280 milligrams for women and 350 milligrams for men, though if you're truly deficient, aiming for 400 to 700 milligrams daily may be better for preventing migraines.

Helpful hint: Roasted pumpkin seeds are among the richest sources of magnesium, with about 151 milligrams per ounce (28 g). Keep a bag in your purse, car, or desk for easy nibbling. Magnesium-rich nuts include Brazil nuts (107 milligrams per ounce/28 g) and almonds (78 milligrams per ounce/28 g). Or try some halibut, which contains 91 milligrams in a 3-ounce (85 g) portion, as well as a smattering of omega-3s.

Make a healing ginger tea in no time. Add about a dozen coin-size slices of fresh gingerroot to a quart (1 l) of water and simmer on the stove for about 20 minutes. If you don't love the taste of fresh ginger, add orange juice and honey to your cup of tea.

NUTRITIONAL SUPPLEMENTS

Magnesium. People often complain that their migraines hit when they're under stress, and a deficiency of magnesium may help explain why. Chronic stress drains our bodies of magnesium, and when levels are low, blood vessels are more likely to spasm. It's estimated that about 50 percent of people who get migraines have low magnesium levels.

When given intravenously, magnesium can completely halt a migraine, often within minutes. Researchers suspect that the mineral relaxes overexcited nerves in the brain and helps serotonin receptors block migraine pain signals. That's also how the newer migraine medications, known as triptans—sumatriptan (Imitrex) and almotriptan (Axert)—work.

Oral magnesium works well, too, but only for preventing migraines. In one three-month study, migraine frequency dropped by 42 percent in people who took 600 milligrams of magnesium, compared to 16 percent in those who took placebos. Supplementing with magnesium can even help triptan medications work better. In one small study of people who reported that Imitrex didn't relieve their migraines, the medication started working when they corrected their magnesium deficiency. The only downside to increasing magnesium is possibly some mild diarrhea. **DOSAGE:** 400 milligrams daily in divided doses. Avoid magnesium hydroxide and magnesium citrate, which are more commonly associated with loose stools.

Riboflavin. Researchers are still sorting out how riboflavin (vitamin B$_2$) prevents migraines, but one theory is that the brains of people with migraines simply require a little extra energy for proper function. Riboflavin increases energy production in all cells, including brain cells. In a recent German study, volunteers taking riboflavin for six months got half the migraines they normally experienced, and they were able to reduce their migraine medication. The only side effect appears to be minor gastric upset. **DOSAGE:** 400 milligrams daily. Since B vitamins work best together, take a B-complex supplement or a multivitamin and, if necessary,

make up the difference in dosage with a riboflavin supplement.

Omega-3 fatty acids. If you can't seem to eat the four weekly servings of fish suggested above, look to fish-oil supplements to fill the omega-3 gap. **DOSAGE:** The University of Cincinnati study used 1 gram of fish oil a day in capsules that contained 300 milligrams of EPA and DHA and 700 milligrams of other oils.

Coenzyme Q10. Like riboflavin, CoQ10 increases cellular energy, and some preliminary research suggests it can prevent migraines. A small double-blind, placebo-controlled study of 42 people done in Switzerland found that over the three months of the study, taking CoQ10 reduced migraine frequency, duration, and accompanying symptoms such as nausea. This beneficial effect on decreasing some of the symptoms of migraine headaches has been verified in more recent studies. **DOSAGE:** 100 milligrams three times daily.

CAUTION

Fatty, greasy, and fried foods. If you're serious about using your diet to help prevent migraines, get serious about cutting back on fat. As we mentioned earlier, eating too much fat increases estrogen levels, which may contribute to migraines. A small three-month study done at Loma Linda University in California found that when participants radically cut their fat intake to about 20 grams per day, they reported a 71 percent decrease in headache frequency, a 66 percent decrease in intensity, and a 74 percent decrease in duration.

This doesn't mean you should cut out fat from fish, however, since omega-3 fatty acids help to reduce inflammation and pain. Instead, take aim at saturated fat (meat, cheese, butter, and ice cream). Choose lower-fat versions of meat, cheese, and ice cream and use olive or canola oil in place of big hunks of butter.

Trigger foods. It used to be that eliminating key foods from your diet was the primary prescription for preventing migraines. Now headache experts are less sure that specific foods per se cause migraines. Rather, it may be that certain foods eaten under certain conditions tip the balance when other factors like stress, lack of sleep, or hormone fluctuations make us more vulnerable to a migraine. It's even possible that making dietary changes—any changes—has a sort of placebo effect. We feel as if we're doing *something,* and that feeling of control has a positive effect.

Still, because food sensitivity is thought to be a factor in 10 to 30 percent of migraines, it can't hurt to do a little sleuthing if you suspect that foods trigger your headaches. Oft-cited culprits include red wine, aged cheese, processed meats, dairy products, citrus fruits, wheat, chocolate, and food additives like monosodium glutamate and artificial sweeteners. Some studies show a connection with migraines; some don't. That may be because migraines are so highly individual; what triggers one person's headache may not trigger someone else's.

The best way to determine if food is affecting your migraines is to keep a food diary. When a headache hits, try to remember what you ate in the previous 12 hours. If you see a pattern, avoid that food for two or more weeks, then add it back to your diet and see if there's a change in your headache episodes. But remember, just as it's important to avoid any foods that may cause migraines, it's equally important not to skip meals, since irregular eating can bring on migraines, too.

Give This Herb a Try

It isn't exactly a food, but since this herb is so potentially useful against migraines, we thought they deserved mention.

Feverfew. Researchers have long debated whether this popular herb really prevents migraines, but the latest study, done in Germany, suggests that it might. When the researchers tested a standardized feverfew extract against a placebo, they found that study volunteers who typically averaged five migraines a month got about two fewer migraines each month when they were taking feverfew. Feverfew preparations vary widely, so follow the package instructions for dosage. Feverfew in low doses—about 50 milligrams a day—has not been shown to cause any serious side effects. Do not take feverfew if you are on an anticoagulant (blood-thinning) medication, however.

NAUSEA

When you're feeling green around the gills, food is probably the last thing you want to think about. In fact, though, your kitchen may hold just the ticket to quell the queasies. The best pantry remedy, ginger, comes in forms you can carry with you to keep you safely away from that deck railing or worry-free in the backseat during a winding car ride. It's even safe for pregnant women.

YOUR FOOD PRESCRIPTION

Ginger

Gingerroot has been used for more than 2,000 years in China to treat nausea. Scientists suspect it blocks the release of hormones that can cause irregular muscle contractions in the gut—the ones that leave you with that heaving feeling. Ginger appears particularly effective against motion sickness and morning sickness. In one study, naval cadets who were new to the open sea took either placebos or 1 gram of powdered ginger prior to a period of sailing through high waves. Those who took the ginger reported much less nausea and vomiting and fewer cold sweats than those who took the placebo.

The National Center for Integrative and Complementary Health (NCCIH) says that ginger may help relieve nausea and vomiting related to pregnancy as well as chemotherapy treatments. When used as a spice, it is considered safe.

Aim for: For motion sickness, chew on 1 gram (about 1 tablespoon or a 1-inch/2.5 cm piece) of peeled raw ginger or candied ginger several hours prior to travel and every 4 hours while traveling. Or take two capsules of powdered ginger every 4 hours for a full day before traveling and throughout the trip. For morning sickness, take 1 gram of fresh or candied ginger daily. You can also drink a cup of ginger tea every few hours. Avoid powdered ginger because it may be less safe in large quantities for pregnant women.

Helpful hint: For some people, ginger is more effective when taken on an empty stomach.

Flat soda and clear fruit juices

Remember staying home from school with the stomach flu while your mother coaxed you to drink ginger ale or flat cola? In small quantities, sweet liquids like these or like apple or grape juice seem to calm the stomach, and they provide some energy when you can't eat. They're absorbed into the bloodstream quickly, yet they have no fiber to activate stomach acid and digestive tract contractions that could stimulate nausea. Coconut water (not to be confused with coconut milk), with its wealth of potassium, is like nature's Gatorade, and island cultures often turn to it as a remedy for nausea. Look for it in health food stores.

Aim for: Small sips. Don't drink too much at once. If carbonation bothers your stomach, let sodas go flat before drinking.

Ice pops

Cold liquids can be a godsend to pregnant women. When you can't keep anything else in your stomach, sucking on frozen fruit juice cubes (make your own in an ice cube tray) or

FEATURED RECIPES

Quick Chicken Noodle Soup *p. 296*
Almond Rice *p. 322*
Pomegranate Ice *p. 334*

fruit-based ice pops can replace some of the liquids and energy that you've lost.

Aim for: A few fruit-based ice pops a day may pave the path to a slightly larger meal. Avoid those that contain artificial sweeteners, some of which may woresn nausea in some people.

Olives and lemons

These quickly dry saliva from the mouth, and that can help tone down nausea. The acid in lemons also triggers the formation of bicarbonate in the stomach, helping to neutralize intestinal acids and calm gas and bloating that may intensify nausea.

Aim for: Suck an olive when nausea strikes or add lemon juice to hot or room-temperature water and sip it.

Clear, salty broths

Chicken broth, vegetable broth, and miso soup all sit easily on the stomach and provide nutrition during episodes when most foods just aren't appealing.

Aim for: 1/2 cup of broth every 2 hours.

Crackers, toast, and dry cereal

These dry snacks soak up the saliva in your mouth and some of the acid in your stomach. Many women in the first trimester of pregnancy can't get out of bed before eating a cracker or two.

Aim for: Eat oyster crackers, saltines, plain toast, and other mild, crunchy foods throughout the day as tiny snacks.

Chamomile, lemon balm, and peppermint teas

Chamomile, known for its muscle-relaxing qualities, can help calm spasms in the stomach. Peppermint can help digestion by calming the stomach's muscle contractions (the reason that after-dinner mints became popular), and its menthol can anesthetize the stomach wall, an ef-

fect that may reduce nausea. Some studies have even shown that sniffing a cloth dotted with peppermint oil can help to reduce postsurgical nausea.

Aim for: Sip tea throughout the day for hydration and nausea relief.

Mints and lemon drops

Many cancer patients undergoing chemotherapy find that sucking on a mint or a piece of hard lemon candy can take the edge off nausea.

Aim for: Use as needed.

NUTRITIONAL SUPPLEMENTS

Vitamin B$_6$. When it comes to morning sickness, a number of studies have shown that vitamin B$_6$ can help calm that green feeling. The vitamin can break down hormones that may lead to nausea and vomiting. Some studies suggest it works best when combined with ginger. *Caution:* Some B vitamin supplements can actually trigger nausea. Take them with food unless directed otherwise. **DOSAGE:** The American College of Obstetrics and Gynecology (ACOG) recommends 10 to 25 milligrams of vitamin B$_6$ three or four times a day to treat nausea and vomiting in pregnancy. Consult your obstetrician about a dose that's appropriate beyond that in your prenatal multivitamin.

CAUTION

Fatty foods. The stomach needs more time to digest foods high in fat, and that means digestive acids linger longer, making symptoms worse for anyone prone to nausea.

Green tea. On an empty stomach, green tea can trigger nausea in some people. Sip it with food if that's true for you, and take a pass on green tea supplements.

Iron supplements. Some people who take iron to treat or prevent iron-deficiency anemia experience nausea as a side effect. If you do, ask your doctor about lowering your dose.

OBESITY

Despite the cliché of jolly fat folks, obesity is not funny. Being obese, defined as having a body mass index (or BMI, a measurement of body fat) of 30 or greater, can lead to heart disease, stroke, high blood pressure, diabetes, and even some forms of cancer. Millions of people are obese, and the number is growing.

You may think the answer is simple: Eat less. But the usual means of weight loss people try—starving themselves or going on fad diets—simply do not work. Some researchers speculate that when we lose weight, fat cells shrink, lessening the amount of leptin, an appetite suppressor, that pours into the blood. When leptin falls below the level genes are programmed for, the brain releases other hormones that increase hunger. This is what dieters know as the rebound effect; they lose weight, only to gain it all back and then some.

In ancient times, such mechanisms helped humans survive famine and predators. Today, the predators chasing us are the marketers who push fast food and other high-calorie, high-fat eats. We're easy targets since we're hardwired to eat (and store) fat.

If you can manage to ignore the siren songs of ever-present vending machines and fast-food joints, though, there's good news: You *can* eat enough to feel plenty full, without taking in too much fat or too many calories. In fact, in a study of 38 common foods, researchers found that high-protein and high-fiber foods were much more satisfying than high-fat foods. Cakes and cookies and other fatty foods were the least satisfying, which may account in part for why we end up gobbling down such big portions when we eat them.

If you want to really enjoy what you're eating, focus on flavorful—and above all, filling—foods. Enjoy fiber- and nutrient-rich whole-grain rice, tabbouleh salad, and vegetable soup instead of nutrient-stripped white rice or bagels, fat-filled potato salad, or cream of corn soup. Losing weight doesn't mean going hungry; it means eating well.

food for thought . . .

"Skipping breakfast isn't as bad as eating 5 pounds of bacon, but day to day, it's one of the worst things someone with a weight problem can do."

— Bruce A. Barton, PhD, president and CEO, Maryland Medical Research Institute, Baltimore

Breakfast

Skipping breakfast is a lot like skipping rope: neither gets you anywhere. Although lots of people think they'll cut calories by cutting breakfast, the opposite is true. Studies show that eating breakfast helps you consume fewer total calories for the day. One national U.S. health and nutrition survey found that men who eat breakfast weigh about 6 pounds (2.7 kg) less than men who skip it; women weigh 9 pounds (4 kg) less. And a 10-year study of almost 2,400 adolescent girls showed that those who ate any kind of breakfast had lower BMIs than girls who did not. People who eat cereal for breakfast have lower BMIs than people who skip breakfast or dine on meat and eggs.

Whole grains, beans, fruits,
and other foods high in fiber

Eat a bowl of brown rice topped with chickpeas and sautéed vegetables for lunch, and it's likely you won't want another bite until supper. High-fiber foods like these have few calories, little fat, and lots of bulk, which keeps you full. They're also digested slowly, which means your blood sugar stays at an even keel instead of rapidly spiking and falling, which leaves you hungry again in no time. Whole grains also provide nutrients, such as magnesium and vitamin B_6, that many weight-loss diets are deficient in. A great way to get a good dose of fiber is to start your day with high-fiber cereal.

Aim for: 25 to 35 grams of fiber per day. A cup of chickpeas has about 12 grams, and 1/2 cup of bran cereal has more than 8.

Helpful hint: If whole grains put you off, ease yourself into the idea by adding them in small amounts. For instance, mix half your usual cereal with a half serving of whole-grain cereal and add some brown rice to white rice. Gradually increase the amount of whole grains as your taste buds adjust.

Fresh greens, raw vegetables,
and other salad foods

Head for the salad bar. Greens and raw vegetables like carrots, zucchini, and broccoli are remarkably low in calories but high in water and slow-digesting fiber, so they tend to fill you up.

Squelching your appetite isn't the only reason to frequent the produce section. In a study of almost 18,000 people, researchers found that those who ate salads often had higher levels of vitamins C and E, folate, and carotenoids, important for overall health, than people who had fewer salads. Researchers have also found that people who eat a vegetarian diet weigh an average of 3 to 20 percent less than meat eaters. And a study at George Washington University School of Medicine found that overweight women on a low-fat plant-based diet who were allowed to eat as much as they wanted lost an average of 12 pounds (5 kg) in 14 weeks compared with 8 pounds (3.6 kg) in the control group.

Aim for: 2 to 3 cups of greens and other non-starchy vegetables a day.

Helpful hint: If you hate vegetables, begin by adding them to foods you like: a handful to a serving of rice or pasta, sliced tomatoes with your eggs, a cup of spinach to noodle soup.

FEATURED RECIPES

Zucchini Frittata *p. 287*
Ultimate Spiced Nuts *p. 288*
Spinach Salad with Chickpeas *p. 293*
Hearty Vegetable Stew *p. 304*
Tuna Kebabs *p. 306*
Chicken in Garlic Sauce *p. 312*
Turkey Cutlets with Grapefruit Salsa *p. 313*
Springtime Quinoa *p. 322*
Frozen Fruit Mousse *p. 334*

Fish, chicken, beans,
and other foods high in protein

Researchers are discovering intriguing information about protein and its effect on weight. A study by British researchers shows that high-protein foods like these help trigger the release of PYY, a hormone known to reduce hunger. In a study of 9 obese and 10 normal-weight men, researchers distributed three types of meals: high protein, high carbohydrate, and high fat. All the men said that the protein meal best satisfied their hunger, and those meals also spurred the highest release of PYY.

We're not advising an extremely high-protein, low-carb diet (short-term studies of these diets do show improved weight loss, but the diets don't seem to have any advantage over other diets in the long term), just that you make it a point to eat some protein with every meal and preferably every snack, too.

Other studies have shown that people on higher-protein diets that are also rich in "slow-burning" carbohydrates low on the glycemic index (such as fruits and vegetables, beans, and whole-wheat pasta) are less hungry and lose more weight than people on low-protein, high-carbohydrate diets.

Getting enough protein when you're dieting also helps you lose fat, not muscle. For instance, in a small 10-week study, one group of women ate 9 to 10 ounces (255 to 283 g) of protein a day for 10 weeks and a reduced amount of carbohydrates. The control group ate about half that amount of protein and about a third more carbohydrates. Although both groups took in the same number of calories and lost about 17 pounds (7.7 g), the women on the higher-protein diet lost 2 more pounds (.9 kg) of fat and 1 less pound (.4 kg) of muscle than the control group.

Don't overdo protein, though. People with type 2 diabetes, which often affects the obese, are at greater risk for kidney disease, and overeating protein may worsen the problem.

Aim for: A good source of protein at every meal. Women should get at least 5 1/2 ounces (155 g) of protein a day and men 6 1/2 ounces (184 g), or about 20 percent of daily calories. One ounce (28 g) of protein is equivalent to 1 ounce (28 g) of chicken, lean cuts of beef and pork, or fish; 1/4 cup of cooked dried beans; one egg; 1 tablespoon of peanut butter; or 1/2 ounce (14 g) of nuts or seeds.

Helpful hint: You can get plenty of protein without upping your intake of saturated fat. Rice and beans, peanut butter and whole-grain bread, and hummus and whole-grain pita bread are all combinations that provide complete protein.

Nuts

Nuts are crunchy, salty—and no longer forbidden. Even though nuts are fatty, they may help you shed pounds, according to a number of studies. Researchers believe that the healthy fat in nuts helps people feel full, and the protein may use up calories as it digests. Large population studies have found that people who eat nuts regularly have lower BMIs than those who don't.

In a study of 65 obese adults at City of Hope National Medical Center in Duarte, California, for example, one group added 3 ounces (85 g) of almonds to a 1,000-calorie liquid diet; another group added complex carbohydrates like popcorn or baked potatoes. Both groups ate roughly the same number of calories and amount of protein, but the almond diet had more than double the fat, primarily healthy monounsaturated fat. Over 24 weeks, the people on the almond diet reduced their weights and body mass indexes by 18 percent compared with 11 percent in the carbohydrate group. Both groups lowered blood sugar, insulin levels, and insulin resistance, which can lead to weight gain—but almost all the diabetic participants in the almond group were able to control their blood sugar on less medication, compared to only half of those in the carb group.

Aim for: 1 ounce (28 g), or a small handful, of unsalted nuts a day in place of a high-carb snack.

Helpful hint: If you crave something sweet and crunchy, mix nuts with dried fruit for a delicious treat.

Dairy products
and other foods high in calcium

Here's a reason to drink milk your mom didn't know: It may help you lose weight. Purdue University researchers found that people who got 1,300 to 1,400 milligrams of calcium a day from dairy products had less body fat after 18 months. And researchers at the University of Tennessee have found much the same thing.

Calcium, it turns out, may play a part in how fat is broken down and stored. The more calcium in a fat cell, the more fat it burns. In a study of obese adults, one group ate three 6-ounce (170-g) servings of fat-free yogurt containing 1,100 milligrams of calcium per day. The other group ate one serving of dairy food containing 400 to 500 milligrams of calcium per day. Both groups also reduced their daily calories by 500. The yogurt group lost an average of more than 14 pounds compared to an average loss of 11 pounds in the low-calcium group. The yogurt group also lost 81 percent more fat from their stomachs. Although studies have found low-fat dairy foods most effective, calcium from other sources, like broccoli or fortified orange juice, works, too.

Despite the positive studies, the jury is still out on this issue. While we wait for final answers, though, eating three servings of low-fat dairy products a day remains a healthy choice.

Aim for: 1,000 to 1,200 milligrams daily, about the equivalent of 1 cup of yogurt plus 2 cups of fat-free milk.

Helpful hint: If a plain glass of milk doesn't tempt you, try other options, such as low-fat cheese on a sandwich, a midmorning latte made with fat-free milk, or oatmeal cooked with low-fat milk instead of water.

Why "Naked" Foods Win

If nuts are good for you, pecan pie must be even better! Sound too good to be true? It is. A handful of pecans contains 200 calories; a slice of pecan pie has 700. Likewise, sweet potatoes, wonderfully healthy on their own, are anything but when smothered in butter and brown sugar. In other words, just because a food in its natural form is good for you doesn't mean it's still good for you when it's sweetened, dressed up, or fried. Fish loses its benefits when battered and fried, as does spinach when creamed. When you dine out, think "naked" food. Ask for fish and meats broiled without butter, steamed vegetables without the sauce, and so on. And if you must have pie, make it pumpkin—without the whipped cream.

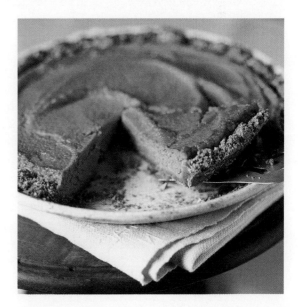

Eggs

Start your day sunny side up. A single egg has 1 ounce (28 g) of high-quality protein and 14 essential nutrients, such as zinc, iron, and vitamins A, D, E, and B$_{12}$. Best of all, it contains only 85 calories. And since eggs are high in protein, it makes sense that they keep you full. In a study at Saint Louis University in Missouri, 30 overweight women ate breakfasts of either two eggs and toast with a bit of jam or a bagel (chock full of "fast-digesting" carbohydrates) with cream cheese and a small serving of yogurt. Both breakfasts contained the same number of calories, but the egg breakfast had more protein and fewer carbohydrates. The egg group reported feeling fuller before lunch and ate 163 fewer calories at lunch than the bagel group, and they ate 418 fewer calories than the bagel group by the end of the day.

Aim for: Even if you have high cholesterol, experts say you can safely eat three or four eggs yolks per week (and all the egg whites you want). Dozens of studies have found that it's saturated fat, not cholesterol, that has the greatest effect on blood cholesterol.

NUTRITIONAL SUPPLEMENTS

Calcium. According to the USDA, most of us don't get enough calcium from our diets, making calcium supplements a smart bet. Calcium in chewable or chelated form, such as calcium citrate, is better absorbed than calcium carbonate but is more expensive. Both types are adequate. Take calcium carbonate with food.
DOSAGE: 1,000 to 1,200 milligrams a day.

CAUTION

Commercial baked goods, fast food, and other processed foods high in fat and sugar. Foods loaded with sugar and refined grains like white flour can cause blood sugar to spike and crash, leaving us hungry again in no time. White potatoes have a similar effect. A survey about fast foods—fatty cheeseburgers and fries and sugar-filled drinks—found that on days when young people ate fast foods, they consumed an average of 187 more calories than those who didn't eat those foods, an addition that amounts to about 6 extra pounds (2.7 kg) a year.

What about those low-fat cookies? Just say no. Manufacturers often add more sugar to replace the fat. Overeating sugary foods, even if they don't contain fat, increases the production of insulin, leading to excess insulin in the blood. Although normal amounts of insulin usually curb appetite, researchers are beginning to understand that the relationship between excess insulin and other hormones that influence appetite may be altered in overweight people in ways that promote both overeating and fat storage.

Sugary drinks. It's easy to drink far more calories than you might think. In one large Harvard study, researchers found that women who went from drinking one or fewer soft drinks per week to one or more a day gained an average of 11 pounds (5 kg) in four years. Even fruit juice—with or without added sugar—can be a problem if you drink too much. You're better off eating whole fruits. According to a study of 2,800 children at the University of Pennsylvania, those already tending toward plumpness who regularly drank fruit juice gained an average of 1/4 pound (113 g) per month, unlike children who ate whole fruits.

If you're a coffee drinker, stick with coffee instead of "coffee drinks." Add sugar and whipped cream to a latte, and you're adding as many as 250 calories. Order a full-fat latte, and you're swigging double the calories of a version made with fat-free milk.

Addicted to Food?

Reaching inside the cookie jar has always been irresistible. Now scientists think they know why. According to researchers, compulsive eating appears to be regulated by the part of the brain that controls emotions, the same part that stirs up cravings in drug addicts. That may explain why some people eat not out of hunger but out of an urge to soothe themselves. Exciting preliminary research suggests that obese people may have significantly more activity in regions of the brain that control sensations in the lips, tongue, and mouth, which may mean that obese people are more sensitive to food's pleasurable qualities, a possible reason for overeating.

Selling Satisfaction

When scientists discover, food companies respond. The new food fad, it appears, spotlights foods—shakes, drinks, snacks—that keep us feeling full. Most combine protein and fiber, two nutrients that keep hunger pangs at bay longer than fat and with far fewer calories. The reason for the fad: Most people feel hungry and deprived when they diet. These foods aim to wipe out those feelings. Of course, you can do this on your own by choosing foods high in fiber and eating some protein with every meal.

OSTEOPOROSIS

A mug of milk and strong bones go hand in hand. But dairy products aren't the skeleton's only pals. To stay strong, bones need other minerals, vitamins, and proteins as well—all of which the right diet can provide in ample amounts.

Our bones are living tissue, constantly breaking down and rebuilding. By about age 30, however, the breakdown of bone outpaces its building, and our bones lose density, particularly a spongy-looking interior structure called trabecular bone that gives bones strength. Over time, bones may become excessively fragile, resulting in fractures related to osteoporosis. Women's risk of the disease is four times higher than men's, in part because they have less bone mass to begin with. Menopausal women lose bone two to four times faster than they did before menopause, the result of a decline in bone-protecting estrogen. That rate slows down eventually, but the decline continues.

Diet won't rev up bone replacement, but along with regular exercise, it can help us hold on to the precious bone we have.

YOUR FOOD PRESCRIPTION

Dairy products
and other foods high in calcium

Our bodies contain 2 to 4 pounds (1 to 1.8 kg) of calcium, 99 percent of it in our teeth and bones. Calcium, along with other minerals, hardens the protein fibers that make up our bones. Eating foods high in calcium—dairy foods, bony sardines and salmon, leafy greens like spinach, and dried beans—may help minimize the inevitable bone loss that comes with aging. For one thing, keeping calcium levels up lowers the amount of calcium our bodies have to borrow from bones to accommodate other essential functions like blood clotting, nerve transmission, and muscle contraction.

Don't worry if you're lactose intolerant, a condition that makes it hard to digest dairy products. Bulk up instead on other calcium-rich foods. Orange juice with added calcium is another good source.

Aim for: 1,000 to 1,200 milligrams of calcium daily, the equivalent of eating the following foods in the course of a day: a cup of low-fat yogurt, a glass of fat-free milk, and a serving each of spinach and canned salmon. Spread your calcium intake throughout the day in amounts of 500 milligrams or less for the best use of the calcium you consume.

Helpful hint: While spinach and chard contain a lot of calcium, they also contain calcium oxalate, a salt that makes the calcium less available to your body.

FEATURED RECIPES

Edamame Hummus with Pita Crisps *p. 288*
Spinach Salad with Chickpeas *p. 293*
Open-Faced Sardine Sandwiches *p. 300*
Mac 'n Cheese Primavera *p. 304*
Roasted Salmon with Sautéed Greens *p. 309*
Baked Chicken with Tomatoes *p. 311*
Orange Beets *p. 323*
Banana-Peanut Bread *p. 326*

Salmon, sardines,
and other foods high in vitamin D

Without vitamin D, our bodies absorb only 10 to 15 percent of the calcium we take in. When calcium levels drop, vitamin D activates to help our bodies absorb more calcium and reduce the amount we excrete.

Many people don't get enough D, especially if they spend less than 10 or 15 minutes a day in the sun without sunscreen. (Sunlight triggers D production in our skin.) But one serving of salmon is all you need for a daily dose.

Aim for: 400 to 800 IU of vitamin D per day; 3 ounces (85 g) of salmon has 425 IU, and a glass of fortified milk or OJ has 100 IU.

Helpful hint: Most milk, cereal, and orange juice are fortified with vitamin D.

Dark green leafy vegetables
and other foods high in vitamin K

Vitamin K, found mostly in green leafy vegetables like kale, spinach, and beet greens, may be important for bone formation. Some studies have found that people who have high levels of K have lower risk of hip fracture, higher bone density, and less loss of calcium in urine. That's because vitamin K activates a bone protein that secures calcium within the bone.

Aim for: 90 to 120 micrograms of vitamin K daily, about the amount in 2 tablespoons of chopped parsley and a quarter of the amount in 1/2 cup of spinach.

Fruits, vegetables, beans, and nuts

Long-term studies at Tufts University in Boston have shown that people who eat plenty of fruits and vegetables—most of which are rich in potassium and magnesium—have significantly less bone loss than those who have lower intakes of these foods. The reason: When the body has an excess of acid—usually the result of eating meat and other animal protein—the body depends on fruits and vegetables full of potassium and magnesium to neutralize it. Without those nutrients, the body borrows calcium from our bones to do that work.

Fruits and vegetables high in potassium, like bananas and tomatoes, also protect bones by counteracting calcium loss caused by high-salt diets. In a University of California study, when 60 women were given a high-salt diet, their calcium loss increased by 42 milligrams a day. But when they added potassium, calcium loss decreased to 8 milligrams. Studies have also shown that if you consume adequate amounts of calcium, you can be less concerned about your salt intake.

Leafy greens, beans, nuts, and whole grains have hefty doses of magnesium, essential for bone strength; 50 percent of your body's magnesium supply lies within your skeleton.

Aim for: *Potassium:* 4,700 milligrams daily. Avocados, bananas, oranges, and tomatoes are just a few of the fruits and vegetables that offer 300 milligrams per serving. *Magnesium:* 320 milligrams daily. Enjoy a cup of cooked oatmeal for breakfast, a handful (1/4 cup) of almonds as an afternoon snack, a 4-ounce (113-g) serving of salmon, and a half cup of sautéed spinach for dinner, and you're all set.

Helpful hint: Eat fresh fruits and vegetables whenever possible instead of canned. Canning destroys some potassium.

Black tea

It turns out that a nice cup of tea isn't as meek as it sounds. In a Chinese study of more than 1,000 people, tea drinkers who'd been indulging in an average of 3 to 4 cups a day for 10 years or more had 0.5 to 5 percent higher bone density than non–tea drinkers, a significant difference when it comes to bones. It turns out that tea contains several compounds, including fluoride and tannins, that may benefit bone. So fire up the kettle and say hip, hip, hurray!

Aim for: 3 to 4 cups a day.

Helpful hint: Add some milk to each cup, and you'll boost bone-building calcium as well.

Soy, fish, chicken,

and other foods high in protein

Several studies have found that people who eat diets moderately rich in protein and take calcium/vitamin D supplements lose less bone density over three years than those with low-protein diets who don't take supplements. The tricky thing is that too much protein—more than 30 percent of daily calories—weakens bones, particularly if calcium intake is low.

Try to get some of your protein from soy (think tofu, edamame, and soy milk). Soy is a rare alkaline protein, which helps lower acid content in the blood—a good thing for your bones. Research also shows that protein from soy foods may help reduce bone loss in menopausal women.

Aim for: About 20 percent of your daily calories should come from protein.

NUTRITIONAL SUPPLEMENTS

Calcium. Scientists are still researching the optimal amount of calcium necessary to slow bone loss. Some studies suggest we need only 550 milligrams a day. Others suggest that a high intake doesn't stop osteoporosis. Longer studies are needed, but for now, the National Academy of Sciences recommends taking the following amount. **DOSAGE:** 1,000 to 1,200 milligrams daily in two doses.

Vitamin D. Those of us who live in sunny climates usually get enough vitamin D by exposing our skin (without sunscreen) to sunlight for about 15 minutes each day or by eating vitamin D–rich foods. But those in less sunny northern climates may need a supplement boost. Ask your doctor if any medication you are taking affects vitamin D absorption. **DOSAGE:** 400 to 800 IU daily. Check your multivitamin; many brands contain up to 400 IU. Many calcium supplements contain vitamin D as well.

Potassium. In 2004, the Institute of Medicine raised the recommended level of potassium to 4,700 milligrams daily, in part to reduce the risk of bone loss. However, experts suggest that no one take supplemental amounts of potassium beyond what's in a multivitamin unless supervised by a doctor. **DOSAGE:** The dose in a multivitamin, which usually doesn't exceed 99 milligrams; take potassium supplements only under medical supervision.

Magnesium. There are various forms of magnesium supplements, and some calcium supplements come with both vitamin D and magnesium. Magnesium chloride and magnesium lactate are the most easily absorbed forms. Many elderly people and those with gastrointestinal diseases may require magnesium supplements, but most people get enough magnesium from a healthy diet. **DOSAGE:** 320 milligrams a day.

CAUTION

Piles of protein. When protein exceeds 30 percent of calories a day, it can hurt your bones, although the type of protein also matters. Sulfur in animal proteins increases the acid content of blood, and without enough alkaline fruits and vegetables, the body rebalances itself by borrowing calcium from bones.

Each evening after dinner, brew yourself a pot of decaf tea. It will stay warm in a ceramic teapot for hours. Sip a cup throughout the evening. It's not only healthy, but wonderfully calming. And it keeps you from noshing as well.

Salty foods. Too much salt pulls calcium out of bones. In fact, according to one study, women on a month-long high-salt (9 grams a day) diet lost 42 milligrams more calcium than they did on a low-salt (2 grams a day) diet. Cut back on processed foods, which are the main source of salt in our diet. Eat lots of potassium-rich foods like bananas, which help offset salt's calcium-leaching effect, and eat plenty of high-calcium foods to replace what's lost. The 2015-2020 Dietary Guidelines for Americans recommends we consume no more than 2,300 milligrams of sodium daily.

Too much alcohol. Drinking to excess undermines bone health. For one thing, too much alcohol can interfere with the body's use of calcium and vitamin D. And it boosts the excretion of magnesium, a mineral essential for bone strength. In men, excess alcohol also lowers testosterone, which can interfere with bone building. In women, frequent overindulgence may lead to irregular menstrual cycles, which raises osteoporosis risk.

Still, you don't always have to skip the wine-and-cheese party. Several studies have found that *moderate* drinking may give bone density a boost. In small amounts, alcohol helps convert testosterone (which women have, too) into estradiol, a form of estrogen that helps prevent bone loss.

Caffeine. You may want to pass on that third or fourth cup of joe. A Swedish study of more than 31,000 women ages 40 to 76 found that 4 or more cups of coffee daily increased the risk of bone fractures, particularly in women who took in too little calcium. Yet another study found that more than 3 cups of coffee a day increased the risk of osteoporosis in both men and women by 82 percent. The reason: Caffeine increases the amount of calcium we lose in urine, and it may also interfere with the absorption of calcium and vitamin D. If you can't give up caffeine, get enough calcium and vitamin D from foods to counteract any losses.

Dieting? You May Be Losing More Than Pounds

Losing and regaining as few as 10 pounds may be a problem for your bones. In a Canadian study of more than 1,000 men and women ages 25 to 96, those whose weight rose and fell several times had significantly greater risk of bone fractures than those whose weight did not fluctuate. Researchers believe that weight loss may lead to decreases in estrogen and progesterone, both of which help preserve bone. Weight loss also increases cortisol, a hormone that, in excess, makes calcium harder for the body to absorb. There are some studies that show if you exercise and consume enough calcium and vitamin D while losing weight, you can minimize bone loss.

PROSTATE CANCER

For men living in Western societies, prostate cancer may seem inevitable. Although it's relatively uncommon in men under 45, by age 80, between 70 and 90 percent of American men have it. In fact, it's the most common type of cancer in men. The average age of diagnosis is 72.

Of course, you can't change your age. You also can't alter your family history (if your father, brother, or son had prostate cancer, your risk is higher) or race (prostate cancer is more prevalent among African Americans). But growing evidence suggests that you can dramatically reduce your risk of this cancer—and slow its progression if you already have it—simply by making moderate changes in your diet. It's worth noting that in Asian countries, where consumption of soy, fish, and produce is high and red meat and dairy consumption is low, rates of prostate cancer are more than 10 times lower than in Western countries, where plates are filled with red meats and fatty dairy foods.

The good news is that most prostate cancers are slow growing. In fact, with early detection, many doctors just take a wait-and-see approach rather than attacking the cancer immediately. The trick is careful monitoring. Screening tests used include the PSA (prostate-specific antigen) blood test and digital rectal exams.

But why sit back and wait for trouble to happen? By improving your diet, you can take a big step toward delaying the cancer's development or inhibiting its growth. In other words, by eating more foods like tomatoes and broccoli, you can make prostate cancer something you live with rather than die from.

YOUR FOOD PRESCRIPTION

Tomatoes and tomato products

If the color pink (think pink ribbons) symbolizes the fight against breast cancer, the color red actually *fights* prostate cancer! An antioxidant called lycopene, which gives tomatoes their fire-engine hue, may help prevent prostate cancer or slow its growth, according to some studies. Lycopene (a member of the carotenoid family, like beta-carotene) does this by preventing free radicals from damaging cells, including the all-important DNA inside. DNA damage is what leads healthy cells to turn cancerous. Some research suggests that the lycopene in about two daily servings of tomato sauce or juice curbs DNA damage by 28 percent. What does that mean for men? Well, in the Health Professionals Follow-Up Study, an ongoing study of the diet and lifestyle habits of 50,000 men, guys who ate at least two servings of tomato sauce a week lowered their prostate cancer risk by 23 percent.

Aim for: A half-cup of cooked tomatoes twice a week may help prevent or slow the progression of prostate cancer. Although about 85 percent of our lycopene comes from tomatoes, watermelon, red grapefruit, and guava are also good sources.

Helpful hint: Although all tomatoes contain lycopene, when they're cooked with a little oil, the lycopene becomes more available, which is why tomato sauce is such a good way to increase your intake. To give your sauce even more cancer-fighting punch, add cruciferous vegetables like broccoli, kale, and cauliflower, which have proven anticancer compounds.

Tofu, soy milk, *and other soy foods*

People in Asian countries tend to eat a lot of soy, and they don't get prostate cancer as often as we do. Coincidence? Probably not. Tofu and other soy foods contain estrogen-like compounds called isoflavones that are thought to delay the development and growth of cancer cells and encourage them to "do the right thing" by destroying themselves.

In a three-month study at the Cancer Research Center of Hawaii, blood levels of prostate-specific antigen (PSA), a marker that signals the possibility of prostate cancer, dropped 14 percent in men who ate two servings of soy a day. Another study of more than 12,000 men conducted at Loma Linda University in California found that men who consumed more than one serving of soy milk each day were 70 percent less likely to have prostate cancer than men who never drank it.

Aim for: At least one to two servings of soy foods daily, such as a cup of soy milk or a half cup of tofu. Unprocessed soy foods like tofu, soy nuts (roasted soybeans), and soy milk retain more of their isoflavones than processed soy products such as soy-based deli "meats" and soy "bacon."

Helpful hint: Edamame, very young soybeans still in their pods, are another excellent way to get more soy into your meals. You can find them in your supermarket freezer section. Steam them lightly and toss them with a little salt for a healthy snack, or add them to stir-fries.

Green tea

In test-tube studies, a powerful compound in green tea called epigallocatechin gallate (EGCG) blocks many processes involved with cancer development and growth. Population studies suggest it may protect against several cancers, including those of the prostate, stomach, colon, and breast. Some research has found no benefit for people with cancer. But a prospective study on 49,920 Japanese men found that men who reported drinking 5 or more cups of green tea a day had a 48 percent decreased risk for advanced prostate cancer compared to men who drank less than 1 cup a day.

The most recent report by the World Cancer Research Fund/American Institute for Cancer Research on diet, nutrition, physical activity, and prostate cancer found limited evidence but no conclusion on green tea and prostate cancer, however.

Aim for: 2 to 4 cups a day if you enjoy the light flavor of this delicate tea, which is also rich in antioxidants.

Tomato sauce isn't just for spaghetti. Use it on chicken, fish, pork, or beef; add it to omelettes or on fried eggs; mix it into soups; stew vegetables in it. You can even add tomato sauce to the cooking liquid for rice, couscous, or lentils!

Pomegranate juice

It makes your mouth pucker—and it may help shield you from cancer. Pomegranate juice is chock-full of colorful plant chemicals called polyphenols, the same chemicals that make grape skins red and lend brilliant colors to autumn leaves. Polyphenols are powerful antioxidants, and that's probably why pomegranate juice is shaping up to be an important cancer fighter.

Studies continue to show that the polyphenols in the juice appear to slow cancer cell growth and encourage cancer cells to kill themselves off. They also lower PSA levels. In a two-year study conducted at UCLA, 48 prostate cancer patients drank 8 ounces (227 ml) of pomegranate juice each day. Researchers found that PSA levels dropped in more than 30 percent of the men—in some cases by up to 85 percent. More significantly, cancer progression was delayed in more than 82 percent of the men.

Aim for: An 8-ounce (227 ml) glass daily.

Helpful hint: Since weight control and reducing sugar consumption are part of prostate cancer prevention, it's best to drink pomegranate juice instead of high-calorie beverages like sodas, not in addition to them.

FEATURED RECIPES

Roasted Cherry Tomatoes in Parmesan Cups p. 289
Tuna Kebabs p. 306
Tomato-Roasted Mackerel p. 308
Turkey Ragu with Spaghetti p. 314
Beef and Broccoli Stew p. 316
Brussels Sprouts with Caramelized Onions p. 319
Roasted Broccoli with Cheese p. 320
Pomegranate Ice p. 334

Salmon, mackerel, sardines, herring, *and other fatty fish*

Surely by now someone's told you to eat more fish—maybe your doctor, who's looking out for your heart. But shopping at the seafood counter more often can also protect your prostate—if you buy the right kinds of fish. In a Swedish study that followed more than 6,000 men for 30 years, those who ate moderate amounts of fatty fish—rich in omega-3 fatty acids—lowered their risk of prostate cancer by 30 percent, while non–fish eaters had a two- to threefold higher risk of developing it. *Note:* Try to get your essential fatty acids from your plate, not a pill. So far, research shows prostate protection from eating fish, but not from taking fish-oil supplements.

Aim for: Three 3- to 4-ounce (85- to 113-g) servings of fatty fish a week. If you've already been diagnosed with early-stage prostate cancer, a recent analysis found that a high consumption of fish could reduce the risk of dying by 63 percent.

Broccoli, brussels sprouts, *and other cruciferous vegetables*

If you're going to grill a steak, be sure to serve a side of broccoli with it. Why? Grilling meat creates cancer-causing substances, such as heterocyclic amines, which damage cells. Vegetables like broccoli, brussels sprouts, and cabbage contain several anticancer compounds that actually help rid the body of these substances before they have a chance to damage cells.

Consider this experiment: In one study, men ate six 1/2-cup servings of broccoli and brussels sprouts each day for 12 days. On the 12th day, the men each had a steak. Next, the guys went 12 days without eating any cruciferous vegetables, and then they each had another steak. After each phase, researchers analyzed the volunteers' urine for heterocyclic amines. What they found was that when the men ate their veggies, they were able to dump more of these carcinogens from their bodies as waste than when they just ate the steaks.

Even if you aren't a big fan of grilling, you'll still do well to get more of these cancer fighters onto your plate. Data from the Health Professionals Follow-Up Study showed that eating five or more servings of cruciferous vegetables a week lowers your risk of developing prostate cancer by up to 20 percent.

Aim for: At least four to five 1/2-cup servings a week.

Helpful hint: Look for broccoli sprouts at the market. They're among the most concentrated amounts of sulforaphane, one of broccoli's cancer-fighting compounds, with 20 to 50 times as much as mature broccoli.

Garlic and onions

Are you a garlic lover? Good! "The stinking rose" does far more than add flavor to food. Garlic, onions, and their cousins (known as allium vegetables), like scallions, shallots, and chives, may help prevent tumors by eliminating cancer-causing substances before they can damage cells. They also encourage cancer cells to self-destruct.

When researchers from the National Cancer Institute looked at how much garlic and other allium vegetables men in Shanghai, China, consumed, they found that those who ate at least 10 grams of these vegetables (1 to 1 1/2 tablespoons of chopped onions or scallions) each day had a 49 percent lower risk of developing prostate cancer compared to men who consumed much less. Men who ate at least five cloves of garlic a week had a 53 percent lower risk.

Aim for: About one garlic clove or 1 to 2 tablespoons of onion most days of the week.

Helpful hint: Put a few garlic cloves through a press, then add them to low-fat salad dressings, tuna salad, and even potato salad. If you'd rather have your garlic cooked, chop the cloves and let them stand for 10 minutes to give the therapeutic compounds a chance to form. Then sauté the garlic and add it to tomato sauce to give it some extra cancer-fighting punch.

NUTRITIONAL SUPPLEMENTS

Vitamin E. Although there was some early evidence that vitamin E supplements may help reduce the risk for prostate cancer in smokers, the most recent report by the World Cancer Research Fund/American Institute for Cancer Research on diet, nutrition, physical activity, and prostate cancer did not find enough evidence to recommend vitamin E supplements to reduce the risk for prostate cancer. In fact, according to the National Institutes of Health Office of Dietary Supplements, daily use of large-dose vitamin E supplements (400 IU) may increase your risk of prostate cancer.

If you are a smoker, consult with your doctor before considering taking supplements of vitamin E.

Selenium. Some scientific evidence suggests that dietary supplements containing selenium may reduce the risk of certain types of cancer, including prostate cancer. Yet recent trials— including a randomized, controlled trial in 35,533 men aged 50 years or older —were

Garlic has a powerful odor when raw, but cooking mellows the flavor considerably. Get in the habit of adding a teaspoon of chopped garlic to almost everything you cook on the stove—be it chicken, fish, vegetables, stir-fries, sauces, soups, or stews.

discontinued after 5 1/2 years when no association between supplementation with 200 micrograms per day of selenium with or without 400 IU per day of vitamin E influenced the risk for prostate cancer. **DOSAGE:** The daily recommendation for selenium is 55 micrograms for adults. If you feel you are not getting enough of this nutrient (see page 83), consider a multivitamin/mineral supplement that provides up to this amount. Do not exceed 400 micrograms a day from supplements, however. This is the upper limit of what is considered a safe dose.

Antioxidant combinations. Antioxidants tend to work better when they work together, and an eight-year study of the health effects of antioxidants in more than 5,000 French men suggested that a combination of vitamin C, vitamin E, beta-carotene, selenium, and zinc may protect men from certain cancers, including prostate cancer. Men who had normal PSA levels when the study started and took this combination of supplements were half as likely to develop prostate cancer as men who were given a placebo. However, among men whose PSA levels were already elevated, the supplement combo seemed to have the opposite effect—the men taking the antioxidants tended to develop more prostate cancer than those taking a placebo.

The most recent report of the World Cancer Research Fund/American Institute for Cancer Research did not find enough evidence to recommend supplements of vitamin C, vitamin E, beta-carotene, and zinc to decrease a man's risk for prostate cancer. **DOSAGE:** Until more research clarifies the safety of this combination of antioxidants, a reliable daily multivitamin/mineral supplement that provides not more than 100 percent of the recommended Daily Value of each of these nutrients might be the best choice. Taking too much of both vitamin E and selenium poses risks, and consuming more than 100 micrograms of zinc a day has been linked to greater prostate cancer risk.

CAUTION

Fatty meats and dairy foods. The scientific jury is still debating whether meat itself is linked with prostate cancer; some research suggests it is, while other studies find no connection. But the way meat is prepared may provide some additional clues. When it's fried, grilled, or otherwise cooked until very well done, carcinogens form, and that could explain meat's tentative link to prostate cancer risk. Indeed, one study found that men who ate more than 2 1/2 ounces (71 g) per week of very well done meat faced a 40 percent greater risk of prostate cancer.

While the meat connection is still likely to be debated for some time, so is the link between dairy foods and prostate cancer. According to the most recent report of the World Cancer Research Fund/American Institute for Cancer Research, there is some, although limited, evidence that suggests a diet high in dairy foods may be linked to an increased risk for prostate cancer. Interestingly, the association was stronger for low-fat milk and cheese and less significant for whole milk and yogurt. Eating a lot of dairy also means consuming a lot of calcium, and there is some, although limited, evidence that excess calcium (more than 1,500 milligrams a day, or about five servings of dairy) may increase prostate cancer risk.

Beyond the calcium link, saturated fat is also known to promote inflammation within the body, which damages cell DNA (remember, damaged DNA can lead to cancer) and stimulates the formation of blood vessels that allow tumors to grow and spread. Inflammation has already been linked with cancers of the stomach, esophagus, and colon, so it's not hard to believe that it contributes to prostate cancer, too. In fact, in one study of more than 1,000 men, higher saturated fat consumption was linked with more than double the risk of aggressive prostate tumors.

Saturated fat also raises cholesterol levels, another cause for concern. High cholesterol provides the raw materials for creating the hormones (like testosterone) that promote prostate cancer growth. Substantially cutting back on saturated fats may lower your risk. A small study recently showed that eating a vegan diet (no meat, dairy foods, or other animal products) that limited fat to just 10 percent of calories helped delay cancer progression among 93 men with early-stage prostate cancer. During the year-long study, PSA levels dropped by an average of 4 percent among the vegans, indicating a slowdown in the cancer's development. But among the control group, PSA levels rose by an average of 6 percent.

Sugar and refined carbohydrates. If you're a big fan of doughnuts, sweet desserts, and "white" foods like white bread and bagels, listen up. These easily digested carbohydrates boost insulin levels, which also raises levels of insulin-like growth factor 1, which in turn promotes tumor growth. An elevated insulin level is also one of the central problems in metabolic syndrome, a collection of symptoms that include a large waist measurement, high blood pressure and triglycerides, and low HDL cholesterol. According to a 13-year Finnish study of 1,880 men, those who had metabolic syndrome at the start of the study were nearly twice as likely to develop prostate cancer as men without metabolic syndrome. Among overweight men, the risk was three times higher. Men with metabolic syndrome are also more likely to die from prostate cancer if they get it.

So far, the evidence for the role of sugar and sugary foods in the development of prostate cancer is limited. But being overweight—overfat, to be more specific—is strongly linked to an increased risk for prostate cancer, according to the most recent report by the World Cancer Research Fund/American Institute for Cancer Research. (See the sidebar on this page for more information.)

One More Reason to Slim Down

The connection's not so obvious, but lugging around extra pounds raises your risk of prostate cancer. Not only does excess body fat produce hormones and inflammation associated with tumor growth (indeed, obesity may promote the development of a more aggressive form of prostate cancer, one that's more likely to recur and more likely to be fatal), but research now suggests that obesity may be connected to more advanced cancer because being overweight makes tumors harder to detect.

Heavy men tend to have larger prostates and lower PSA levels, which can yield false negatives on screening tests; tumors are missed in up to 25 percent of cases. Cancer also recurs more frequently in obese men. A study conducted at the MD Anderson Cancer Center in Houston found that men who were obese at age 40 had more than double the risk of prostate cancer recurrence after surgery than men of average weight.

PROSTATE ENLARGEMENT

If you're like many men over 50, you may have trouble "going"—maybe you go too frequently, or you often feel as if you have to go, but when you try, not much happens.

The problem is most likely an enlarged prostate or, as doctors call it, benign prostatic hyperplasia (BPH). The prostate is a small, walnut-size gland located behind the bladder that adds fluid to semen just before orgasm. After age 50, hormonal changes, such as a drop in testosterone and a rise in other hormones such as prolactin, stimulate the prostate to grow. This puts the squeeze on the urethra, the tube that carries urine out of the bladder, which is why urinating becomes such a problem.

The goal of any treatment is to shrink the prostate and improve urinary function. Prescription medications can accomplish this, but the right diet can also help.

YOUR FOOD PRESCRIPTION

Lean beef, oysters, pumpkin seeds, *and other foods rich in zinc*

The prostate contains more zinc than any other body part. Nutritionally oriented physicians routinely recommend that men with enlarged prostates get more zinc in their diets. Zinc is thought to help by reducing prolactin secretion; this indirectly blocks 5-alpha-reductase, an enzyme that converts testosterone into another form that causes prostate growth. Prescription medications for prostate enlargement inhibit the same enzyme.

Aim for: 11 to 30 milligrams of zinc daily. You can get more than twice this amount in a 3-ounce (85-g) serving of fresh oysters, or try pumpkin seeds, with about 8 milligrams in a half cup.

Helpful hint: You can "roast" pumpkin seeds in your microwave. Put some olive oil in a microwave-safe baking dish and heat for 30 seconds. Then add the pumpkin seeds and cook on high for 7 to 8 minutes, turning them every 2 minutes.

Tofu, edamame, soy milk, and soy nuts

Soy foods are a good source of weak estrogen-like plant compounds called isoflavones, which help prevent prostate growth by blocking 5-alpha-reductase. Choose whole soy foods like tofu, soy milk, and soy yogurt; they contain more isoflavones than processed products like soy lunch meats.

Aim for: There's no set recommendation, but eating a few servings of soy foods a week is a good goal.

FEATURED RECIPES

Edamame Hummus with Pita Crisps *p. 288*
Beef in Lettuce Wraps *p. 302*
Tuna Kebabs *p. 306*
Eggplant Lasagna *p. 305*
Salmon Steaks with Peach Salsa *p. 308*
Pumpkin Streusel Bread *p. 327*

Salmon, flaxseed,
and other sources of omega-3 fatty acids

Omega-3 essential fatty acids are naturally anti-inflammatory. Men who consume adequate amounts tend to have smaller prostates, stronger urine flow, and less urine retention in their bladders.

Aim for: The same foods that promote a healthy heart also promote a healthy prostate—yet another reason to follow the American Heart Association's recommendation to eat at least two fish meals a week.

NUTRITIONAL SUPPLEMENTS

Zinc. Along with getting more zinc in your diet, you might consider a supplement. In one small study of 19 men done at Cook County Hospital in Chicago, zinc supplements reduced prostate size in 14 of the men, and all of them reported improved urinary symptoms. **DOSAGE:** A standard dose is 15 to 30 milligrams. If you're taking a multi and increasing your food sources of zinc, you may not need more. Getting more than 40 milligrams daily for an extended period can depress the immune system and possibly cause urinary problems.

Essential fatty acids. Along with reducing cholesterol and inflammation, both of which appear to contribute to prostate growth, the essential fatty acids (EFAs) gamma-linolenic acid (GLA) and eicosapentaenoic acid (EPA) also block 5-alpha-reductase, the enzyme that triggers prostate growth, according to a test-tube study at the University of California, Davis. **DOSAGE:** There's no established dosage for prostate health, so look for a reputable product and follow label instructions for dosage. Take your EFAs with vitamin E (400 IU) to prevent the fatty acid oxidation that can actually lead to prostate disease.

CAUTION

Foods high in saturated fat, trans fat, cholesterol, and sugar. The same poor eating habits that damage the heart also damage the prostate. Studies suggest that being overweight and having elevated cholesterol, blood pressure, and blood sugar put you at risk for prostate problems. Researchers from the University of California, San Diego, found that obese men were three and a half times more likely to have enlarged prostates than were slimmer men. They also found a strong connection between high blood sugar—which some of these foods contribute to—and prostate growth.

Alcohol. Alcohol, especially beer, is a diuretic, the last thing you want when you're already making many trips to the bathroom. Alcohol also depletes key nutrients for prostate health, like zinc.

Old Man's Friend

Saw palmetto has long been a popular remedy for prostate problems. But despite its reputation for slowing prostate growth, improving urine flow, and reducing urgency, the scientific evidence is mixed. Recently, a study of 225 men published in the *New England Journal of Medicine* reported that saw palmetto was no better than a placebo for alleviating BPH symptoms. But this Florida palm hasn't been known as "old man's friend" for nothing. An earlier analysis of 18 trials with more than 3,000 men showed that, compared to placebos, saw palmetto improved weak urinary flow by up to 50 percent. The typical dosage is 160 milligrams twice a day. Note that the full benefits can take several months to kick in.

Saw palmetto is sometimes used in conjunction with pumpkin seed extract (480 milligrams a day taken in three doses), a natural source of the beta-sitosterols that help improve urinary flow.

PSORIASIS

If anyone's ever told you to "get a thicker skin," they probably weren't thinking about psoriasis. But that's just what the condition does to a person. A faulty immune system tricks the body into producing extra skin cells that build up and create thick, unsightly scaly patches.

Over the course of a month, the top layer of normal skin sloughs off and makes room for fresh new cells. In psoriasis, that new skin growth is speeded up so dramatically that the body has no time to shed the old skin cells, so they pile up like multiple layers of paint that flake and peel on the exterior of a house.

Dermatologists aren't sure just why the immune system causes the body to react this way. There's no cure, which is all the more reason to look to your diet for foods that can help ease symptoms, including natural inflammation fighters and plenty of fresh fruits and vegetables with important nutrients for healthy skin.

YOUR FOOD PRESCRIPTION

Salmon and other fatty fish

Just as creamy moisturizers can help relieve itchy skin, the right fats in your diet are like lotion that you apply from the inside out. Oily fish like salmon, mackerel, and herring provide omega-3 fatty acids that help to quell inflammation. One study from London compared the effect of eating 6 ounces (170 g) of white fish (lacking in omega-3s) daily for six weeks to eating a similar portion of oily fish. The oily fish improved the symptoms of psoriasis in patients by 15 percent, while the white fish provided little to no relief.

Aim for: Two to three 3- to 4-ounce (85- to 113-g) servings of fatty fish per week.

FEATURED RECIPES

Ginger Butternut Squash Soup p. 298
Tuna Kebabs p. 306
Tomato-Roasted Mackerel p. 308
Roasted Salmon with Sautéed Greens p. 309
Brown Rice Risotto p. 321
Orange Beets p. 323
Pumpkin Streusel Bread p. 327

Tomatoes, carrots, spinach,
and other vegetables high in beta-carotene

When researchers in Italy compared the diets of 316 people with psoriasis to the diets of 366 people without it, they found that eating carrots, tomatoes, and other foods high in beta-carotene helped decrease the risk of developing psoriasis. Beta-carotene is converted to vitamin A in the body, where it helps maintain the tissues that make up skin. Other good sources are pumpkin, sweet potatoes, winter squash, cantaloupe, and beet greens.

Aim for: Follow the advice to eat 4 to 6 cups of fruits and vegetables a day, and make sure as many as possible are rich in beta-carotene.

The Mediterranean diet

Call it the Fountain of Youth, but the Mediterranean diet, consisting mainly of fresh fruits and vegetables, fish, chicken, whole grains, and olive oil, has been linked to a number of health benefits, including relieving psoriasis. Researchers in Hawaii tracked the symptoms of psoriasis in five patients who followed a diet featuring many of the foods in the Mediterranean diet.

After six months, all five had improved significantly.

Aim for: In the study, the patients ate fresh fruits and vegetables and moderate amounts of fish, chicken, and olive oil, and they avoided highly processed foods like potato chips as well as refined carbohydrates like white bread.

Turmeric

Studies have linked turmeric, the spice that gives curry its yellow hue, to reduced inflammation in a number of conditions, including psoriasis.

Aim for: 1 tablespoon daily. Add it to stews, soups, and stir-fries.

Lemon juice

Could squeezing lemon juice into the water you drink help your skin? Some natural health practitioners think so.

By way of some rather complicated chemistry, weak acids like lemon juice (despite its mouth-puckering taste, it is actually a weak acid) are thought to create a friendly environment for beneficial bacteria in the intestinal tract that help support a healthy immune system and lessen its burden. These acids may help against autoimmune conditions in other ways as well. On the other hand, some people report that *avoiding* lemons, oranges, and pineapples, among other acidic fruits, helps improve their psoriasis.

Aim for: Squeeze lemon juice into your drinking water for several weeks to see how it affects your skin. If it seems to make things worse, take it off the menu.

Have an indoor Mediterranean picnic for dinner. Put out platters of raw vegetables, olives, low-fat cheese, good-quality tuna, dry-roasted nuts, and pita bread. Then nibble to your health's and heart's content.

NUTRITIONAL SUPPLEMENTS

Omega-3 fatty acids. Studies keep stacking up on the benefits of omega-3s—especially the type known as EPA—for skin conditions. **DOSAGE:** Most studies indicate that 6 grams per day will produce results. Make sure the product you buy contains EPA. It may take several months to see an effect.

A multivitamin/mineral. Studies have shown that people with psoriasis are often deficient in the antioxidant mineral selenium as well as vitamin D. Taking a multivitamin will help reverse any problems associated with inadequate intake of either nutrient. It's best to stick with a multi for selenium, as it can be toxic at high doses. **DOSAGE:** One a day.

CAUTION

Bread and other foods made with gluten-containing grains. Some people who have an allergy to gluten, a protein in wheat, oats, rye, and barley, have flare-ups of psoriasis after eating anything made from these grains. Avoid foods with gluten for at least three weeks to see if it makes a difference in your skin.

Red meat. Excess saturated fat in high-fat cuts of meat can worsen inflammation.

Alcohol. Heavy drinkers have a higher incidence of psoriasis than moderate drinkers or people who abstain from alcohol.

SINUSITIS

If there's ever a time to grate some ginger or chop up some chile peppers, it's when you have a sinus infection. Get these infections often? Serve yourself more fruits and vegetables to take advantage of their immunity-boosting antioxidants.

If you've suffered through sinus infections, just thinking about them can make your face tender and your head ache. Sinuses, the air-filled cavities in your forehead and cheeks and behind the bridge of your nose, produce thin mucus that drains through narrow ducts into the nasal cavity. Because of their many delicate blood vessels, sinuses are particularly vulnerable to inflammation. Sinusitis is actually inflammation of the membrane that lines the sinus and nasal passages. It can spring from hay fever, a cold, or just about anything that irritates your nasal passages.

The inflammation alone can cause painful, tender eyes, cheeks, and nasal passages; headaches; and even earaches. When congestion builds up along with it, mucus can't drain into the nasal cavity. The lingering congestion provides a perfect breeding ground in the sinuses for infectious bacteria and viruses. Not only are sinus infections painful, they are also notoriously long-lived and difficult to clear up, even with antibiotics—a good reason to thin the mucus and encourage drainage with foods.

YOUR FOOD PRESCRIPTION

Chiles, onions, horseradish,
and other foods that make your nose run

Draining mucus is a sure way to relieve sinus pressure and pain, and these foods should do the trick. Chiles, in their many varieties, can make grown men weep and sniffle. The fire comes from capsaicin, a compound so powerful it can numb pain receptors. It can also numb nerve receptors, helping to arrest inflammation. You can add chiles to your meals or simply sprinkle on some cayenne pepper.

Onions and garlic have "bite" and contain compounds that reduce inflammation. Horseradish, a pungent root that makes great cocktail sauce for boiled shrimp, is also a terrific sandwich spread. Radishes, round little flavor bombs from the mustard family, have a sharp bite that packs a punch in salads. If you get sinus infections often, consider planting radish seeds in your garden. They sprout quickly and tend to be the first crop harvested from the spring garden. Plant a row every few weeks for a continuous supply.

Also opt for spicy dishes that are traditional to Indian or Cajun cooking. A good old-fashioned bowl of spicy chili can do the trick, too.

Aim for: Enough to make your nose run.

Helpful hint: If you overdo the heat from chile peppers at a meal, eat bread with butter or drink milk to relieve the burning. The fat in these foods breaks down the capsaicin and coats the mouth, blocking the burn.

FEATURED RECIPES

Red bell peppers, kiwifruit,
and other foods rich in vitamin C

Vitamin C is crucial for keeping the immune system in top form, and better immune function means fewer colds, flus, and even allergies that can provoke congestion and sinusitis. Studies suggest that people who are prone to sinus infections have low blood levels of antioxidants. So keep your kitchen stocked with citrus fruits and red bell peppers as well as C-rich greens, including broccoli and brussels sprouts. Papayas and raspberries are other good sources of C.

Aim for: Five to six 1/2-cup servings of vegetables and three to four 1/2-cup servings of fruits every day.

Hot liquids

Sip hot tea with lemon or a steaming bowl of chicken soup (or any soup made with clear broth) to get the "juices" in your head flowing. While you're at it, breathe in the steam for the benefits of warm, moist heat without taking a shower. Grate ginger, an anti-inflammatory, into your tea or broth for an added benefit. To make ginger tea, grate a large piece of ginger into a pot containing 1 pint (1/2 l) of water and simmer for 15 minutes. Strain, then drink. You can also use the tea and a clean cloth to make a hot, moist compress to apply to your sinuses.

Aim for: Several cups a day.

Tea and water

The more fluids you take in, the thinner the mucus in your nasal passages will be. It's best to avoid sugary liquids like juice because they can promote the growth of yeast, linked to sinusitis.

Aim for: 8 to 10 glasses of liquids every day.

Nuts, greens, sweet potatoes,
and other foods rich in vitamin E

Of the many antioxidants recently found to boost health, vitamin E has proven particularly effective in helping to reduce inflammation. You can get it from kale, sweet potatoes, canola oil, almonds, wheat germ, and sunflower seeds—all foods that have a bevy of health benefits, so eat up.

Aim for: At least 15 milligrams of vitamin E daily (roughly the amount in 1 ounce (28 g) of almonds plus a cup of cooked spinach).

NUTRITIONAL SUPPLEMENTS

Vitamin C. Because it boosts the immune system, vitamin C can be a true ally in preventing the triggers that lead to sinusitis, like colds and hay fever. Choose a C supplement with bioflavonoids for even more immunity-boosting power. **DOSAGE:** 200 milligrams per day, the amount that many experts say is adequate to saturate tissues.

Vitamin E. It can be difficult to get much vitamin E from your diet unless you eat a lot of nuts, seeds, and vegetable oils. **DOSAGE:** 15 IU daily, the amount found in many multivitamin supplements.

CAUTION

Dairy products. Some people find that milk, cheese, and other dairy foods are mucus forming, although science has yet to prove this. If you feel that dairy products make your congestion worse, skip them when you have sinus problems. If you find you have to permanently cut them from your diet to get relief, be sure to make up your calcium needs with other calcium-rich foods and a supplement.

Alcohol. Alcohol swells nasal and sinus membranes, the last thing you want when you have a sinus infection.

STROKE

You know that a diet of butter, bacon, burgers, and processed foods puts you on a fast track to a heart attack, but it also increases your risk of a stroke, which is also caused by narrowed arteries—in this case, blood vessels that feed the brain. (A small percentage of strokes, called hemorrhagic strokes, are caused not by clogged arteries but by ruptured ones.) Since the underlying problems are similar, so are the solutions, like not smoking, renewing your gym membership, and of course, changing your diet, which, by the way, can help control high blood pressure, considered the leading modifiable risk factor for stroke. (Also, as with heart disease, there are some factors, like age, gender, and race, that you can't do anything about—so why not act on the ones you *can* influence?)

A massive study of thousands of women, called the Nurses Health Study, showed that eating the typical Western-style diet increased stroke risk by 58 percent, whereas consuming more whole grains, fruits, vegetables, and fish—the same foods that guard against so many other diseases—lowered that risk by 30 percent. Here's where to start. (Hint: Buy a bunch of bananas at the store and plan a spinach salad topped with tuna for tomorrow's lunch.)

YOUR FOOD PRESCRIPTION

The DASH Diet

One of the most important ways to protect yourself from stroke is to lower your blood pressure. When your pressure is higher than 140/90 mmHg (millimeters of mercury), your stroke risk doubles. And for every 20 mmHg increase in systolic pressure (the first number in your blood pressure reading) or 10 mmHg increase in diastolic pressure (the second number), your risk doubles yet again.

The DASH (Dietary Approaches to Stop Hypertension) Diet, which is low in saturated fat and cholesterol and high in fiber, low-fat and fat-free dairy foods, and fruits and vegetables, has been shown to decrease blood pressure by 5.5/3.0 mmHg, which is enough to cut your stroke risk by 27 percent. Go a step further and reduce your sodium intake to about 2/3 teaspoon of salt a day, and you can lower your pressure by 8.9/4.5 mmHg. That's about the same reduction you can get by taking a single blood pressure medication.

Even on their own, the foods that make up the DASH Diet are potent stroke fighters. Eating plenty of whole-grain fiber lowers risk by about 40 percent, and other research shows that eating fruit and vegetables daily reduces it by 20 to 40 percent. While you're "doing the DASH," you can lower your blood pressure another 4 points or so by getting some regular exercise, maintaining a healthy weight, and moderating your alcohol intake (see Caution on page 272). For more information about this diet, see the High Blood Pressure entry on page 191.

Oats, almonds, soy foods, and cholesterol-lowering margarine

How does a nice, steaming bowl of cholesterol-lowering oatmeal sound, or a snack of crunchy almonds (excellent sources of vitamin E)? Have you discovered soy milk or edamame—young green soybeans, great in soups and salads or eaten right out of their pods—yet? These are three of the foods that make up a cholesterol-

Blueberries are extraordinarily healthy, but their growing season is short. The solution: Buy large amounts when in season, wash thoroughly, then freeze in airtight containers. Use the berries year-round as a topping, in smoothies, or in your cooking.

lowering regimen known as the Portfolio Diet, developed by researchers in Toronto. When eaten as part of a total diet that's low in saturated fat, this combination of foods appears to reduce LDL ("bad") cholesterol levels by 28 percent, almost as much as a statin drug does. (For more information on the meal plan as well as recipes, visit http://stmichaelshospital.com/media/hospital_news/2018/0706.php).

It's not clear whether high cholesterol levels contribute as much to strokes as they do to heart attacks, but there's good reason to suspect they may. Some research suggests that lowering cholesterol levels with statin medications can reduce stroke risk by about 25 percent. It follows that lowering your cholesterol through diet would also help.

High cholesterol contributes to plaque buildup in blood vessels around the brain, paving the way for an ischemic stroke, the most common kind. In fact, for women under age 55, having high cholesterol seems to increase the risk of dying from a stroke by about 23 percent, even if they don't have cardiovascular disease. Even more frightening: Elevated cholesterol increased stroke deaths among younger African American women by a whopping 76 percent.

Now, to get your LDL cholesterol below the 100 mg/dl level that's recommended for people with multiple risks for cardiovascular disease (below 70 mg/dl for those at very high risk), you may still need a statin, but following a cholesterol-lowering diet is a good place to start.

Aim for: The Portfolio plan calls for eating the following each day: about a handful of almonds; 20 grams of soluble fiber from foods such as oats, barley, and certain fruits (to get there, you'll need to eat 1 cup each of oatmeal,

beans, strawberries, and mashed sweet potatoes and one apple); 50 grams of soy protein (the equivalent of a whopping five or more servings of soy foods); 2 grams of plant sterols from sterol-enriched margarine; and five to nine daily servings of fruits and vegetables. Of course, even if you don't follow this plan exactly, you're bound to see benefits from adding more of these foods to your diet.

Blueberries, sweet potatoes, artichokes, *and other foods rich in antioxidants*

One reason fruits and vegetables are so helpful against stroke is that they're such good sources of antioxidants, which help reduce inflammation and prevent plaque buildup in the arteries. They also improve blood flow by helping blood vessels dilate.

Aim for: 4 to 6 cups of fruits and vegetables a day. One serving is one medium piece of fruit; 1/2 cup of fruit or vegetable juice; 1/2 cup of chopped fruit or cooked vegetables, beans, or legumes; or 1 cup of leafy vegetables.

FEATURED RECIPES

Buckwheat Pancakes with Fruit Sauce *p. 286*
Updated Waldorf Salad *p. 290*
Tuna and White Bean Salad *p. 295*
Sweet Potato Soup *p. 297*
Mac 'n Cheese Primavera *p. 304*
Roasted Salmon with Sautéed Greens *p. 309*
Creamed Spinach *p. 320*
Blueberry-Oat Scones *p. 324*
Pumpkin Streusel Bread *p. 327*

Bananas, baked potatoes, white beans, *and other foods rich in potassium*

Here's a great reason to pack a banana with your lunch: Bananas are loaded with potassium, and experts think one of the reasons the DASH Diet works so well is that it provides plenty of this mineral. Research shows that eating a diet low in potassium (less than 1.5 grams a day) increases stroke risk by 28 percent. The Health Professionals Follow-Up Study found that participants who ate nine daily servings of potassium-rich fruits and vegetables, like potatoes, prunes, and raisins, as well as the foods listed above, lowered their stroke risk by 38 percent compared to people who ate just four servings daily.

Aim for: 4.7 grams (4,700 milligrams) of potassium daily, an amount you can get by eating 7 to 10 servings of potassium-rich fruits and vegetables each day. One baked potato, a cup of white beans, a cup of canned tomatoes, and a cup of winter squash contain about 1,000 milligrams.

Beans, spinach, *and other foods rich in folate*

Beans aren't just good for your heart; they're also good for protecting your brain. That's because they're rich in the B vitamin folate (a.k.a. folic acid). According to a 20-year study of nearly 10,000 adults, eating a diet rich in folate lowers the risk of stroke by 20 percent. Here's more intriguing evidence: Researchers who looked at the number of strokes in the United States before and after food manufacturers began fortifying flour with folic acid to prevent birth defects found 10 to 15 percent fewer stroke deaths in the three years after fortification began than in the three years before.

Aim for: 400 micrograms of folate daily, which you can get from a half cup of pinto beans plus a cup of cooked spinach.

Low-fat milk

If you've stopped drinking milk, it may be time to start again. There's an excellent reason that low-fat and fat-free dairy foods are mainstays of the DASH Diet—they're good sources of potassium, magnesium, and calcium, all of which naturally lower blood pressure. Indeed, a study of men in Puerto Rico found that hypertension was half as prevalent among milk drinkers as among those who didn't drink it. So it makes sense that if milk (and dairy foods) lowers blood pressure, it would also reduce the risk of stroke. In fact, a 22-year study of more than 3,100 Japanese men in the Honolulu Heart Study found that those who drank at least two 8-ounce (236-ml) glasses of milk a day had half the risk of stroke compared to non–milk drinkers.

Aim for: Two to three 8-ounce (236-ml) servings daily.

Helpful hint: Not everyone loves a glass of cold milk, so if you'd prefer not to drink

Few vegetables contain as many healing nutrients as spinach. At least once a week, sauté fresh spinach and garlic in olive oil and season with pepper and a dash of lemon juice. It's the perfect dinner side dish, for both taste and health.

yours straight, remember that all the milk you consume—in coffee and on cereal, for example—counts toward your daily goal. And because saturated fat is linked to cardiovascular disease in general, opt for 1 percent or fat-free milk.

Barley, buckwheat, cornmeal,
and other magnesium-rich foods

The same study that found that potassium-rich foods decreased stroke risk also showed that a diet higher in magnesium-rich foods reduced risk by 30 percent, even if you don't have high blood pressure.

Aim for: 420 milligrams for men and 320 milligrams for women of magnesium a day. You can get there by eating a cup of black beans, a cup of spinach, a serving of halibut, and an ounce (28 g) of pumpkin seeds.

Salmon *and other fatty fish*

You know it's good for your heart, so you should be eating fish like salmon anyway. If you are, you're probably protecting yourself from stroke. For starters, by eating more fish, you're automatically eating less red meat and processed meats like sausage, hot dogs, bacon, or lunch meat, and that means you're eating less arterty-clogging saturated fat.

It's also possible that the omega-3 fats in fish like tuna, mackerel, and salmon improve blood flow by reducing inflammation in the arteries and making blood less likely to clot. A 12-year study done at Harvard Medical School of nearly 5,000 adults age 65 and older found that eating fish one to four times a week lowered stroke risk by 27 percent.

Aim for: The American Heart Association recommends at least two servings of oily fish (8 to 12 ounces/227 to 340 g total) a week. Since mercury contamination is a concern, opt for types lower in mercury, such as salmon and canned light tuna, and steer clear of highly contaminated fish such as shark, swordfish, king mackerel, and tilefish.

Getting the Salt Out

Trying to cut back on sodium? The good news is that you can still add some salt to your food when you prepare it. As long as you're not dumping a shakerful into every dish, table salt isn't that much of a worry. Rather, it's processed foods that are the big concern, since they account for about 75 percent of the sodium we consume. In fact, many foods that you wouldn't even think of as "salty," like cereals, contain more sodium than potato chips! The best way to curb your sodium intake is to steer clear of these high-sodium processed foods. You can also follow this rule of thumb: When you check the calorie and sodium content per serving on product labels, the number of milligrams of sodium should be less than or at most equal to the number of calories.

NUTRITIONAL SUPPLEMENTS

Omega-3 fatty acids. Although fish-oil supplements aren't specifically recommended to prevent strokes, there's reason to suspect they may be helpful because they lower levels of triglycerides. These blood fats, which contribute to blood vessel blockages, are shaping up to be an independent risk factor for stroke. Research indicates that heart patients who have triglyceride levels above 200 mg/dl have a 30 percent increased risk of stroke. **DOSAGE:** The American Heart Association recommends taking 2 to 4 grams of eicosapentaenoic acid (EPA) and docosahexaenoic acid (DHA) a day to lower elevated triglycerides under your doctor's supervision, of course. Taking the supplements with food can help reduce the burping often associated with fish oils. So can choosing a fish-oil supplement that contains citrus essence.

Folic acid and vitamin B$_{12}$. These B vitamins may lower stroke risk by reducing levels of homocysteine, an amino acid that can damage arteries. While high doses aren't recommended, if you're not getting enough from your diet, make sure your multivitamin fills the gap. **DOSAGE:** *Folic acid:* 400 micrograms daily. *Vitamin B$_{12}$:* 2 micrograms daily.

CAUTION

Sodium. Excess sodium raises blood pressure, which in turn increases stroke risk. In a study of more than 29,000 adults in Japan, men whose diets were highest in sodium had more than twice the risk of dying from strokes compared to men who ate low-sodium diets. For women, the death rate from stroke was 70 percent higher in those who consumed the most sodium than in those who ate less.

Reducing your sodium intake substantially lowers both your blood pressure *and* your stroke risk. Both the American Heart Association and the National Heart, Lung, and Blood Institute recommend limiting sodium intake to no more than 2,300 milligrams each day—the equivalent of 1 teaspoon of salt. According to research from studies on the DASH Diet, doing so lowers blood pressure by 2.1/1.1 mmHg. Cut back even more—to about 2/3 teaspoon daily—and you can drop your blood pressure by 8.9/4.5 mmHg. That's helpful because even a 5-point drop in pressure reduces your stroke risk by 27 percent. See "Getting the Salt Out" on page 271 for tips on lowering your sodium intake.

Saturated fat, cholesterol, refined sugar, and refined flour. In other words, the stuff that makes up the typical Western diet. All of these are known contributors to heart disease, so it's no surprise that they boost stroke risk as well—by as much as 58 percent. The grease factor increases fatty deposits in the arteries that can lead to blockages. Refined flour and sugar raise blood sugar and insulin levels, which in turn raise stroke risk by increasing fat levels in the blood, thickening artery walls, and increasing blood pressure and inflammation. If you're overweight or have high blood pressure, a Western-style diet becomes even more problematic: The Nurses Health Study found that obese women who followed such a diet had double the risk of stroke; women with high blood pressure had triple the risk, and smokers had quadruple the risk.

Heavy drinking. Alcohol is tricky, and whether it raises your stroke risk depends largely on your drinking habits. Light to moderate drinking (two drinks daily for men and one for women) actually lowers stroke risk by 28 percent, probably by boosting HDL cholesterol—the good kind—and making blood less likely to clot. Yet, if you have three or four drinks a day, your risk suddenly goes up by 42 percent. Toss back five, and it jumps by 69 percent. Heavy drinking raises blood pressure, thickens the blood, interferes with heart rhythm, and reduces blood flow to the brain. If you've already had a stroke, it may be best to give up the goblet and stick to club soda.

Insulin Resistance: A Hidden Stroke Risk

Do you have a spare tire around your middle? Have high blood sugar, high triglycerides, or high blood pressure? You may have a condition called insulin resistance syndrome, which puts you at significantly increased risk for a stroke. If you do have it, your stroke risk increases by 78 percent if you're a man and 100 percent if you're a woman.

Insulin resistance is typically associated with developing diabetes (see the Diabetes entry on page 144). But now research suggests that being insulin resistant (even without diabetes) raises stroke risk by increasing the assault on the arteries.

What is insulin resistance syndrome (which also goes by the names metabolic syndrome and syndrome X)? Rather than being a single disease, it's a collection of health problems that include excess belly fat (a measurement of more than 35 inches (89 cm) around the waist for women and 40 inches (102 cm) for men); elevated triglycerides (over 150 mg/dl) and blood sugar (over 110 mg/dl); high blood pressure (over 130/85 mmHg); and low HDL cholesterol (under 40 mg/dl for women and 50 mg/dl for men). If you have any three of these conditions, you have insulin resistance syndrome. And while there may be some debate about what to call this condition, there's no doubt about its dangers.

Eating more fruits, vegetables, and whole grains—the core formula for stroke prevention—will also help you combat insulin resistance.

ULCERS

Before you reach for a glass of milk to soothe your ulcer pain, read this: Much of what we used to "know" about ulcers has been proven wrong. Most ulcers aren't caused directly by stress but by the bacterium *Helicobacter pylori*, which is why ulcers today are often treated with antibiotics along with an acid suppressor. Spicy foods don't cause ulcers either—in fact, chile peppers are used in some countries to treat them—although these foods can worsen the pain if you're not used to eating them. And milk, once considered an ulcer soother, won't do any good and may even make things worse.

H. pylori, a bug with a spiral shape, can screw itself into the mucosal lining that protects the digestive tract. Once there, it weakens the mucus produced by the stomach and the duodenum (the first part of the small intestine) and exposes the delicate lining to digestive acids. What begins as irritation can quickly develop into sores along the walls of the esophagus, small intestine, and stomach. In advanced ulcers, sores can become so severe that they burn a hole in the tissue.

Researchers estimate that almost 80 percent of the people in the world carry *H. pylori* in their bodies. Obviously, not all of them develop ulcers. Sometimes it takes another factor to pave the way. An all-too-common one is the regular use of painkillers such as aspirin and ibuprofen, known as nonsteroidal anti-inflammatory drugs (NSAIDs). Over time, these can inflame and irritate the linings in the GI tract and often trigger *H. pylori* into action. Because NSAIDs also block the production of hormones that protect the stomach lining, digestive acids can begin their damage, and soon afterward, ulcers make themselves known. Once an ulcer takes up residence, stress, diet, alcohol, caffeine, and smoking can aggravate it.

While antibiotics are often necessary to kill off *H. pylori,* certain foods also wield power against the bugs. Others can help strengthen the digestive tract's own protective bacteria, making it less inviting to *H. pylori*. And once an ulcer has taken hold, foods that help to rebuild the lining of the stomach can aid in healing.

Tired of the same old salad? Cut the amount of lettuce in half and replace with thinly sliced cabbage. Add broccoli or cauliflower crowns, berries, grapes, or pear slices. Then change to a yogurt-based dressing. Your new salad will be as delicious as it is healthy.

Honey

Modern medicine has finally caught on to a folk remedy that has been used for centuries. Because honey fights bacteria, hospitals and clinics sometimes apply it to burns and other open wounds. For the same reason that it can help heal a skin ulcer, honey may help thwart *H. pylori*. Researchers from New Zealand tested honey made from the nectar of the Manuka flower on bacteria from biopsies of gastric ulcers and found that the honey inhibited bacterial growth. Other researchers have been successful in using other types of honey to halt the growth of *H. pylori*.

Aim for: The research on honey is young, so a specific recommendation has yet to be made. Start by taking a tablespoon of raw, unprocessed honey in the morning and at night to calm a fiery belly. Spread it on toast or a cracker to keep it in the stomach longer. Because *H. pylori* is slow growing, be sure to keep up your honey regimen until ulcer symptoms are long gone.

Slippery elm tea

Slippery elm coats the stomach just as it does a sore throat, bringing some relief, albeit short-lived, from ulcer pain.

Aim for: Several cups throughout the day.

Broccoli, brussels sprouts, cauliflower, and kale

These cruciferous vegetables all contain sulforaphane, a compound that appears to squelch *H. pylori*. In one study, after patients who tested positive for the bacteria ate a half cup of broccoli sprouts twice daily for seven days, 78 percent tested negative for the bacteria. Other studies, on mice, have shown that sulforaphane extracts can successfully destroy the bacteria in the mice's digestive tracts.

Aim for: We'll have to wait for studies to show just how much broccoli you would have to eat to help cure ulcers. Until then, consider eating a cup a day of broccoli, raw or cooked, or broccoli sprouts. Not only will the broccoli begin to battle your ulcer, but it will also provide more than a day's worth of vitamin C and a generous amount of fiber, two more allies in the fight against ulcers.

Cabbage

Scientists think that it may be the amino acid glutamine that gives cabbage its anti-ulcer punch. Glutamine helps to fortify the mucosal lining of the gut and to improve blood flow to the stomach, meaning it not only helps prevent ulcers but can also speed healing of existing sores.

Aim for: Eat cabbage a few times a week. Add it to salads, coleslaw, and wraps. You can also drink raw cabbage juice, sold in health food stores.

Yogurt with active cultures

Foods like yogurt and kefir (fermented milk) contain "good" bacteria that can inhibit *H. pylori* and may help ulcers heal faster. In one large study in Sweden, people who ate fermented milk products like yogurt at least three times a week were much less likely to have ulcers than people who ate yogurt less often.

Aim for: Have a cup of yogurt, kefir, or another fermented milk product with live, active cultures at least once a day. Avoid sweetened varieties, which are less effective.

FEATURED RECIPES

Coleslaw with Orange-Sesame Vinaigrette *p. 290*
Broccoli Salad *p. 291*
Hearty Vegetable Stew *p. 304*
Chicken-Barley Bake *p. 312*
Springtime Quinoa *p. 322*
Blueberry-Oat Scones *p. 324*

Plantain

This large, green, banana-like fruit is starchy and sticky in texture. It helps to soothe inflamed and irritated mucous membranes and has some antibacterial properties to boot. Studies on rats with ulcers caused by daily aspirin use have shown that unripe green plantain can both prevent the formation of ulcers and help to heal them. Plantain works its magic best when it's unripe.

Aim for: Until human studies determine the amount that might help, use the fruit as they do in Latin America, where green plantain is eaten boiled like a potato. Avoid fried plantain, as the fat can aggravate ulcers.

Fruits, vegetables, whole grains, *and other foods high in fiber*

Add another star to fiber's crown. Besides keeping you regular, fiber has a role in keeping ulcers at bay, especially those in the duodenum. A number of studies have found that people who eat high-fiber diets have a lower risk of developing ulcers. In the Physicians Health Study from Harvard, researchers looked at the diets of 47,806 men and found that those who ate 11 grams or more of fiber from vegetables had a 32 percent lower risk of developing duodenal ulcers.

Scientists aren't sure how fiber helps, but it may be thanks to the fact that it slows the emptying of the stomach and thus reduces the amount of time the stomach lining and duodenum are exposed to digestive acids. Soluble fiber, the kind found in oats, beans, barley, peas, and pears, also forms a slippery goo in the stomach that acts as a barrier between the stomach lining and corrosive stomach acids.

Aim for: General health guidelines suggest getting 25 to 35 grams of fiber a day.

NUTRITIONAL SUPPLEMENTS

DGL tablets or wafers. Strong-tasting licorice made from the root of the licorice plant contains a number of compounds that help soothe irritated, inflamed mucosal tissue. Licorice also stimulates the lining of the stomach and small intestine to produce more mucus, which may help sores heal faster. It may also have some antibacterial properties against *H. pylori.*

In a recent animal study on rats with ulcers, licorice-coated aspirin cut the number of ulcers in half. A separate study compared the effect of licorice extract with that of cimetidine (Tagamet), a common ulcer medication, on 100 patients with chronic ulcers. The researchers found that both treatments cured 90 percent of the ulcers after 12 weeks.

Unfortunately, the licorice candy most commonly sold today won't do the trick because it contains little or no real licorice, so you'll need to go to a health food store for chewable supplements (not capsules). Because real licorice can cause high blood pressure, it's important to get deglycyrrhizinated licorice (DGL), which has been processed to eliminate the problem. **DOSAGE:** One or two tablets or wafers before meals and at bedtime.

Probiotics. Probiotics—the "good" bacteria found in yogurt and other fermented milk products—may help heal your ulcer faster and could even help prevent future ulcers. Several studies have shown that one bacterium in particular, *Lactobacillus gasseri,* is especially effective in helping to protect the gastrointestinal tract.

If you're taking antibiotics for your ulcer, it's a good idea to take probiotics as well, since antibiotics wipe out both the bad and good bacteria in your system, and eliminating good bacteria can have unwanted side effects, such as diarrhea. **DOSAGE:** Take no more than one to two billion live organisms once a day. Higher doses sometimes cause intestinal discomfort. Choose a supplement with multiple strains, including *L. gasseri.*

CAUTION

Milk. It was once considered the perfect therapy for ulcers because it was thought to coat and soothe the stomach. Although the calcium in milk can buffer the strong acids in the stomach, studies have shown that milk may also stimulate stomach acid production. No need to eliminate milk entirely; just avoid it if it causes pain.

Spicy foods. People who eat spicy diets loaded with chile peppers are actually less likely to develop ulcers, probably because many spices contain compounds that kill bacteria. But if you already have an ulcer, it's best to steer clear of the fiery stuff, which may increase ulcer pain because it can irritate the exposed sores.

Fatty foods. The higher the fat content of your dinner, the more stomach acid is needed to digest it, and the acids can irritate ulcers.

Coffee and alcohol. Caffeine and alcohol stimulate the release of stomach acids that can crank up ulcer pain. (Nicotine has the same effect, so add this to your reasons to quit smoking.) Alcohol can also irritate and wear down the mucosal lining of the stomach.

Calcium carbonate supplements. Ironically, the very acids that stimulate ulcer pain help protect your gut from *H. pylori* when you don't have an ulcer, so taking antacids such as calcium carbonate supplements (the form found in Tums) may work against you in the long run. If you want to take calcium for your bones, take it in the form of calcium citrate, which doesn't cause these problems.

Say Hello to Aloe?

If you're looking around your kitchen for ways to help soothe and heal an ulcer, consider the aloe plant on the counter. Better yet, go to the health food store for some aloe vera juice, which helps heal the lining of the digestive tract. Take 1/4 to 1/2 cup three times a day for a month. Make sure you don't get the leaf exudate (sometimes just called aloe), which is a laxative. Aloe juice may also help stop the bleeding of a bleeding ulcer because of its astringent, or drying, effects.

URINARY TRACT INFECTIONS

No one thinks much about their personal plumbing until something goes awry. If that something is a urinary tract infection, or UTI, you don't need a plumber—but you may need antibiotics. See your doctor if you suspect you have a UTI. If you get frequent UTIs, there are steps you can take to help prevent them.

UTIs start at the end of the urinary tract. The urethra, a tube only about 2 inches (5 cm) long, carries urine from your bladder out of the body. The trouble starts when gastrointestinal bacteria, often of the *Escherichia coli* variety, stick to the walls of the urethra and begin to multiply, leading to an infection. The result is a burning sensation when you urinate, along with the urge to urinate even when you don't need to go. You may also feel pressure above your pubic bone or in the rectum. If the infection moves up the urinary tract into the bladder or even farther, into the kidneys, the condition becomes trickier and more serious, causing pain in the sides and back as well as nausea and fever.

The best way to prevent a UTI is to prevent problem bacteria from clinging to the lining of the urethra. Your doctor will explain that one way to do this is to urinate after sex. Two simple beverages can also do the trick (read on for details).

YOUR FOOD PRESCRIPTION

Cranberry and blueberry juice

Doctors used to think that it was acidity that made cranberries so effective in treating UTIs, but other acidic juices like pineapple don't work. (And increasing the acidity of urine by taking vitamin C supplements also appears to have little or no effect, although the practice became popular in recent years.) Now research hints that an antioxidant compound in cranberries and blueberries called epicatechin may work directly on bacteria like *E. coli,* affecting the tendrils on their surface. The bacteria essentially become boats without anchors and are no longer able to attach to the lining of the urethra walls. Cranberry compounds also appear to weaken bacteria cells.

A study from Finland involving 150 women prone to UTIs found that those who drank cranberry juice daily for 12 months experienced a 20 percent reduction in infections. In a study in Massachusetts, scientists found that more intense cranberry products like whole cranberries and pure cranberry juice (rather than cranberry juice cocktail) were particularly effective at quashing the bacterial threat.

If you have kidney stones made of oxalate, note that one small study suggests that cranberry extract tablets may contribute to the stones. Also, drinking more than a liter of juice a day over a long period may increase the risk of uric acid kidney stones. Check with your doctor before starting a cranberry regimen.

Aim for: 4 to 8 ounces (118 to 236 ml) of cranberry or blueberry juice. To avoid the added sugar that bacteria thrive on, choose unsweetened or "light" varieties. Because the unsweetened stuff is so tart, some people prefer to take cranberry extract tablets (see Nutritional Supplements on page 279).

Helpful hint: Like all acidic juices, cranberry juice can erode tooth enamel. Be sure to brush your teeth after drinking it.

Water

Drinking plenty of water keeps urine diluted so bacteria have less chance to group together and cause problems. It also stimulates you to urinate more often, helping to flush the walls of the urethra, where bacteria may be clinging.

Aim for: At least 8 to 10 eight-ounce glasses (2 to 2 1/2 l total) of water per day. If you exercise or live in a humid, hot environment, drink even more.

Plain yogurt with active cultures

Yogurts that contain live bacterial cultures help keep up your gut's population of "good" bacteria, which in turn keep "bad" bacteria in check. Studies on whether yogurt and other natural sources of "good" bacteria, like kefir (fermented milk), can help to prevent UTIs have had mixed results. It may be that the abundant added sugar in some yogurts cancels the effect of the probiotic bacteria. But eating some yogurt every day can't hurt, and if you have to take antibiotics for a UTI, it may help you avoid a yeast infection, which antibiotics sometimes trigger. Keep eating yogurt for two weeks following your last dose of antibiotics to keep up with the continued effect of the medication.

Aim for: A cup a day. Stick to plain yogurt with live, active cultures.

NUTRITIONAL SUPPLEMENTS

Cranberry extract. Although most of the studies that offer evidence to support the power of cranberry in preventing UTIs have been conducted using cranberry juice, a recent study from Finland suggests that cranberry extract tablets work just as well. **DOSAGE:** One 400-milligram tablet twice daily.

Probiotics. *Acidophilus* and *bifidobacteria* are the two main probiotics ("good" bacteria) that can help support a healthy immune system if you're not eating enough yogurt. They're sometimes combined in supplements. **DOSAGE:** Follow the dosage instructions on the label.

CAUTION

Sugary foods and beverages. Cookies, candy, soda, and other foods and drinks made with refined sugar or high-fructose corn syrup create an environment in which bacteria thrive and multiply, making infection more likely. Try to stick to natural sources of sugar like fresh fruits.

Coffee, tea, cola, and alcohol. All of these beverages can irritate the bladder and make a UTI more likely.

If you find cranberry juice hard to drink on its own, then dilute it with an equal amount of club soda and add a squeeze of lime or lemon juice for flair. Or you can mix it with other fruit juices that will counter its tart, unsweetened flavor.

WRINKLES

A face can tell a thousand stories, both happy and sad, but most of us would rather not have our histories written out in wrinkles.

As we age, the surface layer of the skin thins. The layer beneath the surface also loses collagen—skin's scaffolding—and elastin, fibers that give skin its bounce. Far beneath the surface, fat cells also shrink. The result? Wrinkling and sagging. You can blame some of this on exposure to the sun. Ultraviolet rays damage the skin and generate unstable molecules called free radicals that wreak further havoc by breaking down collagen. Smoking and air pollution have a similar effect.

The body fights back with its own antioxidants, which neutralize free radicals, but getting more antioxidants from foods as sweet and delicious as berries increases your protection when the damage starts to overwhelm the body's natural defenses.

YOUR FOOD PRESCRIPTION

Skinless chicken, fish, beans, nuts, *and other lean protein foods*

Protein helps repair cells that have suffered free radical damage. When protein is digested, it breaks down into amino acids, the building blocks of cells. Having plenty of amino acids available helps to speed the repair and regeneration of skin cells and collagen.

Aim for: Lean protein at every meal.

Olive oil

Olive oil is chock-full of oleic acid, one of the fatty acids that keep cell membranes fluid and therefore make skin supple. Olive oil also has small amounts of other essential fatty acids that fight inflammation. Yet another benefit comes in the form of vitamin E and polyphenols, a class of antioxidants that protect skin from free radical damage.

Aim for: Choose olive oil for most of your dishes that include oil.

Helpful hint: Opt for 100 percent extra-virgin oil, which is the least refined and has the most antioxidants. Drizzle it over sautéed and steamed vegetables. Heating the oil as little as possible helps retain its healing properties.

Garlic

The "stinking rose" offers much more than essential flavor for cooking; it also brings a wealth of skin-protective polyphenols to your plate.

Aim for: Keep a clean garlic press at the ready and add minced garlic—especially raw—to as many of your dishes as possible. You can also eat a garlic clove, chopped into several pill-size pieces, every day.

Helpful hint: After you chop garlic, let it stand for 10 to 15 minutes before using it in cooking. The waiting period allows the garlic's active compounds to develop.

FEATURED RECIPES

Tropical Fruit Salad *p. 286*
Spinach Salad with Chickpeas *p. 293*
Tuna and White Bean Salad *p. 295*
Salsa Tuna Salad Sandwiches *p. 300*
Three-Bean Chili *p. 306*
Salmon Steaks with Peach Salsa *p. 308*
Roasted Salmon with Sautéed Greens *p. 309*
Mixed Berry Tart *p. 335*

Blueberries, blackberries, raspberries, and strawberries

For tiny fruits, berries pack more antioxidant punch than any other fruit or vegetable tested. Next in line? Red apples with the peel. All these fruits work beautifully to help protect skin from the damage that leads to wrinkles. Citrus fruits are also rich in antioxidants.

Aim for: A cup of berries a day. Blend them into fruit smoothies, add them to breakfast cereal, and use them in pancake or muffin batter.

Green tea

Thanks to its impressive storehouse of polyphenols, green tea is high on the list of skin-friendly beverages.

Aim for: 4 cups throughout the day. If you're sensitive to caffeine, drink your last cup before 3:00 in the afternoon.

Salmon, mackerel, *and other fatty fish rich in omega-3 fatty acids*

No doubt you've already heard what omega-3 fatty acids can do for your heart, but a nice piece of broiled salmon can also do wonders for your skin. The omega-3s provide a wealth of protection by keeping cell membranes fluid.

Aim for: At least two 4-ounce (113 g) servings of fatty fish per week.

Vegetables and beans

Add these foods to the fish and olive oil we already mentioned, and you're really feeding your skin the foods it needs to achieve that youthful smoothness. When researchers in Australia compared the diets and wrinkles of hundreds of people in Australia, Greece, and Sweden, they found that those who ate more vegetables, beans, fish, and olive oil had the fewest wrinkles. The researchers suspect it was a combination of monounsaturated fats, antioxidants, and lean protein that did the trick.

Aim for: Five to six 1/2-cup servings of a range of vegetables daily. In addition, sprinkle beans on salads, enjoy bean-based soups, and plan a bean-based meal such as chili once a week.

Water

Skin cells need a bounty of fluid to keep their membranes supple and receptive to the nutrients that keep them healthy. Take out a half-gallon (2 l) pitcher and fill it with water. That's the very least you ought to drink in a day to keep your skin smooth and hydrated. If you're sweating because of physical activity or being outside in hot weather, you should drink even more.

Aim for: At least 8 to 10 eight-ounce glasses (2 to 2 1/2 l total) per day.

NUTRITIONAL SUPPLEMENTS

Vitamin E. Vitamin E has long been linked to a glowing complexion because its protective antioxidants help to heal damaged skin. Parents rub vitamin E oil on their babies' sensitive skin and bottoms for the same reason that cosmetic companies add it to lotions and other facial products. **DOSAGE:** Up to 400 IU a day.

Omega-3 fatty acids. These fatty acids, especially EPA, combat skin inflammation, and one study showed that EPA applied topically helped to improve collagen and elastin fibers in the skin. We're not suggesting that you apply EPA to your skin; more research is needed before dermatologists can make that kind of recommendation. But taking fish-oil supplements may go a long way toward preventing wrinkles. **DOSAGE:** 1,000 milligrams a day.

CAUTION

Coffee. Some health professionals believe that coffee contributes to wrinkles by increasing stress hormones like adrenaline and noradrenaline.

Sugar. It's time to kick that cake and candy bar habit. Several studies indicate that consuming excess amounts of sugary foods and beverages like sodas can damage collagen, the protein that supports skin.

YEAST INFECTIONS

Ask a baker about yeast, and you'll hear stories of the miracles it creates in the oven—airy pastries and crusty breads that can make you swoon. But ask a woman who has had a yeast infection, and you'll hear a very different tale. Having too much of a certain type of yeast in your body can make you miserable, leaving you itching and irritated in the most intimate places.

The moist, dark areas of your body—the mouth, vagina, and rectum—are full of beneficial bacteria that help protect against infection, as well as fungi that normally cause no problems. But certain conditions change that balance, killing off beneficial bacteria that keep yeast populations in check. Common culprits include pregnancy and diabetes, both of which can change the acidity of the vagina, making it more vulnerable to infection, and antibiotics, which can wipe out the good bacteria that protect the body from more harmful bacteria. The result? Fungus of the *Candida* variety, the type behind most yeast infections, can take over. Oral thrush, a white, itchy, sensitive rash in the mouth, and vaginal yeast infections, with their burning itch and discharge, commonly crop up as a result.

Yeast infections can be stubborn, recurring even after successful treatment with medicines and antifungal creams. For that reason, prevention is the best option, and you can start with that yogurt in the refrigerator. Eating foods that strengthen the immune system is also smart because it may help fortify your body against many types of infection, so you might avoid the antibiotics that make you vulnerable to yeast infections. (See the Immune Weakness entry on page 192 for more advice.)

YOUR FOOD PRESCRIPTION

Garlic

Garlic's a powerful bacteria fighter—in fact, it was used to help wounds heal back in World War I. But the "stinking rose" also fights fungi. When scientists in Iran added extracts of pure garlic and onion to samples of *C. albicans*, the fungus that causes most yeast infections, the garlic and onion kept it from growing.

Only recently have scientists discovered that garlic's little bulbs are packed with antioxidants, so eating plenty of garlic should also help keep your immune system running at full steam.

Aim for: Two cloves per day. Garlic is most effective when eaten raw, so chop some and add it to salads, salsa, and pasta dishes, or simply chew the cloves if you can bear it.

Yogurt with active cultures

This fermented dairy product is chock-full of "good" bacteria. When more of these bugs take up residence in your body, there's less

FEATURED RECIPES

Edamame Hummus with Pita Crisps *p. 288*
Greens with Creamy Garlicky Dressing *p. 292*
Simple Broccoli Soup *p. 298*
Chicken in Garlic Sauce *p. 312*

room for yeast to multiply and cause trouble. In one study on women with recurring yeast infections, yogurt proved particularly helpful. For six months, the women ate a daily 8-ounce (227-g) serving of yogurt with the active culture *Lactobacillus acidophilus*. For the next six months, they ate no yogurt at all. During the yogurt period, the women experienced 30 percent fewer yeast infections.

Aim for: 8 ounces (227 g) of plain yogurt a day. Make sure you choose yogurt with live, active cultures, particularly *L. acidophilus*.

NUTRITIONAL SUPPLEMENTS

Garlic. If you don't want to risk the scent-ual side effects of garlic, consider a no-odor garlic supplement. A word of warning: Theoretically, garlic may increase the risk of bleeding and should be used under a doctor's supervision by anyone taking a blood-thinning medication, such as warfarin (Coumadin). Garlic can also irritate the gastrointestinal tract and should be used with caution by people with infectious or inflammatory GI conditions. **DOSAGE:** 500 milligrams three times a day for up to six weeks.

Probiotics. If you can't eat enough yogurt, or if it doesn't seem to be working as quickly as you'd like, try supplementing with probiotics, the very bacteria found in yogurt. Probiotics teem with live, active cultures that aid digestion and keep the body's population of good bacteria at healthy numbers. They have shown such promise in fighting yeast infections in both the vagina and mouth that some doctors recommend taking them whenever you start a course of antibiotics that may make you vulnerable to yeast infections.

Several studies have found particular benefits from the probiotic *L. rhamnosus*, often listed on labels as *Lactobacillus GG*, which can survive the digestive acids in the gut better than others. *L. acidophilus*, which is more common and much less expensive, has also shown promise.

A study on premature babies found that when their breast milk was supplemented with probiotics for the first six weeks of life, the infants' risk of yeast infections in their mouths, a common problem, decreased by 20 percent. **DOSAGE:** Usually 1 tablespoon of liquid probiotic culture or one or two capsules a day. Take the dose between meals when digestive acid production is at its lowest and be sure to follow the product's dosing instructions for best results. Check with your pediatrician before giving your infant probiotics.

Probiotics should be taken for at least two weeks after finishing a course of antibiotics to ensure that your good bacteria reach effective levels.

CAUTION

Sugary foods, sugary drinks, and alcohol. Yeasts love sugars—in fact, they thrive on them. To starve the troublemakers, make a conscious effort to cut back. That means avoiding fruit juices, sweetened breakfast cereals, ice cream, and desserts as well as anything made with high-fructose corn syrup, like soft drinks and packaged cookies or candy. Try to satisfy your sweet tooth with fruits like cherries, grapes, and fresh apricots or, better yet, have some sweet, crunchy carrots.

You should also avoid alcohol if you have a yeast infection, because yeasts feed on it.

White bread, white rice, and white potatoes. Refined grains and starches raise the level of blood sugar (glucose) in the body, and yeasts feed on glucose. Switch to high-fiber foods like whole-wheat bread, brown rice, and whole-grain pasta and cereal. Choose sweet potatoes over white potatoes whenever possible because they have less effect on blood sugar.

WHAT ABOUT YEASTY FOODS?

Contrary to what you may think, yeasts in food are an entirely different species from the pathogen *Candida albicans,* most associated with yeast infections in the body. Yeasts in foods like mushrooms and yeast breads are "friendly fungi" and therefore don't seem to pose a problem for most people.

Healing Recipes

Medicine never tasted this delicious! We threw just about every healing ingredient into the recipes that follow, but what you'll notice is an explosion of flavor.

Tropical Fruit Salad Serves 6

Prep Time • 20 minutes

1 cup low-fat vanilla yogurt

1 teaspoon grated lime zest

2 red grapefruits

2 kiwifruits, peeled and cut into thin wedges

2 bananas, sliced

1 small cantaloupe or large papaya, seeded and cut into chunks

2 tablespoons crystallized ginger

Fresh and flavorful, this salad features antioxidant-rich fruits blended with ginger and lime for a scrumptious breakfast treat. Don't forget that bananas and cantaloupe are both loaded with blood pressure–lowering potassium.

1. In a small bowl, combine the yogurt and lime zest.

2. Over a large bowl, cut the grapefruits into sections, then place in the bowl. Squeeze the membranes over the bowl to release the juice. Add the kiwis, bananas, cantaloupe, and ginger. Toss to blend.

3. To serve, divide the fruit among 6 bowls. Top each with 1 1/2 table-spoons of the yogurt mixture.

164 calories, 4 g protein, 37 g carbohydrates, 7 g fiber, 1 g total fat, 1 g saturated fat, 39 mg sodium

Buckwheat Pancakes with Fruit Sauce Serves 5

Prep Time • 5 minutes
Cook Time • 20 minutes

3 apples, pears, or plums, cored and sliced

1/3 cup pure maple syrup

1 cup buckwheat flour

1/3 cup brown rice flour

2 tablespoons brown sugar

1 teaspoon baking powder

1/2 teaspoon baking soda

1/2 teaspoon salt

1/2 teaspoon cinnamon

3/4 cup milk

2 tablespoons canola oil

2 eggs

Here's a gluten-free recipe that tastes great! Buckwheat isn't a cereal like wheat and rice but actually a fruit seed related to rhubarb and sorrel. Its nutty flavor makes these a step up from plain white pancakes.

1. Heat a nonstick skillet coated with cooking spray over medium heat. Add the apples and cook, turning, until just tender, 5 minutes. Add the syrup and reduce the heat to low to keep warm.

2. In a large bowl, whisk together the buckwheat flour, rice flour, brown sugar, baking powder, baking soda, salt, and cinnamon. In a measuring cup, whisk together the milk, oil, and eggs. Stir into the flour mixture just until blended.

3. Heat a griddle or nonstick skillet coated with cooking spray over medium heat. Drop the batter by 2 tablespoons onto the griddle to form pancakes. Cook until browned on the bottom and bub-bles form on top, 3 minutes. Turn and cook until the bottoms are browned and the pancakes are firm to the touch, 3 minutes. Place on a plate and cover to keep warm. Repeat with the remaining batter. Serve with the fruit syrup.

328 calories, 7 g protein, 54 g carbohydrates, 7 g fiber, 10 g total fat, 2 g saturated fat, 283 mg sodium

Zucchini Frittata Serves 6

Prep Time • 5 minutes
Cook Time • 15 minutes

4 eggs

4 egg whites

1/4 cup grated Parmesan cheese

1/4 teaspoon salt

2 tablespoons olive oil

1 clove garlic, minced

2 small zucchini, shredded

2 roasted red peppers, cut into thin strips

Eggs, a stellar source of protein, will start your day off right. Here, only half the yolks are used to keep down the cholesterol and fat.

1. Preheat the oven to 400°F (200°C). In a medium bowl, whisk together the eggs, egg whites, cheese, and salt.

2. Heat the oil in a large ovenproof nonstick skillet over medium heat. Add the garlic and cook just until tender, 1 minute. Add the zucchini and peppers and cook 1 minute. Pour in the egg mixture and cook until the bottom of the frittata is set, 3 minutes. Bake until set, 10 minutes.

138 calories, 9 g protein, 5 g carbohydrates, 1 g fiber, 9 g total fat, 2 g saturated fat, 331 mg sodium

Edamame Hummus with Pita Crisps Serves 8

Prep Time • 20 minutes
Cook Time • 10 minutes

4 pita breads, halved crosswise

1/2 teaspoon cumin

2 cups shelled edamame

1/4 cup sesame tahini

3 tablespoons lemon juice

2 cloves garlic, mashed

1/2 teaspoon salt

2 tablespoons extra-virgin olive oil

This unique hummus features edamame (green soybeans) instead of the traditional chickpeas. Tahini is a paste made from ground sesame seeds that's similar to peanut butter. Sesame seeds are a great source of manganese and copper and a good source of magnesium as well as sterols, plant compounds that help lower cholesterol.

1. Preheat the oven to 350°F (180°C). Place the pita halves on a cutting board and lightly coat with cooking spray. Sprinkle with the cumin and cut each into 8 wedges. Place on a baking sheet and bake until lightly browned, 10 minutes. Transfer to a rack and let cool.

2. Meanwhile, place the edamame in a medium saucepan, add enough water to cover, and bring to a boil over medium-high heat. Cook until very tender, 10 minutes. Drain and rinse under cold water. Let cool slightly.

3. In a food processor, combine 1/3 cup water and the edamame, tahini, lemon juice, garlic, and salt. Process until smooth. With the motor running, gradually add the oil and blend until combined. Serve with pita wedges.

212 calories, 9 g protein, 24 g carbohydrates, 5 g fiber, 10 g total fat, 1 g saturated fat, 333 mg sodium

Ultimate Spiced Nuts Serves 18

Prep Time • 5 minutes
Cook Time • 20 minutes

1 medium egg white

2 cups mixed nuts, such as Brazil nuts, walnuts, pecans, and almonds

1/2 cup pumpkin seeds

1 tablespoon brown sugar

2 teaspoons ground ginger

1/2 teaspoon ground nutmeg

1/2 cup dried cranberries

Just 1/4 cup of this high-protein snack will give you the afternoon boost to get through the day. But don't reserve nuts just for snacking. Try sprinkling some on a tossed salad, fruit salad, or frozen yogurt.

1. Preheat the oven to 350°F (180°C). In a large bowl, whisk the egg white, then add the nuts and seeds. With a rubber spatula, toss to coat. Add the brown sugar, ginger, and nutmeg and stir until well blended. Stir in the cranberries. Spread onto 2 ungreased baking sheets with sides and bake until browned, 20 minutes.

129 calories, 4 g protein, 6 g carbohydrates, 2 g fiber, 11 g total fat, 1 g saturated fat, 0 mg sodium

Roasted Cherry Tomatoes in Parmesan Cups Serves 4

Prep Time • 10 minutes
Cook Time • 16 minutes

3/4 cup coarsely shredded
  Parmesan cheese

2 cups cherry tomatoes

2 tablespoons extra-virgin olive oil

1/4 cup basil leaves, cut into
  thin strips

Be sure to use Parmesan cheese for this recipe; a richer cheese such as pecorino or Romano may have too much fat to hold a shape. When shredding the cheese, use the section of your shredder with the largest holes.

1. Preheat the oven to 375°F (190°C). Line a baking sheet with parchment paper. Place 3 tablespoons cheese on the paper and, with a spoon, spread into a 6-inch (15 cm) circle. Repeat with the remaining cheese to make 4 circles. Bake until lightly browned around the edges, 6 minutes.

2. Meanwhile, place 4 custard cups or small shallow bowls upside down on a countertop. Working one at a time, carefully remove the hot cheese circles from the baking sheet and place over the cups. Let stand to form cups and cool completely.

3. Place the tomatoes in a roasting pan and drizzle with the oil. Roast until the tomatoes split, 10 minutes. Add the basil, tossing to blend.

4. Place a Parmesan cup on each of 4 plates. Divide the tomatoes equally among the cups and serve immediately.

173 calories, 10 g protein, 4 g carbohydrates, 1 g fiber, 14 g total fat, 5 g saturated fat, 394 mg sodium

Updated Waldorf Salad Serves 6

Prep Time • 15 minutes

1/2 cup low-fat Greek yogurt

3 tablespoons pure maple syrup

1 1/2 tablespoons Dijon mustard

1/4 teaspoon salt

4 medium apples, quartered, cored, and cut into chunks

1 small head fennel, coarsely chopped

1/4 cup dried cranberries

1/3 cup toasted nuts, such as walnuts or almonds

Forget the fat-laden, mayonnaise-coated salads of days gone by. Here you'll find a delicious dressing made from low-fat yogurt spiked with mustard and maple syrup. Turn this tasty salad into a light meal or lunch by adding 3 cups cooked chicken, turkey, or fish.

1. In a medium bowl, whisk together the yogurt, syrup, mustard, and salt. Add the apples, fennel, cranberries, and nuts and toss to coat well.

169 calories, 3 g protein, 32 g carbohydrates, 5 g fiber, 4 g total fat, 1 g saturated fat, 196 mg sodium

Coleslaw with Orange-Sesame Vinaigrette Serves 6

Prep Time • 50 minutes

1/4 cup fresh orange juice

2 tablespoons rice wine vinegar

1 tablespoon grated fresh ginger

1 clove garlic, minced

1/2 teaspoon salt

2 tablespoons dark sesame oil

1 head Napa cabbage, shredded

3 carrots, shredded

1 bunch scallions, thinly sliced

2 tablespoons sesame seeds, toasted

Like broccoli, cabbage is a strong anticancer food, and here's a delicious way to eat more. Napa cabbage, also known as Chinese cabbage, differs from the round, waxy heads of green and red cabbage. Napa cabbage heads are elongated, with tender, ruffled leaves and a mild flavor.

1. In a large bowl, stir together the orange juice, vinegar, ginger, garlic, and salt. Whisk in the oil. Add the cabbage, carrots, and scallions and toss to coat well. Let stand for 30 minutes or refrigerate for 2 hours. Sprinkle with the sesame seeds before serving.

98 calories, 2 g protein, 9 g carbohydrates, 3 g fiber, 6 g total fat, 1 g saturated fat, 229 mg sodium

Broccoli Salad Serves 6

Prep Time • 20 minutes

1/4 cup balsamic vinegar

2 tablespoons Dijon mustard

2 tablespoons honey

1/4 teaspoon salt

1/4 teaspoon black pepper

2 tablespoons flaxseed oil

2 tablespoons extra-virgin olive oil

2 heads broccoli

1 small red onion, cut into thin
   wedges

1/2 cup whole almonds, toasted
   and coarsely chopped

1/2 cup dried cranberries

4 ounces (113 g) chèvre goat
   cheese, crumbled

If raw broccoli florets are too strong for you, steam them for 4 minutes, then rinse in cold water and drain well before adding to the salad.

1. In a large bowl, whisk together the vinegar, mustard, honey, salt, and pepper. Whisk in the flaxseed and olive oils until well blended. Set aside.

2. Remove the florets from the broccoli and add to the vinaigrette. Trim the ends of the stalks and, with a vegetable peeler, peel off the thick outer layer. Shred the stalks with a food processor or by hand.

3. Add the shredded stalks, onion, almonds, and cranberries to the bowl and toss to coat well. Top with the cheese.

333 calories, 12 g protein, 33 g carbohydrates, 7 g fiber, 20 g total fat, 4 g saturated fat, 303 mg sodium

Corn, Tomato, and Quinoa Salad Serves 4

Prep Time • 20 minutes
Cook Time • 15 minutes

1 cup quinoa, rinsed well

1/2 teaspoon salt

1/4 cup lime juice

1 tablespoon olive oil

1 tablespoon flaxseed oil

1 teaspoon honey (optional)

1/8–1/2 teaspoon crushed
 red pepper

1 cup fresh or thawed frozen
 corn kernels

1 tomato, seeded and chopped

1 avocado, peeled, seeded,
 and chopped

Known as the super grain, quinoa is considered a complete protein and is higher in unsaturated fat and lower in carbohydrates than other grains. When preparing quinoa, be sure to rinse it well to remove the bitter saponin coating.

1. Heat 2 cups water in a medium saucepan over medium heat. Add the quinoa and salt and bring to a simmer. Reduce the heat to low, cover, and simmer until the liquid is absorbed and the quinoa is tender, 15 minutes. Transfer to a large bowl and let cool for 15 minutes.

2. Meanwhile, in a measuring cup, whisk together the lime juice, olive oil, flaxseed oil, honey, if desired, and red pepper.

3. Add the corn, tomato, and avocado to the quinoa. Drizzle with the vinaigrette and toss to coat well.

345 calories, 8 g protein, 44 g carbohydrates, 7 g fiber, 17 g total fat, 2 g saturated fat, 310 mg sodium

Greens with Creamy Garlicky Dressing Serves 6

Prep Time • 20 minutes

1/2 cup low-fat Greek yogurt

1 tablespoon extra-virgin olive oil

1 tablespoon balsamic vinegar

1 tablespoon lemon juice

2 tablespoons minced fresh herbs,
 such as basil, cilantro, or
 parsley

2 cloves garlic, minced

1/4 teaspoon salt

3 cups mixed greens

3 cups baby kale

No need to give up creamy salad dressings. Yogurt, rich in beneficial bacteria, forms the base of this dressing, and flavorful ingredients—garlic, basil, and balsamic vinegar—make it delicious.

1. Place the yogurt in a small bowl and whisk in the oil, vinegar, lemon juice, herbs, garlic, and salt.

2. Place 1 cup greens and kale on each of 6 salad plates. Top with 2 tablespoons of the dressing.

59 calories, 3 g protein, 5 g carbohydrates, 1 g fiber, 3 g total fat, 1 g saturated fat, 141 mg sodium

Spinach Salad with Chickpeas Serves 4

Prep Time • 10 minutes
Cook Time • 20 minutes

2 medium onions, cut into
   1/2-inch (1.25-cm) slices

1 can (15.5 ounces/439 g)
   chickpeas, drained, rinsed, and
   patted dry

1/4 cup lemon juice

2 tablespoons flaxseed oil

1 tablespoon olive oil

1 clove garlic, minced

1/2 teaspoon salt

1/4 cup crumbled feta cheese

1 package (5 ounces/142 g) baby
   spinach

2 apples, cored and sliced

2 tablespoons ground flaxseed

Forget the heavy spinach salads loaded with fat and cholesterol. Fresh and delicious, this crunchy salad is packed with antioxidants, fiber, and cancer-fighting ingredients.

1. Preheat the oven to 400°F (200°C). Coat a baking sheet with sides with olive oil cooking spray. Add the onion slices and coat each with the spray. Roast for 10 minutes. Add the chickpeas and roast until the onions are tender and browned, 10 minutes.

2. Meanwhile, in a measuring cup, whisk together the lemon juice, flaxseed oil, olive oil, garlic, and salt. Stir in the cheese.

3. Place the spinach in a large bowl and toss with the onions, chickpeas, apples, and flaxseed. Drizzle with the vinaigrette.

292 calories, 9 g protein, 37 g carbohydrates, 10 g fiber, 14 g total fat, 3 g saturated fat, 476 mg sodium

Shrimp and Grapefruit Salad Serves 4

Prep Time • 15 minutes

1 red grapefruit

1 teaspoon Dijon mustard

1/2 teaspoon salt

1/4 teaspoon black pepper

2 tablespoons olive oil

1 large head romaine lettuce, shredded (about 6 cups)

1 Hass avocado, peeled, pitted, and chopped

1 pound (454 g) peeled deveined cooked large shrimp

Grapefruit isn't just for breakfast. It helps boost the antioxidants in this salad while forming a delicious vinaigrette.

1. Working over a large bowl, section the grapefruit, letting the juice drip into the bowl. Place the sections in a small bowl. Squeeze the membranes over the large bowl to release any juice (you should have 1/4 cup).

2. Whisk the mustard, salt, and pepper into the juice. Whisk in the oil. Add the lettuce, avocado, shrimp, and grapefruit. Toss gently to coat well.

317 calories, 31 g protein, 15 g carbohydrates, 7 g fiber, 16 g total fat, 2 g saturated fat, 656 mg sodium

Citrus Chicken Salad Serves 4

Prep Time • 3 hours, 10 minutes
Cook Time • 18 minutes

1/4 cup orange juice

2 tablespoons lemon juice

2 tablespoons lime juice

1 clove garlic, minced

4 boneless skinless chicken breast halves

2 tablespoons olive oil

1 package (5 ounces/142 g) mixed baby greens

1 red bell pepper, seeded and cut into thin strips

1 orange, cut into sections

Citrus makes the calcium in greens like spinach more available to the body. Here, citrus juices—orange, lemon, and lime—blend with garlic to make a delicious marinade. While the chicken grills, the marinade is thickened, creating a flavorful salad dressing.

1. In a zipper-seal plastic bag, combine the orange juice, lemon juice, lime juice, and garlic. Add the chicken and turn to coat. Seal the bag and refrigerate for 1 to 3 hours.

2. Preheat the broiler or grill. Coat a broiler pan or grill rack with cooking spray. Remove the chicken from the marinade, reserving the marinade. Broil or grill the chicken until a thermometer inserted in the center of the breasts reaches 160°F (71°C), 15 minutes.

3. Meanwhile, in a small saucepan over high heat, bring the marinade to a boil and cook for 3 minutes. Remove from the heat and whisk in the oil.

4. Divide the greens, bell pepper, and orange equally among 4 plates. Slice the chicken, place on the salads, and drizzle with the marinade.

241 calories, 29 g protein, 13 g carbohydrates, 4 g fiber, 9 g total fat, 1 g saturated fat, 123 mg sodium

Chicken Pasta Salad Serves 4

Prep Time • 10 minutes
Cook Time • 10 minutes

6 ounces (168 g) whole-wheat
pasta shells

2 tablespoons low-fat mayonnaise

2 tablespoons low-fat plain yogurt

2 tablespoons red wine vinegar

2 tablespoons grated
Parmesan cheese

1 clove garlic, minced

3 cups shredded cooked
chicken breasts

1 cup grape or cherry
tomatoes, halved

1/4 cup Kalamata olives, cut
into thin strips

2 cups baby arugula

Pasta salad gets a healthy makeover with whole-wheat pasta and nutri-ent-rich vegetables like tomatoes and arugula. Opt for canola mayonnaise the next time you shop to add omega-3 and omega-6 fatty acids to your diet.

1. Cook the pasta according to package directions. Drain well but do not rinse.

2. Meanwhile, in a large bowl, whisk together the mayonnaise, yogurt, vinegar, cheese, and garlic. Add the chicken, tomatoes, olives, and arugula and toss gently to coat.

3. When the pasta has drained, let cool slightly, about 2 minutes. Add to the chicken mixture and toss to coat.

408 calories, 36 g protein, 36 g carbohydrates, 5 g fiber, 13 g total fat, 2 g saturated fat, 228 mg sodium

Tuna and White Bean Salad Serves 4

Prep Time • 15 minutes

1/3 cup tomato juice

3 tablespoons lemon juice

2 tablespoons olive oil

1 tablespoon chopped fresh basil
or 1 teaspoon dried basil

1/4 teaspoon salt

1 can (5 ounces/142 g) tuna,
drained

1 can (15.5 ounces/439 g) white
beans, drained and rinsed

1 medium cucumber, peeled,
seeded, and chopped

1/4 cup pitted Kalamata olives,
chopped

1 package (5 ounces/142 g) mixed
greens

Delicious salad dressings don't have to be laden with fat. Vitamin-rich tomato juice is the base for this delightful dressing.

1. In a measuring cup, whisk together the tomato juice, lemon juice, oil, basil, and salt.

2. In a medium bowl, toss the tuna, beans, cucumber, olives, and 1 ta-blespoon of the vinaigrette.

3. Divide the greens equally among 4 plates. Top each with 1/4 of the tuna mixture and drizzle with the vinaigrette.

206 calories, 18 g protein, 20 g carbohydrates, 7 g fiber, 9 g total fat, 1 g saturated fat, 597 mg sodium

Quick Chicken Noodle Soup Serves 6

Prep Time • 10 minutes
Cook Time • 25 minutes

2 tablespoons olive oil

3/4 pound (340 g) boneless skinless chicken breasts, cut into 1-inch (2.5-cm) pieces

1 large onion, chopped

2 cloves garlic, chopped

2 carrots, chopped

1 red bell pepper, chopped

1 teaspoon dried thyme

1 carton (32 ounces/907 g) chicken broth

8 ounces (224 g) whole-grain spaghetti, broken into 2-inch (5 cm) pieces

Perfect for a last-minute supper or to ward off a winter cold, this flavorful soup will hit the spot. Garlic, onion, carrots, and bell pepper add flavor and healing properties, while the spaghetti is reminiscent of the noodle soup of days gone by.

1. Heat the oil in a large saucepan over high heat. Add the chicken and cook, stirring, until browned, 5 minutes. With a slotted spoon, transfer to a bowl.

2. Add the onion to the saucepan and cook until lightly browned, 5 minutes. Add the garlic, carrots, bell pepper, and thyme. Cook, stirring, until lightly browned, 3 minutes. Add the broth and 1 cup water, the chicken, and any drippings in the bowl and bring to a boil. Add the spaghetti and cook for 8 minutes or until tender.

275 calories, 20 g protein, 37 g carbohydrates, 7 g fiber, 6 g total fat, 1 g saturated fat, 345 mg sodium

Chicken Curry Soup Serves 6

Prep Time • 15 minutes
Cook Time • 30 minutes

2 tablespoons olive oil

2 onions, chopped

4 large carrots, chopped

1 russet potato, peeled and finely chopped

1 tablespoon mild curry powder

1 carton (32 ounces/907 g) low- sodium chicken broth

1 pound (454 g) boneless skinless chicken breasts, cut into thin strips

1/2 small head cauliflower, cut into florets (2 cups)

1 cup frozen peas, thawed

You'll want to eat this warming soup because it's comforting and delicious, but you'll get a bonus: the anticancer properties of turmeric, found in curry powder, and cauliflower. With its creamy carrot base, this soup is a meal in itself. Round it out with a whole-grain pita or bread.

1. Heat the oil in a large saucepan over medium heat. Add the onions and carrots and cook, stirring, until lightly browned, 5 minutes. Add the potato, curry powder, 1 cup broth, and 1 cup water. Cover and cook for 10 minutes or until the vegetables are tender.

2. Remove from the heat and let cool slightly, 5 minutes. Place in a food processor or blender and process until smooth.

3. Return the mixture to the saucepan and add the remaining broth and the chicken and cauliflower. Bring to a boil, reduce the heat to medium-low, and simmer until the chicken is cooked and the cauliflower is tender, 15 minutes. Add the peas and cook until heated through, 3 minutes.

260 calories, 25 g protein, 26 g carbohydrates, 6 g fiber, 7 g total fat, 1 g saturated fat, 230 mg sodium

Sweet Potato Soup Serves 6

Prep Time • 10 minutes
Cook Time • 30 minutes

2 tablespoons olive oil

2 cloves garlic, minced

1 large onion, chopped

1 red bell pepper, seeded and chopped

1 teaspoon ground ginger

1 teaspoon allspice

4 cups low-sodium vegetable or chicken broth

2 large sweet potatoes, peeled and cut into 1-inch (2.5-cm) pieces

1 can (14.5 ounces/411 g) diced tomatoes

1/2 cup natural peanut or almond butter

1 package (16 ounces/454 g) frozen shelled edamame

1 package (5 ounces/142 g) baby spinach or kale

This rich, creamy dish is thickened with peanut butter, which adds delicious flavor and stellar nutrition. Packed with chunks of vegetables and seasoned with ginger and allspice, it's sure to become a favorite.

1. Heat the oil in a large saucepan over medium-high heat. Add the garlic, onion, and bell pepper and cook until lightly browned, 5 minutes. Add the ginger and allspice and cook for 1 minute.

2. Stir in the broth, sweet potatoes, and tomatoes and bring to a boil. Reduce the heat to low, cover, and simmer until the potatoes are just tender, 15 minutes.

3. Place the peanut butter in a small bowl. Whisk in about 1 cup of the simmering broth. Return to the saucepan and add the edamame and spinach. Cook until the edamame is cooked through, 10 minutes.

405 calories, 20 g protein, 40 g carbohydrates, 10 g fiber, 20 g total fat, 3 g saturated fat, 303 mg sodium

Ginger Butternut Squash Soup Serves 4

Prep Time • 20 minutes
Cook Time • 45 minutes

2 tablespoons olive oil

1 large onion, chopped

2 cloves garlic, minced

1 teaspoon turmeric

1 butternut squash
   (2–2 1/2 pounds/900-1,200 g),
   peeled, seeded, and cubed

4 cups vegetable or chicken broth

2 large apples, peeled, cored,
   and chopped

1 tablespoon grated fresh ginger or
   1 teaspoon ground ginger

1/2 teaspoon salt

Sweet butternut squash is delicious pureed with apple and ginger, and this soup is a perfect way to get the inflammation-fighting properties of ginger and turmeric. For a lovely presentation, swirl a dollop of plain yogurt on top before serving.

1. Heat the oil in a large saucepan over medium heat. Add the onion and cook, stirring, until lightly browned, 4 minutes. Stir in the garlic and turmeric and cook for 1 minute. Add the squash and broth and bring to a boil.

2. Reduce the heat to low, cover, and simmer until the squash is just tender, 20 minutes. Add the apples, ginger, and salt and cook until the squash and apples are very tender, 10 to 20 minutes. Remove from the heat and let cool for about 10 minutes.

3. Working in batches, place the mixture in a food processor or blender and process until smooth.

267 calories, 4 g protein, 51 g carbohydrates, 10 g fiber, 8 g total fat, 1 g saturated fat, 762 mg sodium

Simple Broccoli Soup Serves 4

Prep Time • 20 minutes
Cook Time • 1 hour, 45 minutes

1 bulb garlic

1 bunch broccoli

2 tablespoons olive oil

1 large onion, chopped

1 carton (32 ounces/907 g)
   vegetable or chicken broth

1 russet potato, peeled
   and chopped

1/2 cup low-fat plain yogurt

You'd never know this vitamin-rich soup is low in fat. Instead of heavy cream, a potato and roasted garlic thicken it. If you'd like to make it really special, top with a sprinkling of low-fat cheddar cheese.

1. Preheat the oven to 400°F (200°C). Cut the top 1/4 inch (.5 cm) off the garlic to expose the cloves. Wrap in a double thickness of foil and bake until very tender and browned, 1 hour.

2. Meanwhile, remove the florets from the broccoli and chop coarsely. Peel and chop the stalks.

3. Heat the oil in a large saucepan over medium heat. Add the onion and cook until lightly browned, 5 minutes. Add 3 cups broth, the broccoli, and the potato. Bring to a boil, then reduce the heat to low, cover, and simmer until the broccoli stalks and potato are very tender, 30 minutes.

4. Squeeze the garlic into a food processor. Add the hot broccoli mixture and puree until smooth. Return to the saucepan and add the remaining broth and 1 cup water. Simmer to blend flavors, 10 minutes. Top each serving with a dollop of yogurt.

247 calories, 9 g protein, 37 g carbohydrates, 7 g fiber, 8 g total fat, 1 g saturated fat, 512 mg sodium

Lentil-Tomato Soup Serves 8

Prep Time • 10 minutes
Cook Time • 50 minutes

6 teaspoons olive oil

3 ounces (85 g) sliced Canadian bacon, cut into matchsticks

3 carrots, sliced

2 celery stalks, sliced

1 onion, chopped

2 cloves garlic, minced

1 teaspoon chili powder

1/2 teaspoon dried oregano

1/2 teaspoon ground cumin

1/2 teaspoon salt

1 can crushed tomatoes (28 ounces/794 g), with juice

1 1/2 cups lentils, sorted and rinsed

2 cups low-fat plain yogurt

Low-fat Canadian bacon adds smoky flavor to tomato soup packed with lycopene and studded with high-fiber, protein-rich lentils.

1. Heat 1 teaspoon oil in a stockpot over medium heat. Add the bacon and cook, stirring constantly, until well browned, 3 minutes. Transfer to a plate.

2. Add the remaining 5 teaspoons oil to the pot and heat. Add the carrots, celery, and onion and cook, stirring, until well browned, 5 minutes. Add the garlic, chili powder, oregano, cumin, and salt. Cook for 2 minutes, stirring constantly.

3. Add the tomatoes and juice, lentils, and 6 cups water and bring to a boil. Reduce the heat to medium-low, partially cover, and simmer until the lentils are tender, 30 to 40 minutes.

4. To serve, ladle the soup into 8 bowls and top each with 1/4 cup yogurt and a few strips of bacon.

256 calories, 15 g protein, 38 g carbohydrates, 9 g fiber, 6 g total fat, 1 g saturated fat, 506 mg sodium

Minestrone with Fava Beans Serves 8

Prep Time • 10 minutes
Cook Time • 25 minutes

2 tablespoons olive oil

2 carrots, sliced

2 celery stalks, sliced

1 medium onion, chopped

2 zucchini, halved and sliced

1 red bell pepper, chopped

1 carton (32 ounces/907 g) vegetable or chicken broth

2 cans (14.5 ounces/411 g each) diced tomatoes with basil, garlic, and oregano

2 cups whole-grain rotelle, penne, or shell pasta

1 can (19 ounces/538 g) fava beans, drained and rinsed

Parmesan cheese (optional)

Using flavored diced tomatoes saves you time when making this hearty soup. The flavors are rich and make a lovely base for vegetables, pasta, and beans.

1. Heat the oil in a stockpot over medium heat. Add the carrots, celery, and onion and cook, stirring, until the onion is soft and translucent, 5 minutes. Add the zucchini and bell pepper and cook, stirring, until lightly browned, 2 minutes.

2. Add the broth, tomatoes, and 2 cups water and bring to a boil. Add the pasta, then reduce the heat to low and simmer until the pasta is cooked, 12 minutes.

3. Stir in the beans and cook until heated through, 2 minutes. Sprinkle each serving with cheese, if desired.

229 calories, 9 g protein, 42 g carbohydrates, 7 g fiber, 4 g total fat, 1 g saturated fat, 634 mg sodium

Salsa Tuna Salad Sandwiches Serves 2

Prep Time • 20 minutes

1/2 cup salsa

2 tablespoons low-fat mayonnaise

1/2 teaspoon lime or lemon juice

1 can (5 ounces/142 g)
  water-packed tuna, drained

4 slices whole-grain bread

1/2 avocado, peeled, pitted,
  and sliced

Salsa adds flavor and moisture to canned tuna without any added fat. The avocado adds unexpected creaminess and richness—not to mention "good" fats.

1. Drain the salsa by placing it in a sieve over a bowl for about 10 minutes. Shake the sieve to release any remaining liquid.

2. In a small bowl, stir together the salsa, mayonnaise, and lime or lemon juice. Add the tuna and mix well.

3. Spread 1/2 of the tuna mixture onto 2 slices of bread. Top each with 1/2 of the avocado slices and top with another slice of bread.

350 calories, 27 g protein, 35 g carbohydrates, 14 g fiber, 13 g total fat, 1 g saturated fat, 644 mg sodium

Open-Faced Sardine Sandwiches Serves 2

Prep Time • 5 minutes
Cook Time • 3 minutes

1 tablespoon low-fat mayonnaise

1/2 teaspoon fresh lemon juice

1/4 teaspoon grated lemon zest

2 slices (each 3/4 inch/2 cm thick)
  whole-grain bread, such as
  12-grain

1 small tomato, cut into 4 slices

1 can (3.75 ounces/106 g)
  sardines in olive oil

2 slices low-fat Jarlsberg cheese

Here's a sandwich that features sardines—one of the best nondairy sources of calcium if you buy them with the bones, and an excellent source of omega-3 fatty acids. The lemon's fresh flavor blends with the nutty taste of the cheese to create a delicious warm sandwich.

1. Preheat the broiler. In a small bowl, combine the mayonnaise, lemon juice, and zest. Spread half of the mixture onto each slice of bread.

2. Top each slice with 1/2 of the tomatoes, sardines, and cheese. Place on a broiler pan or baking sheet and broil until the cheese melts, about 3 minutes.

228 calories, 20 g protein, 17 g carbohydrates, 5 g fiber, 9 g total fat, 1 g saturated fat, 637 mg sodium

Curried Chicken Salad Sandwiches Serves 4

Prep Time • 10 minutes

1/4 cup low-fat plain yogurt

2 tablespoons low-fat mayonnaise

1 1/2 teaspoons curry powder

1 teaspoon honey

1/4 teaspoon salt

2 cups chopped cooked chicken

1 apple, cored and chopped

2 celery stalks, chopped

4 lettuce leaves

2 whole-grain pita breads, halved

Make all your creamy salads healthier by replacing most of the mayonnaise with low-fat yogurt, leaving just 2 tablespoons of mayo. Here, blended with curry powder and honey, tender chicken is combined with apple and celery for a delicious light lunch.

1. In a large bowl, whisk together the yogurt, mayonnaise, curry powder, honey, and salt. Add the chicken, apple, and celery.

2. Place a lettuce leaf in each pita half and fill with 1/4 of the chicken salad.

253 calories, 23 g protein, 27 g carbohydrates, 4 g fiber, 6 g total fat, 1 g saturated fat, 440 mg sodium

Salmon Cake Sandwiches Serves 4

Prep Time • 45 minutes
Cook Time • 6 minutes

1/4 cup mild salsa

2 egg whites

1/4 cup low-fat canola mayonnaise

1/2 teaspoon ground cumin

1/4–1 teaspoon hot red pepper sauce

3 pouches (5 ounces/142 g each) salmon, patted dry

1 cup fresh whole-wheat bread crumbs

4 lettuce leaves

4 whole-wheat sandwich rolls

1 large tomato, cut into 4 slices

If you find the flavor of salmon a bit too strong, try this sandwich made with salmon sold in a pouch, which has a mild, subtle flavor. If, however, you love the bold flavor of canned salmon, use a 14.75-ounce/418 g can instead of the pouches.

1. Drain the salsa by placing it in a sieve over a bowl for about 10 minutes. Shake the sieve to release any remaining liquid.

2. Line a baking sheet with parchment paper. In a medium bowl, whisk the egg whites. Stir in the salsa, mayonnaise, cumin, and red pepper sauce. Add the salmon and bread crumbs and gently fold in just until combined. Shape the mixture into 4 cakes, place on the baking sheet, and refrigerate for at least 30 minutes.

3. Coat a nonstick skillet with cooking spray. Add the cakes and cook over medium heat, turning once, until browned and crisp, about 6 minutes.

4. Place a lettuce leaf on each roll. Top with a salmon cake and a tomato slice.

367 calories, 30 g protein, 39 g carbohydrates, 6 g fiber, 11 g total fat, 1 g saturated fat, 779 mg sodium

Beef in Lettuce Wraps Serves 4

Prep Time • 5 minutes
Cook Time • 11 minutes

3 tablespoons hoisin sauce

2 tablespoons wine vinegar

1 tablespoon soy sauce

1 teaspoon toasted sesame oil

1/2 teaspoon ground ginger

1 pound (454 g) lean ground beef

4 scallions, chopped

2 carrots, shredded

1 clove garlic, minced

12 Bibb or Boston lettuce leaves

What fun—using lettuce in place of bread to hold this warm, flavorful filling. Great for when you're looking for a light lunch, and kids will love them, too!

1. In a small bowl, whisk together the hoisin sauce, vinegar, soy sauce, oil, and ginger.

2. In a nonstick skillet over medium heat, cook the beef until browned, 5 minutes. Add the scallions, carrots, and garlic and cook until tender, 3 minutes. Stir in the hoisin mixture and cook until it thickens and flavors are blended, 3 minutes.

3. Place 3 lettuce leaves on each of 4 plates and fill with the beef mixture.

201 calories, 24 g protein, 13 g carbohydrates, 3 g fiber, 6 g total fat, 2 g saturated fat, 619 mg sodium

Mac 'n Cheese Primavera Serves 8

Prep Time • 15 minutes
Cook Time • 1 hour

16 ounces (448 g) whole-grain pasta, such as penne, rotelle, or elbows

2 bunches broccoli, cut into florets (4 cups)

1 large red bell pepper, chopped

2 carrots, sliced

4 cups low-fat milk

1/4 cup cornstarch

1 teaspoon mustard powder

16 ounces (448 g) shredded low-fat (2%) extra-sharp cheddar cheese

1/4 cup wheat germ

Here's a low-fat dish bursting with richness, flavor—and calcium. Tossing high-fiber vegetables with whole-grain pasta makes this comfort food good for your health as well as your soul.

1. Preheat the oven to 350°F (180°C). Coat a 9 x 13-inch (23 x 33-cm) baking pan with cooking spray.

2. Cook the pasta according to package directions, adding the broccoli, bell pepper, and carrots during the last 2 minutes of cooking. Drain and return to the pot.

3. Meanwhile, in a medium saucepan, whisk together the milk, cornstarch, and mustard. Bring to a simmer over medium heat. Add the cheese and cook until the cheese melts and the sauce thickens, 3 minutes. Pour over the pasta and toss to coat. Pour into the pan and sprinkle with the wheat germ. Bake until bubbling, 45 minutes.

427 calories, 27 g protein, 61 g carbohydrates, 7 g fiber, 8 g total fat, 5 g saturated fat, 94 mg sodium

Hearty Vegetable Stew Serves 6

Prep Time • 15 minutes
Cook Time • 30 minutes

2 tablespoons olive oil

2 onions, chopped

2 celery stalks, chopped

2 carrots, chopped

2 cloves garlic, minced

1 tablespoon balsamic vinegar

1 1/2 pounds (680 g) precut, preseeded butternut squash

8 ounces (227 g) green beans

3 1/2 cups chicken broth

1/2 teaspoon rubbed sage

1 red bell pepper, chopped

2 cups sliced shiitake mushrooms

1 tablespoon Dijon mustard

1 tablespoon honey

This nourishing stew is a snap to make because you can chop some of the vegetables while it's cooking. The stew will be almost ready by the time you're finished chopping.

1. Heat the oil in a large saucepan or Dutch oven over medium heat. Add the onions and celery and cook until lightly browned, 3 minutes. Add the carrots and garlic and cook for 2 minutes. Add the vinegar and stir to break up the brown bits, 1 minute.

2. Add the squash, beans, broth, and sage and bring to a simmer. Cook until the squash is almost tender, 15 minutes. Add the bell pepper and mushrooms and simmer until the vegetables are tender, 5 to 10 minutes.

3. In a small bowl, whisk together the mustard and honey. Stir into the stew until well blended.

170 calories, 4 g protein, 31 g carbohydrates, 7 g fiber, 5 g total fat, 1 g saturated fat, 325 mg sodium

Eggplant Lasagna Serves 12

Prep Time • 15 minutes
Cook Time • 1 hour, 45 minutes

2 tablespoons olive oil

1 large onion, chopped

2 cloves garlic, minced

1 tablespoon Italian seasoning

2 cans (14.5 ounces/411 g each) diced tomatoes

1 can (28 ounces/794 g) tomato sauce

1 small eggplant, peeled and cut into 1-inch (2.5-cm) pieces

1/4 teaspoon salt

1 package (16 ounces/454 g) lite silken tofu, drained

2 large eggs

1 cup grated Parmesan cheese

9 no-boil lasagna noodles

1 package (8 ounces/227 g) shredded part-skim mozzarella cheese

Even though it's not especially rich in vitamins and minerals, eggplant is surprisingly high in antioxidants. It's also an excellent replacement for meat. Here, the eggplant is roasted to mellow any bitterness, blending beautifully with garlic, onions, and tomato for a wholesome, stick-to-your-ribs meal.

1. Preheat the oven to 400°F (200°C). Heat the oil in a large saucepan over medium-high heat. Add the onion and cook until tender, about 5 minutes. Add the garlic and Italian seasoning and cook for 1 minute. Add the tomatoes and tomato sauce and bring to a simmer. Reduce the heat to low and simmer until the flavors are blended, 20 minutes.

2. Meanwhile, coat a baking sheet with sides with olive oil cooking spray. Add the eggplant, coat with cooking spray, and sprinkle with the salt. Roast, turning occasionally, until browned, 30 minutes.

3. In a food processor, combine the tofu, eggs, and Paremesan cheese and puree until smooth.

4. Coat a 9 x 13-inch (23 x 33-cm) baking dish with cooking spray. Spread 1 cup sauce on the bottom of the dish and arrange 3 lasagna noodles on top. Spread 1/2 of the tofu filling over the noodles, followed by 1/2 of the eggplant. Top with 1 1/2 cups sauce and 1/2 cup mozzarella. Repeat with another layer, then top with the remaining noodles, sauce, and mozzarella.

5. Cover with foil and bake for 1 hour. Remove the foil and bake until heated through, about 15 minutes. Let cool slightly before serving.

229 calories, 15 g protein, 23 g carbohydrates, 3 g fiber, 10 g total fat, 4 g saturated fat, 852 mg sodium

Three-Bean Chili Serves 8

Prep Time • 10 minutes
Cook Time • 7 hours, 15 minutes

3 carrots, sliced

3 celery stalks, sliced

2 cloves garlic, minced

1 large onion, chopped

1 can (28 ounces/794 g) crushed tomatoes

1 jar (16 ounces/454 g) salsa

2 teaspoons chili powder

1 teaspoon ground cumin

1 can (15.5 ounces/439 g) kidney beans, drained and rinsed

1 can (15.5 ounces/439 g) black beans, drained and rinsed

1 can (15.5 ounces/439 g) white beans, drained and rinsed

1 green bell pepper, chopped

1 red bell pepper, chopped

Every ingredient here is loaded with vitamins, minerals, antioxidants, and fiber. Even better, this simple dish cooks in a slow cooker while you're off living life! To change the flavors, vary the types of salsa—chipotle for a spicy, smoky flavor; roasted garlic for pungent flavor; or mild for just a hint of spice.

1. Place the carrots, celery, garlic, onion, tomatoes, salsa, chili powder, and cumin in a 4- to 6-quart (1- to 1 1/2-liter) slow cooker. Cover and cook on high until the vegetables are tender, 5 to 7 hours.

2. Stir in the beans and bell peppers and cook, uncovered, on high until the chili thickens slightly and the peppers are tender, 15 minutes.

299 calories, 19 g protein, 58 g carbohydrates, 20 g fiber, 2 g total fat, 0 g saturated fat, 712 mg sodium

Tuna Kebabs Serves 4

Prep Time • 35 minutes
Cook Time • 5 minutes

1/4 cup lime juice

1 tablespoon olive oil

1 clove garlic, minced

1 teaspoon grated fresh ginger

1/4 teaspoon salt

1 1/2 pounds (680 g) tuna steaks, cut into 1 1/2-inch (4 cm) cubes

2 cups cherry tomatoes

6 scallions, cut into 2-inch (5 cm) pieces

These mouthwatering kebabs cook up in a jiffy and look pretty on your plate. Fresh tuna, abundant in omega-3s, is very different from the canned variety. Firm and dense, tuna steaks have meaty texture and a milder taste.

1. In a small shallow dish, combine the lime juice, oil, garlic, ginger, and salt. Add the tuna and turn to coat. Let stand 30 minutes, turning once. Place 8 wooden skewers in water and soak for 30 minutes.

2. Preheat the broiler or grill. Lightly coat a broiler pan or grill rack with cooking spray. Alternately thread the tuna, tomatoes, and scallions onto the skewers. Broil or grill, turning once, until the tuna is opaque, 5 minutes.

304 calories, 40 g protein, 7 g carbohydrates, 2 g fiber, 12 g total fat, 3 g saturated fat, 226 mg sodium

Fish Tacos Serves 4

Prep Time • 20 minutes
Cook Time • 7 minutes

1 tablespoon olive oil

2 cloves garlic, minced

1 teaspoon ground cumin

1/2 teaspoon salt

3 tablespoons lime juice

1 1/2 pounds (680 g) halibut fillets

1 ripe mango, peeled, seeded, and chopped

1/2 small red bell pepper, seeded and finely chopped

1/2 jalapeño pepper, seeded, deveined, and finely chopped (wear gloves when handling; they burn)

1/4 cup chopped cilantro (optional)

8 soft corn tortillas (6 inches/15 cm)

1 cup shredded lettuce

Here's a truly fun way to enjoy fish. The mango's sweetness marries well with spicy peppers, creating a refreshing salsa. Mangoes are deliciously rich in beta-carotene, vitamin C, potassium, and fiber and contain an enzyme with stomach-soothing properties. Even the corn tortillas are rich in antioxidants.

1. Preheat the broiler. Coat a broiler pan with cooking spray. In a medium bowl, combine the oil, garlic, cumin, salt, 1 tablespoon lime juice, and the fish and toss to coat. Let stand 15 minutes.

2. In a small bowl, combine the mango, bell pepper, jalapeño, cilantro, if desired, and the remaining 2 tablespoons lime juice. Set aside.

3. Wrap the tortillas in foil. Remove the fish from the marinade and place on the broiler pan. Broil until opaque, 3 to 6 minutes. Transfer to a plate and place the tortillas in the oven to warm slightly, 1 minute. Flake the fish.

4. Top the tortillas with equal amounts of lettuce, fish, and salsa.

380 calories, 39 g protein, 36 g carbohydrates, 5 g fiber, 9 g total fat, 1 g saturated fat, 430 mg sodium

Salmon Steaks with Peach Salsa Serves 4

Prep Time • 15 minutes
Cook Time • 8 minutes

2 peaches, peeled, seeded, and chopped

1 red bell pepper, seeded and chopped

1 jalapeño pepper, seeded, deveined, and minced (wear gloves when handling; they burn)

1 clove garlic, minced

1/2 teaspoon salt

1/2 teaspoon black pepper

2 tablespoons honey

2 tablespoons lime juice

4 salmon steaks (about 1 1/2 pounds/680 g)

2 tablespoons olive oil

If peaches aren't in season, substitute frozen (not in syrup) peaches or another seasonal fruit, such as cantaloupe, plums, pears, grapes, or pineapple.

1. In a small bowl, combine the peaches, bell pepper, jalapeño, garlic, 1/4 teaspoon salt, 1/4 teaspoon black pepper, and the honey and lime juice. Toss to coat well and set aside.

2. Sprinkle both sides of the salmon with the remaining 1/4 teaspoon salt and 1/4 teaspoon black pepper. Heat the oil in a large nonstick skillet over high heat. Add the salmon and cook, turning once, until browned and seared, 4 minutes. Reduce the heat to medium-low and cook until opaque, 3 to 4 minutes. Serve with the salsa.

439 calories, 35 g protein, 17 g carbohydrates, 2 g fiber, 26 g total fat, 5 g saturated fat, 393 mg sodium

Tomato-Roasted Mackerel Serves 4

Prep Time • 5 minutes
Cook Time • 10 minutes

1 pound (454 g) mackerel, cod, or flouder fillets

2 tablespoons low-fat mayonnaise

1/4 cup basil leaves

2 large tomatoes, sliced

1/2 teaspoon salt

1/4 teaspoon black pepper

Tired of salmon? Mackerel is also a fantastic source of omega-3 fatty acids. Its strong flavor is mellowed by mayo and flavorful tomato and basil. Baking the tomatoes brings out more of their lycopene.

1. Preheat the oven to 400°F (200°C). Place the fish on a baking sheet and spread with the mayonnaise. Layer the basil and tomatoes on top of each fillet and sprinkle with the salt and pepper. Bake until the fish is just opaque, 5 to 10 minutes depending on thickness.

268 calories, 22 g protein, 4 g carbohydrates, 1 g fiber, 18 g total fat, 4 g saturated fat, 450 mg sodium

Roasted Salmon with Sautéed Greens Serves 4

Prep Time • 5 minutes
Cook Time • 10 minutes

1/4 cup balsamic vinegar

2 tablespoons brown sugar

1 teaspoon mustard powder

1/2 teaspoon salt

1 1/4 pounds (567 g) salmon, cut into 4 pieces

1 tablespoon olive oil

1 large red onion, cut into thin strips

8 ounces (227 g) baby spinach

Balsamic vinegar adds natural sweetness to savory dishes. It gets its dark color and sweetness from aging in barrels, like wine. For dishes where you'd like the flavor without the dark brown color, opt for white balsamic vinegar.

1. Preheat the broiler or grill. In a small bowl, combine the vinegar, brown sugar, mustard, and salt. Brush 1/2 of the mixture over the salmon. Broil or grill until opaque, 4 to 5 minutes, brushing with the vinegar mixture after 2 minutes.

2. Meanwhile, heat the oil in a large skillet over medium heat. Add the onion and cook until lightly browned, 2 minutes. Cover and cook until tender, 2 minutes. Add the spinach and cook, stirring, until almost wilted, 1 minute. Add the remaining vinegar mixture and cook, stirring, until the spinach is wilted and the sauce thickens slightly, 1 minute.

3. Divide the spinach mixture equally among 4 dinner plates. Top each serving with a piece of salmon.

356 calories, 31 g protein, 13 g carbohydrates, 2 g fiber, 20 g total fat, 4 g saturated fat, 428 mg sodium

Curry-Seared Scallops Serves 4

Prep Time • 5 minutes
Cook Time • 15 minutes

1/2 cup low-fat plain yogurt

2 teaspoons cornstarch

1 1/2 pounds (680 g) sea scallops

1 tablespoon curry powder

1/2 teaspoon salt

3 tablespoons olive oil

1 box (10.5 ounces/297 g) grape or cherry tomatoes, halved

6 scallions, sliced

You'll never believe this creamy dish is good for you! Antioxidants abound in this dish of delicately sweet sea scallops cooked in curry with tomatoes and scallions. Healthful yogurt creates a sauce you'd swear was made with heavy cream. Serve over cooked brown rice or quinoa if you like.

1. In a small bowl, combine the yogurt and cornstarch and set aside. Place the scallops in a medium bowl, sprinkle with the curry powder and salt, and toss to coat well.

2. Heat 2 tablespoons oil in a large nonstick skillet over medium-high heat. Add the scallops and cook, turning to brown all sides, until well browned and opaque, 3 to 6 minutes. With tongs or a slotted spoon, transfer to a plate.

3. Add the remaining 1 tablespoon oil to the skillet and reduce the heat to low. Add the tomatoes and scallions and cook until tender and lightly browned, about 4 minutes.

4. Return the scallops to the skillet along with the yogurt mixture. Cook until thickened and heated through, 2 minutes.

287 calories, 31 g protein, 12 g carbohydrates, 2 g fiber, 13 g total fat, 2 g saturated fat, 595 mg sodium

Thai Roasted Shrimp Serves 4

Prep Time • 5 minutes
Cook Time • 15 minutes

1 can (13.5 ounces/400 mL) lite coconut milk

1 cup low-sodium vegetable or chicken broth

2 tablespoons low-sodium soy sauce

1/4–1/2 teaspoon green curry paste

1 pound (454 g) peeled deveined shrimp

8 scallions, thinly sliced

1 large tomato, seeded and chopped

1 tablespoon lime juice

2 cups cooked brown rice or quinoa

Lite coconut milk varies from the thick, sweet crème of coconut used in desserts and cocktails. Lower in fat but full of rich flavor, it cools the heat of spicy curry paste and creates a quick, flavorful shrimp dish in minutes.

1. In a large saucepan, whisk together the coconut milk, broth, soy sauce, and curry paste. Bring to a boil over medium-high heat. Add the shrimp and scallions and cook until the shrimp is opaque, 5 minutes.

2. Remove from the heat and stir in the tomato and lime juice. Serve over the rice.

311 calories, 23 g protein, 31 g carbohydrates, 3 g fiber, 9 g total fat, 6 g saturated fat, 516 mg sodium

Baked Chicken with Tomatoes Serves 4

Prep Time • 10 minutes
Cook Time • 18 minutes

1 egg

1/2 teaspoon salt

1/2 cup toasted Brazil nuts or blanched almonds, finely chopped

1/3 cup wheat germ

4 boneless skinless chicken breast halves

2 tablespoons olive oil

2 cups grape or cherry tomatoes, halved

1 teaspoon dried basil

Extraordinarily rich in the antioxidant trace mineral selenium, Brazil nuts add crunch and health to chicken breast crust. Here, they're blended with wheat germ, which is loaded with vitamin E and folate, for a flavorful, rich crust.

1. Preheat the oven to 425°F (220°C). Coat a baking sheet with cooking spray.

2. Place the egg and salt in a shallow dish and whisk with 1 tablespoon water. In another shallow dish, combine the nuts and wheat germ. Dip the chicken breasts into the egg and then the nut mixture. Place on the baking sheet and coat with cooking spray. Bake, turning once, until a thermometer inserted in the center reaches 160°F (71°C), 15 minutes.

3. Meanwhile, heat the oil in a large skillet over medium-high heat. Add the tomatoes and basil and cook until just browned, 3 minutes. Serve with the chicken.

371 calories, 34 g protein, 10 g carbohydrates, 4 g fiber, 22 g total fat, 5 g saturated fat, 391 mg sodium

Chicken-Barley Bake Serves 4

Prep Time • 5 minutes
Cook Time • 1 hour, 5 minutes

2 tablespoons olive oil

1 onion, chopped

1 clove garlic, minced

1 cup pearled barley

1 1/2 cups chicken broth

1 cup orange juice

1 teaspoon dried thyme, crushed

1/2 teaspoon salt

4 skinless bone-in chicken breast halves

1/2 cup dried cranberries

1 orange, washed and sliced (optional)

With a robust nutty flavor, barley's so high in soluble fiber that it can lower high cholesterol and even help stabilize blood sugar. Blended here with orange and cranberry, it becomes a tasty base for roasted chicken breasts.

1. Preheat the oven to 350°F (180°C). Coat a 9 x 13-inch (23 x 33-cm) baking pan with cooking spray.

2. Heat the oil in a large skillet over medium heat. Add the onion and garlic and cook until tender, 2 minutes. Add the barley and cook for 2 minutes. Add the broth, orange juice, thyme, and salt and bring to a boil. Carefully pour into the baking pan. Top with the chicken breasts, cover, and bake for 45 minutes.

3. Uncover and stir the cranberries into the barley mixture. If desired, top each chicken breast with 1 or 2 orange slices. Bake until the chicken is cooked and the barley is tender, 15 minutes.

451 calories, 34 g protein, 58 g carbohydrates, 10 g fiber, 10 g total fat, 2 g saturated fat, 548 mg sodium

Chicken in Garlic Sauce Serves 4

Prep Time • 5 minutes
Cook Time • 13 minutes

2 tablespoons olive oil

4 boneless skinless chicken breast halves

4 cloves garlic, minced

1/4 cup white wine or white balsamic vinegar

1 3/4 cups chicken broth

Help prevent heart disease with this dish bursting with garlic. Serve over brown rice with steamed broccoli on the side for a scrumptious meal in minutes.

1. Heat the oil in a large skillet over medium heat. Add the chicken and cook until browned on both sides, 5 minutes. Transfer to a plate.

2. Add the garlic to the skillet and cook until tender, 2 minutes. Add the wine or vinegar and cook, stirring to loosen the brown bits, 3 minutes. Add the broth and return the chicken and any accumulated juices to the skillet. Cook until a thermometer inserted in the center of the chicken reaches 160°F (71°C), about 5 minutes.

214 calories, 28 g protein, 3 g carbohydrates, 0 g fiber, 8 g total fat, 1 g saturated fat, 268 mg sodium

Turkey Cutlets with Grapefruit Salsa Serves 4

Prep Time • 10 minutes
Cook Time • 3 minutes

2 ruby red grapefruits, sectioned and chopped

1/2 small red bell pepper, seeded and minced

4 scallions, chopped

1 tablespoon olive oil

1/2 teaspoon sugar

1 pound (454 g) turkey breast cutlets

1/4 teaspoon salt

1/4 teaspoon black pepper

Always reach for red grapefruits, which are not only a great source of vitamin C but are also rich in lycopene. Here, they blend with crunchy bell pepper and pungent scallions for a flavorful medley that's perfect atop browned turkey cutlets.

1. In a small bowl, combine the grapefruit, bell pepper, scallions, oil, and sugar. Set aside.

2. Season the cutlets with the salt and pepper. Coat a large skillet with cooking spray and heat over medium heat. Add the cutlets, in batches if necessary, and cook until browned on both sides and cooked through, 3 minutes. Transfer to a plate and top with the salsa.

203 calories, 29 g protein, 13 g carbohydrates, 3 g fiber, 4 g total fat, 0 g saturated fat, 256 mg sodium

Turkey Ragu with Spaghetti Serves 6

Prep Time • 15 minutes
Cook Time • 1 hour, 15 minutes

2 tablespoons olive oil

2 carrots, finely chopped

1 onion, finely chopped

1 red bell pepper, finely chopped

2 cloves garlic, minced

1 pound (454 g) ground turkey breast

1/2 cup white wine or chicken broth

1 can (28 ounces/794 g) crushed tomatoes

1 can (6 ounces/170 g) tomato paste

1 teaspoon Italian seasoning

12 ounces (336 g) whole wheat spaghetti

1/2 cup low-fat milk

Where's the beef? You'll never miss it in this hearty tomato sauce studded with vegetables and ground turkey. Ground turkey, a low-fat substitute for ground beef, works best when bathed in a healthful, flavorful sauce.

1. Heat the oil in a large saucepan over medium heat. Add the carrots, onion, and bell pepper and cook until lightly browned, 5 minutes. Add the garlic and turkey and cook, stirring, until the turkey is no longer pink, 5 minutes. Add the wine or broth and cook until the liquid is absorbed, 4 minutes.

2. Add the tomatoes, tomato paste, and Italian seasoning. Reduce the heat to low, cover, and simmer until well blended, 1 hour.

3. About 15 minutes before serving, cook the spaghetti according to package directions.

4. Remove the sauce from the heat and stir in the milk. Serve over the hot pasta.

437 calories, 32 g protein, 66 g carbohydrates, 13 g fiber, 7 g total fat, 1 g saturated fat, 470 mg sodium

Barbecued Flank Steak Serves 4

Prep Time • 6 hours, 5 minutes
Cook Time • 13 minutes

2 cloves garlic, grated

1 small onion, grated

1/2 cup tomato sauce

2 tablespoons red wine vinegar

2 tablespoons brown sugar

1 tablespoon Worcestershire sauce

1/4 teaspoon salt

1 pound (454 g) flank steak

It may be lower in fat than many other cuts of beef, but flank steak, an excellent source of protein, vitamins, and minerals, is bursting with rich flavor. Marinated in a healthy homemade barbecue sauce, it's sure to be a crowd pleaser.

1. In a large zipper-seal bag, combine the garlic, onion, tomato sauce, vinegar, brown sugar, Worcestershire, and salt. Add the steak, seal the bag, and turn to coat. Refrigerate for 6 hours or overnight.

2. Preheat the broiler or grill. Remove the steak from the marinade, reserving the marinade. Broil the steak 2 to 3 inches (5 to 8 cm) from the heat source or grill until a thermometer inserted in the center reaches 145°F (63°C) for medium-rare, 13 minutes. Transfer to a cutting board.

3. Meanwhile, place the marinade in a small saucepan, bring to a boil, and cook for 4 minutes. Slice the steak and serve with the sauce.

219 calories, 25 g protein, 11 g carbohydrates, 1 g fiber, 8 g total fat, 3 g saturated fat, 415 mg sodium

Herb-Crusted Roast Beef Serves 12

Prep Time • 15 minutes
Cook Time • 1 hour, 5 minutes

1 top round beef roast (about
  3 pounds/1.4 kg), trimmed of all
  visible fat

5 cloves garlic, minced

1 tablespoon olive oil

1 teaspoon dried basil

1 teaspoon dried thyme

1 teaspoon mustard powder

1 teaspoon salt

1 teaspoon black pepper

Yes, roast beef can be healthy! Top round is a very tender yet lean roast—delicious topped with garlic, basil, thyme, and mustard.

1. Preheat the oven to 350°F (180°C). Rinse the meat and pat dry. Place on a rack in a large roasting pan.

2. In a small bowl, combine the garlic, oil, basil, thyme, mustard, salt, and pepper. Rub the mixture over the meat.

3. Roast until a thermometer inserted in the center reaches 145°F (63°C) for medium-rare or 160°F (71°C) for medium, 55 to 65 minutes. Transfer to a cutting board and let stand for 10 minutes before slicing.

169 calories, 26 g protein, 1 g carbohydrates, 0 g fiber, 6 g total fat, 2 g saturated fat, 644 mg sodium

Beef and Broccoli Stew Serves 4

Prep Time • 10 minutes
Cook Time • 25 minutes

4 tablespoons olive oil

1 pound (454 g) top round steak, cut into 1-inch (2.5 cm) pieces, then halved

1/4 teaspoon black pepper

1/4 teaspoon cayenne pepper

2 onions, cut into wedges

1 clove garlic, mashed

1 tablespoon minced fresh ginger

1/4 cup low-sodium soy sauce

3 1/2 cups low-sodium beef broth

3 carrots, cut into julienne strips

1 bunch broccoli, cut into florets

2 tablespoons cornstarch mixed with 2 tablespoons water

This hearty stew contains an unexpected taste twist—inflammation-fighting ginger—and cooks in no time, making it a favorite for weeknight meals. Serve with cooked brown rice or crusty whole-grain bread.

1. Heat 2 tablespoons oil in a large saucepan over high heat. Season the meat with the black pepper and cayenne. Add 1/2 of the meat to the saucepan and stir-fry until no longer pink, 2 minutes, then transfer to a bowl. Repeat with the remaining meat.

2. Add the onions to the saucepan and cook until lightly browned, 4 minutes. Stir in the garlic and ginger and cook for 1 minute.

3. Add the soy sauce and broth and bring to a boil over high heat. Reduce the heat to medium-low, add the carrots and broccoli, and cook until crisp-tender, 10 minutes.

4. Add the beef and any drippings from the bowl. Stir in the cornstarch mixture and cook until thickened, 2 minutes.

429 calories, 31 g protein, 29 g carbohydrates, 7 g fiber, 22 g total fat, 5 g saturated fat, 997 mg sodium

Pork Chops with Dried Fruits Serves 4

Prep Time • 5 minutes
Cook Time • 20 minutes

4 boneless pork chops (about 1 pound/454 g)

1/4 teaspoon salt

1/4 teaspoon black pepper

2 tablespoons olive oil

1 medium onion, finely chopped

1 1/4 cups apple cider or juice

1 package (6 ounces/170 g)) dried sliced apple rings

1/2 cup pitted prunes

1 tablespoon fresh thyme or 1 teaspoon dried thyme

Simmering boneless pork chops and dried fruits in apple cider creates a succulent, creamy sauce. Lovely enough to serve to guests, this simple dish is rich in fiber and low-fat protein.

1. Sprinkle the chops with the salt and pepper. Heat 1 tablespoon oil in a large skillet over medium-high heat. Add the chops and cook, turning once, until browned on both sides, 4 minutes. Transfer to a plate and keep warm.

2. Add the remaining 1 tablespoon oil to the skillet. Add the onion and cook until lightly browned, 4 minutes. Add the cider and bring to a simmer, stirring to loosen the browned bits. Return the chops to the skillet and add the apples, prunes, and thyme. Reduce the heat to medium-low, cover, and simmer until the chops reach 150°F (65°C) on an instant-read thermometer, about 10 minutes.

404 calories, 21 g protein, 51 g carbohydrates, 4 g fiber, 12 g total fat, 3 g saturated fat, 491 mg sodium

Harvest Pork Roast Serves 8

Prep Time • 30 minutes
Cook Time • 1 hour, 15 minutes

1 butternut squash (about
    2 pounds/908 g), peeled,
    seeded, and cut into 2-inch (5
    cm) pieces

2 red onions, cut into wedges

2 large red bell peppers, seeded
    and cut into 2-inch (5-cm)
    pieces

2 tablespoons olive oil

1 teaspoon salt

1 teaspoon black pepper

1 teaspoon ground ginger

1/2 teaspoon ground allspice

1/2 teaspoon ground cinnamon

1 boneless pork loin roast (about
    2 pounds/908 g)

2 cups apple cider

When company's coming, serve this roast spiked with health benefits from the vegetables as well as the spices. Red onions, red bell peppers, and butternut squash tossed in ginger olive oil are a powerhouse of nutrients and are bursting with great flavor.

1. Preheat the oven to 400°F (200°C). Place the squash, onions, and peppers in a large roasting pan. Drizzle with the oil, sprinkle with 1/2 teaspoon salt and 1/2 teaspoon black pepper, and toss to coat well. Set aside.

2. In a small bowl, combine the ginger, allspice, and cinnamon and stir to blend well. Remove 1 teaspoon spice mixture, place in a small saucepan, and set aside.

3. Add the remaining 1/2 teaspoon salt and 1/2 teaspoon black pepper to the bowl with the spice mixture. Rub the mixture over the meat and place the meat in the same pan. Roast until the vegetables are tender and an instant-read thermometer inserted in the center of the pork reaches 150°F (65°C), about 1 hour.

4. Meanwhile, add the cider to the saucepan with the spice mixture. Bring to a boil over high heat and cook until thick and syrupy and reduced to about 1/2 cup, about 40 minutes.

5. When the meat is cooked, transfer to a cutting board and let stand for 10 minutes. Pour 1/2 of the cider mixture over the vegetables in the pan and toss to coat well. Roast for 5 minutes. Serve with the meat. Use the rest of the cider mixture as gravy.

294 calories, 25 g protein, 25 g carbohydrates, 4 g fiber, 11 g total fat, 3 g saturated fat, 360 mg sodium

Shiitake Green Beans Serves 4

Prep Time • 5 minutes
Cook Time • 12 minutes

1 pound (454 g) green beans, trimmed

2 tablespoons olive oil

8 ounces (224 g) shiitake mushrooms, cleaned and stems removed

1 clove garlic, minced

1 tomato, seeded and chopped

1/2 teaspoon salt

Shiitake mushrooms deserve a place on your plate thanks not only to their rich, earthy flavor but also to their immunity-boosting qualities. Here, they blend with tomato to turn ordinary green beans into a tasty dish.

1. Bring 2 inches (5 cm) of water to a boil in a large saucepan over high heat. Insert a steamer basket and add the beans. Cover and cook over medium heat until bright green and crisp-tender, 4 minutes. Transfer to a serving plate and keep warm.

2. Meanwhile, heat the oil in a large skillet over medium-high heat. Add the mushrooms and cook, stirring, until browned and tender, 5 minutes. Add the garlic, tomato, and salt and cook, stirring, until the tomato is tender and the mixture forms a sauce, 3 minutes. Spoon over the green beans.

109 calories, 3 g protein, 11 g carbohydrates, 5 g fiber, 7 g total fat, 1 g saturated fat, 300 mg sodium

Roasted Root Vegetables Serves 4

Prep Time • 10 minutes
Cook Time • 40 minutes

1 pound (454 g) carrots, peeled and sliced diagonally into 1/2-inch (1 cm) pieces

1 pound (454 g) parsnips, peeled and sliced diagonally into 1/2-inch (1 cm) pieces

2 tablespoons olive oil

1 tablespoon grated fresh ginger

1 teaspoon ground cinnamon

1/2 teaspoon salt

Parsnips and carrots are related, and although both are good sources of fiber, they're nutritionally different. Carrots burst with beta-carotene, while parsnips are rich in potassium. Roasting with ginger and cinnamon lends them both an especially savory flavor.

1. Preheat the oven to 400°F (200°C). Place the carrots, parsnips, oil, ginger, cinnamon, and salt in a large roasting pan and toss to coat well. Roast, turning occasionally, until tender and browned, 40 minutes.

199 calories, 3 g protein, 33 g carbohydrates, 9 g fiber, 7 g total fat, 1 g saturated fat, 361 mg sodium

Brown Rice Risotto Serves 4

Prep Time • 10 minutes
Cook Time • 1 hour

2 tablespoons olive oil

1 medium onion, chopped

1 medium red bell pepper, seeded and chopped

1 cup brown rice, preferably short or medium grain

1 clove garlic, minced

1/2 teaspoon turmeric

3 1/2 cups low-sodium chicken broth

1/3 cup grated Romano cheese

Whole-grain brown rice mimics Arborio rice in this hearty dish reminiscent of risotto. The turmeric adds great color as well as anti-inflammatory benefits.

1. Preheat the oven to 425°F (220°C). Heat the oil in a large oven-proof saucepan or Dutch oven over medium heat. Add the onion and bell pepper and cook for 3 minutes. Add the rice, garlic, and turmeric and cook until the rice is shiny and coated with oil, 2 minutes. Add the broth and bring to a boil.

2. Cover and bake until the broth is absorbed and the rice is just tender, about 55 minutes. Top with the cheese, then cover and let stand for 5 minutes.

305 calories, 8 g protein, 43 g carbohydrates, 3 g fiber, 11 g total fat, 3 g saturated fat, 220 mg sodium

Almond Rice Serves 6

Prep Time • 5 minutes
Cook Time • 55 minutes

2 tablespoons olive oil

1 medium onion, chopped

1 clove garlic, minced

1 cup brown rice

1/2 cup wild rice

1 cup orange juice

1 teaspoon ground ginger

1/2 cup toasted almonds, chopped

1/2 cup raisins

For a change of pace, try short-grain brown rice in this dish. It has a chewier texture and nuttier flavor than long-grain brown rice and can be used interchangeably with it.

1. Heat the oil in a medium saucepan over medium heat. Add the onion and garlic and cook until just beginning to brown, 3 minutes.

2. Add the brown and wild rice, 1 1/2 cups water, and the orange juice and ginger. Bring to a boil, then reduce the heat to low, cover, and simmer until the rice is tender, 50 minutes. Stir in the almonds and raisins.

317 calories, 7 g protein, 53 g carbohydrates, 4 g fiber, 10 g total fat, 1 g saturated fat, 8 mg sodium

Springtime Quinoa Serves 6

Prep Time • 10 minutes
Cook Time • 25 minutes

1 cup quinoa, rinsed and drained

1/2 teaspoon salt

1 tablespoon olive oil

1 small red onion, halved and cut into thin slices

1/2 cup vegetable or chicken broth

1 pound (454 g) asparagus, cut into 2-inch (5 cm) pieces

1 cup fresh or thawed frozen peas

High-fiber, protein-rich quinoa has a nutty flavor and a creamy, fluffy texture. It can easily replace white rice in dishes and cooks in half the time as brown rice. Here, it's tossed with healthful vegetables that are most delicious when fresh in the spring.

1. In a small saucepan over high heat, bring the quinoa, salt, and 2 cups water to a boil. Reduce the heat to low, cover, and simmer until all the water is absorbed, 15 minutes.

2. Meanwhile, heat the oil in a large nonstick skillet over medium heat. Add the onion and cook until lightly browned, 4 minutes. Add the broth, asparagus, and peas and cook until crisp-tender, 5 minutes. Stir in the quinoa.

171 calories, 8 g protein, 28 g carbohydrates, 5 g fiber, 4 g total fat, 1 g saturated fat, 262 mg sodium

Pasta with Walnut Cream Sauce Serves 4

Prep Time • 10 minutes
Cook Time • 10 minutes

8 ounces (224 g) whole-grain penne, fusilli, or farfalle pasta

1 cup walnuts, toasted

1–3 cloves garlic, mashed

1/4 cup basil leaves

2 tablespoons olive oil

1/2 cup low-fat evaporated milk

1/4 cup grated Parmesan cheese

Walnuts are the base of this creamy pesto-like sauce that's so rich and delicious you'd swear it was loaded with heavy cream. Serve over whole-grain pasta, and you have a high-fiber, omega-3–rich side dish that's sure to become a favorite.

1. Cook the pasta according to package directions.

2. Meanwhile, place the nuts, garlic, and basil in a food processor or blender and process until the nuts are finely chopped. Add the oil and milk and pulse until well blended.

3. Toss the sauce with the hot pasta and sprinkle with the cheese.

479 calories, 16 g protein, 49 g carbohydrates, 4 g fiber, 26 g total fat, 4 g saturated fat, 115 mg sodium

Orange Beets Serves 6

Prep Time • 15 minutes
Cook Time • 55 minutes

1 1/2 pounds (680 g) beets with greens (about 4 medium beets)

1 tablespoon olive oil

1 clove garlic, minced

1/2 teaspoon salt

3 tablespoons orange marmalade

1 tablespoon white wine vinegar

1/4 teaspoon black pepper

If you've only had beets from a can, give fresh ones a chance. They're mild, delicious, and sure to become a favorite. Here, flavorful, folate-rich beets are tossed with sautéed beet greens, high in beta-carotene, and bathed in a sweet marmalade sauce.

1. Preheat the oven to 350°F (180°C). Trim the greens from the beets and set aside. Fold a 36-inch piece (91-cm) of foil in half crosswise. Scrub the beets and place in the center of the foil. Sprinkle with 1 teaspoon water and seal the foil around the beets. Roast until tender, about 45 minutes. Let cool for 15 minutes, then remove the skins and cut each beet into 8 wedges.

2. Meanwhile, trim the stems from the beet greens, wash the greens, and cut into 1-inch (2.5-cm) strips. While the beets are cooling, heat the oil in a skillet over medium-high heat. Add the garlic and cook for 1 minute. Add the greens and 1/4 teaspoon salt and cook, stirring constantly, until wilted, 2 minutes. Transfer to a serving dish.

3. Add the marmalade, vinegar, pepper, and the remaining 1/4 teaspoon salt to the skillet and cook until hot and bubbling. Add the beets and toss to coat well. Transfer to the serving dish and toss with the greens.

75 calories, 1 g protein, 13 g carbohydrates, 2 g fiber, 2 g total fat, 0 g saturated fat, 253 mg sodium

Blueberry-Oat Scones Serves 12

Prep Time • 10 minutes
Cook Time • 15 minutes

1 cup whole oats, ground

1 cup whole-wheat pastry flour

1/4 cup sugar

2 teaspoons baking powder

1/2 teaspoon baking soda

1/2 teaspoon salt

1 cup low-fat plain yogurt

2 tablespoons canola oil

2 cups blueberries

1 teaspoon grated lemon zest

A great way to add the fiber and wholesomeness of whole oats to foods is by grinding them into flour. Here, half of the wheat flour is replaced by ground oats.

1. Preheat the oven to 400°F (200°C). Lightly coat a baking sheet with cooking spray.

2. In a large bowl, whisk together the ground oats, flour, sugar, baking powder, baking soda, and salt. In a measuring cup, stir together the yogurt and oil.

3. Make a well in the center of the flour mixture and add the yogurt mixture. Add the blueberries and lemon zest and stir just until blended.

4. Drop by 1/4 cups onto the baking sheet. Bake until lightly browned, 12 to 15 minutes.

112 calories, 3 g protein, 18 g carbohydrates, 2 g fiber, 3 g total fat, 0 g saturated fat, 255 mg sodium

Raspberry-Almond Muffins Serves 12

Prep Time • 10 minutes
Cook Time • 20 minutes

2 cups whole-wheat pastry flour

1 cup almonds, toasted and finely chopped

2 tablespoons wheat germ

1 tablespoon baking powder

1/2 teaspoon salt

1 cup soy milk

1/2 cup honey

1 egg

3 tablespoons canola oil

1 teaspoon vanilla extract

1/4 teaspoon almond extract (optional)

1 cup fresh or frozen raspberries

Use baked goods like these scrumptious muffins, bursting with antioxidants (almonds are a surprising source), to sneak some soy milk into your diet. You can substitute it equally for dairy milk.

1. Preheat the oven to 400°F (200°C). Lightly coat a 12-cup muffin pan with cooking spray.

2. In a large bowl, whisk together the flour, almonds, wheat germ, baking powder, and salt. In a medium bowl, whisk together the milk, honey, egg, oil, and vanilla. Add the almond extract, if desired.

3. Make a well in the center of the flour mixture and add the milk mixture. Stir just until blended, then gently fold in the raspberries. Pour the batter into the muffin pan.

4. Bake until a wooden pick inserted in the center of a muffin comes out clean, 20 minutes.

198 calories, 5 g protein, 29 g carbohydrates, 4 g fiber, 8 g total fat, 1 g saturated fat, 246 mg sodium

Blueberry-Oat Scones and Raspberry-Almond Muffins Breads and Baked Goods 325

Banana-Peanut Bread Serves 10

Prep Time • 10 minutes
Cook Time • 50 minutes

3 very ripe medium bananas, mashed (about 1 cup)

1/2 cup natural peanut butter

2 eggs

1 tablespoon canola oil

1 1/2 cups whole-wheat pastry flour

1/2 cup whole oats, ground

1/4 cup sugar

2 tablespoons ground flaxseed

2 teaspoons baking powder

1/2 teaspoon baking soda

1/2 teaspoon salt

Spice up your banana bread with peanut butter! It adds protein, vitamins, monounsaturated fat, and great flavor to this bread, also a good source of fiber.

1. Preheat the oven to 350°F (180°C). Lightly coat a 5 x 9-inch (12 x 23 cm) loaf pan with cooking spray.

2. In a medium bowl, stir together the bananas, peanut butter, eggs, and oil. In a large bowl, whisk together the flour, oats, sugar, flaxseed, baking powder, baking soda, and salt.

3. Make a well in the center of the flour mixture, add the banana mixture, and stir just until moistened. Place in the pan.

4. Bake until a wooden pick inserted in the center comes out clean, 40 to 50 minutes. Transfer to a rack and let cool for 5 minutes, then remove from the pan and let cool completely.

234 calories, 7 g protein, 31 g carbohydrates, 4 g fiber, 9 g total fat, 1 g saturated fat, 351 mg sodium

Zesty Cornbread Serves 8 *(See photograph, p. 35)*

Prep Time • 20 minutes
Cook Time • 30 minutes

4 tablespoons canola oil

1 small red bell pepper, seeded and chopped

1 jalapeño pepper, seeded, deveined, and minced (wear gloves when handling; they burn)

1 small onion, chopped

1 clove garlic, minced

1 cup cornmeal

1 cup whole-wheat pastry flour

2 teaspoons baking powder

1/2 teaspoon salt

1 cup soy milk

1 egg, beaten

Cornmeal is a grain (a whole grain if you buy whole cornmeal) that's quite rich in folate and iron. Try preparing this bread the old-fashioned way—baked in a cast-iron skillet. Not only is cooking in cast iron delicious and easy, but it adds iron to the food.

1. Preheat the oven to 375°F (190°C). Coat a 9-inch (23-cm) square baking pan with cooking spray.

2. Heat 1 tablespoon oil in a medium skillet over medium heat. Add the bell pepper, jalapeño, and onion and cook until lightly browned, 4 minutes. Add the garlic and cook for 1 minute. Remove from the heat.

3. In a large bowl, stir together the cornmeal, flour, baking powder, and salt. In a measuring cup, combine the milk, egg, and remaining oil. Make a well in the center of the cornmeal mixture, add the milk and pepper mixtures, and stir just until blended. Place in the pan.

4. Bake until a wooden pick inserted in the center comes out clean, 30 minutes.

205 calories, 6 g protein, 27 g carbohydrates, 3 g fiber, 9 g total fat, 1 g saturated fat, 310 mg sodium

Pumpkin Streusel Bread
Makes 2 loaves

Prep Time • 25 minutes
Cook Time • 50 minutes

Topping

1/3 cup pumpkin seeds

2 tablespoons packed brown sugar

2 teaspoons canola oil

Bread

1 can (15 ounces/425 g) pumpkin puree

1 cup soy milk

1/2 cup canola oil

4 large eggs

1 cup packed brown sugar

3 1/2 cups whole-wheat pastry flour

1/4 cup ground flaxseed

4 teaspoons baking powder

2 teaspoons ground cinnamon

1 teaspoon ground ginger

1/2 teaspoon freshly ground nutmeg

3/4 teaspoon salt

You'd never know this delicious, sweet bread offers so many health benefits. Pumpkin seeds, also known as pepitas, are loaded with magnesium, and canned pumpkin is just about the best source of beta-carotene on Earth. We've even sneaked some flaxseed into this bread.

1. Preheat the oven to 350°F (180°C). Coat two 4 x 8-inch (10 x 20-cm) loaf pans with cooking spray.

2. *To make the topping:* In a small bowl, stir together the pumpkin seeds, brown sugar, and oil. Set aside.

3. *To make the bread:* In a medium bowl, combine the pumpkin, milk, oil, eggs, and brown sugar. In a large bowl, combine the flour, flaxseed, baking powder, cinnamon, ginger, nutmeg, and salt.

4. Make a well in the center of the flour mixture, add the pumpkin mixture, and stir just until blended. Place in the pans and top with the pumpkin seed mixture, pressing the seeds gently into the top.

5. Bake until a wooden pick inserted in the center comes out clean, 50 minutes. Transfer to a rack and let cool for 10 minutes, then remove from the pans and let cool completely.

226 calories, 5 g protein, 31 g carbohydrates, 3 g fiber, 9 g total fat, 1 g saturated fat, 252 mg sodium

Cinnamon-Raisin Coffee Cake Serves 12

Prep Time • 10 minutes
Cook Time • 30 minutes

1 cup low-fat granola with almonds

1 cup Greek yogurt

1 cup sugar

3 eggs

1/3 cup canola oil

1 tablespoon vanilla extract

1 teaspoon ground cinnamon

1 1/2 teaspoons baking powder

1 teaspoon baking soda

1/2 teaspoon salt

2 1/4 cups whole-wheat pastry flour

1/2 cup raisins

Nutrient-rich yogurt replaces the butter of typical coffee cakes, but you'll never notice in this moist, tender treat. The cinnamon helps lower blood sugar, and the raisins offer blood pressure–lowering potassium.

1. Preheat the oven to 350°F (180°C). Coat a Bundt pan with cooking spray. Sprinkle the granola into the bottom of the pan.

2. In a large bowl, whisk together the yogurt, sugar, eggs, oil, vanilla, and cinnamon. Stir in the baking powder, baking soda, and salt. Add the flour and whisk until well blended, then fold in the raisins. Pour into the pan.

3. Bake until a wooden pick inserted in the center comes out clean, 30 minutes. Transfer to a rack and let cool for 10 minutes, then remove from the pan and let cool completely.

279 calories, 7 g protein, 45 g carbohydrates, 3 g fiber, 8 g total fat, 1 g saturated fat, 333 mg sodium

Chocolate-Almond Biscotti Makes 4 dozen

Prep Time • 3 hours
Cook Time • 1 hour

2 1/2 cups whole-wheat pastry flour

3/4 cup sugar

2 teaspoons baking powder

1 teaspoon ground cinnamon

1 teaspoon salt

1 1/2 cups whole almonds

6 ounces (170 g) bittersweet chocolate (60% or higher cocoa content), chopped

4 large eggs

These low-fat cookies are bursting with flavor. Packed with almonds, which are a great source of vitamin E, and drizzled with antioxidant-rich chocolate, they're perfect with an after-dinner cup of coffee.

1. Preheat the oven to 350°F (180°C). Line a baking sheet with parchment paper. In a large bowl, whisk together the flour, sugar, baking powder, cinnamon, and salt. Stir in the almonds and 2/3 of the chocolate.

2. Beat the eggs in a small bowl, then stir into the flour mixture. Place the dough on a lightly floured surface and knead until smooth. Cut in half and shape each piece into a log 12 inches (30 cm) long and 3 inches (8 cm) thick. Place on the baking sheet and bake until the outside seems firm and puffed, 30 minutes. Transfer to a rack and let cool, 2 hours.

3. With a serrated knife, cut the logs crosswise into slices about 1/2 inch (1 cm) thick. Place the slices on their sides on the parchment-lined baking pan and bake, turning once, until crisp and lightly browned, 30 minutes. Transfer to a rack and let cool for 30 minutes.

4. Meanwhile, place the remaining chocolate in a small bowl and microwave on low until almost melted, 1 minute. Stir until melted completely. Drizzle over the biscotti.

80 calories, 2 g protein, 10 g carbohydrates, 1 g fiber, 4 g total fat, 1 g saturated fat, 75 mg sodium

Chock-Full Chocolate Chip Cookies Makes 5 dozen

Prep Time • 15 minutes
Cook Time • 50 minutes

1 1/2 cups whole-wheat pastry flour

1 cup whole oats, ground

1/3 cup cocoa powder

1 teaspoon baking soda

1/2 teaspoon salt

1 cup butter

1/2 cup granulated sugar

1 cup packed light brown sugar

2 eggs

1 tablespoon vanilla extract

1 cup bittersweet chocolate chips
    (60% or higher cocoa content)

1 cup raisins

1 cup walnuts, coarsely chopped

Yes, you can have your chocolate and eat it, too! The darker the chocolate, the healthier it is, so these cookies boast both cocoa powder and 60% cocoa chips. To make them even tastier and healthier, raisins and nuts are added with the chocolate chips.

1. Preheat the oven to 350°F (180°C). In a medium bowl, whisk together the flour, oats, cocoa, baking soda, and salt.

2. In a large bowl, with an electric mixer at medium speed, beat the butter with the granulated and brown sugar until light and fluffy, 2 minutes. Add the eggs and vanilla and beat until smooth. Beat in the flour mixture until combined. Stir in the chocolate chips, raisins, and walnuts. Drop by teaspoons onto a baking sheet.

3. Bake until browned, 10 minutes. Repeat with remaining dough. Let cool on the baking sheet for 2 minutes, then transfer to a rack and let cool completely.

97 calories, 1 g protein, 12 g carbohydrates, 1 g fiber, 5 g total fat, 2 g saturated fat, 77 mg sodium

Chocolate-Pecan Torte Serves 16

Prep Time • 2 hours, 20 minutes
Cook Time • 40 minutes

1 1/2 cups pecan halves

1 cup sugar

6 ounces (170 g) bittersweet
chocolate (60% or higher cocoa
content)

6 eggs, separated

1/4 cup cocoa powder

1/3 cup orange juice

1 teaspoon grated orange zest

Confectioners' sugar (optional)

Orange sections (optional)

This rich cake, loaded with antioxidants, tastes best the day after baking, so whenever possible, make it ahead of time. Store, covered, at room temperature for a few days or freeze any extra for future use.

1. Preheat the oven to 350°F (180°C). Coat a 10-inch (25-cm) spring-form pan with cooking spray. Place the pecans and 1/2 cup sugar in a food processor and pulse until finely ground. Add the chocolate and pulse until ground. Set aside.

2. In a large bowl, with an electric mixer on high speed, beat the egg whites until foamy. Continue to beat, gradually adding the remaining 1/2 cup sugar, until stiff, glossy peaks form.

3. In another bowl, with the same beaters, beat the egg yolks until thick, about 4 minutes. Add the cocoa, orange juice, and zest and beat until well blended. Fold in the pecan mixture. Stir in 1/4 of the egg whites, then fold in the rest in 2 batches. Pour into the pan.

4. Bake until a knife inserted in the center comes out clean, 40 minutes. Transfer to a rack and let cool completely, 2 hours, then cut around the cake and release the sides of the pan. Sprinkle the torte with confectioners' sugar and top with oranges, if desired.

205 calories, 4 g protein, 21 g carbohydrates, 2 g fiber, 14 g total fat, 4 g saturated fat, 25 mg sodium

Chocolate Fondue Serves 10

Prep Time • 5 minutes
Cook Time • 10 minutes

1 cup low-fat evaporated milk

1/4 cup sugar

1/4 cup cocoa powder

1 tablespoon vanilla extract

1/2 package (5 ounces/142 g)
bittersweet chocolate chips
(60% or higher cocoa content)

Fruit is only made healthier when dipped in this fondue, made with antioxidant-rich bittersweet chocolate. Serve surrounded by apple or pear wedges, thick banana slices, orange sections, whole strawberries, and pineapple chunks for dipping.

1. In a small saucepan, whisk together the milk, sugar, cocoa, and vanilla until well blended. Add the chocolate chips.

2. Place over low heat and cook, stirring occasionally, until melted, 10 minutes. Pour into a fondue pot or small slow cooker set on low.

128 calories, 3 g protein, 20 g carbohydrates, 1 g fiber, 5 g total fat, 3 g saturated fat, 33 mg sodium

Carrot Cake with Cream Cheese Glaze Serves 12

Prep Time • 1 hour, 20 minutes
Cook Time • 35 minutes

1/2 cup applesauce

2/3 cup granulated sugar

2 large eggs

2 tablespoons canola oil

1 teaspoon vanilla extract

1 1/4 cups whole-wheat pastry flour

1 teaspoon baking soda

1 teaspoon ground cinnamon

1/2 teaspoon salt

1 1/2 cups shredded carrots
(3 large)

1/2 cup chopped walnuts

1 ounce (28 g) low-fat
cream cheese

2 tablespoons low-fat milk

2–3 tablespoons confectioners' sugar

You'll never notice that this dense, flavorful cake is low in fat and made with healthful ingredients. What you will notice is how delicious and moist it is and how quickly it disappears from the plate.

1. Preheat the oven to 350°F (180°C). Coat a 9-inch (23-cm) round cake or bundt pan with cooking spray. In a small bowl, whisk together the applesauce, sugar, eggs, oil, and vanilla.

2. In a large bowl, whisk together the flour, baking soda, cinnamon, and salt. Make a well in the center, add the applesauce mixture, and stir just until blended. Stir in the carrots and walnuts. Pour the batter into the pan.

3. Bake until a wooden pick inserted in the center comes out clean, 35 minutes. Transfer to a rack and let cool for 10 minutes, then remove from the pan and let cool completely, 1 hour.

4. Meanwhile, in a small bowl, whisk together the cream cheese and milk until well combined. Add 2 tablespoons confectioners' sugar and whisk until smooth, adding more sugar if the glaze is too thin. Place the cake on a serving plate and drizzle with the glaze.

160 calories, 3 g protein, 23 g carbohydrates, 2 g fiber, 6 g total fat,
1 g saturated fat, 236 mg sodium

Pear Crisp Serves 6

Prep Time • 10 minutes
Cook Time • 30 minutes

4 cups sliced pears (about 5
medium)

1/2 cup prunes, chopped

1/4 cup packed brown sugar

1 tablespoon chopped
crystallized ginger

1 tablespoon lemon juice

2 cups low-fat granola

3 tablespoons pure maple syrup

A great way to sneak prunes into a dessert, this sweet, flavorful crisp is bursting with fiber, with pears being a terrific source. The prunes are blended with the pears, sugar, and ginger and topped with a simple crunchy topping.

1. Preheat the oven to 350°F (180°C). In a large bowl, combine the pears and prunes. Sprinkle with the brown sugar, ginger, and lemon juice and toss gently to coat. Place in a 9-inch (23-cm) pie plate.

2. In a small bowl, toss the granola with the maple syrup. Sprinkle over the pear mixture, pressing into the pears. Bake until bubbling in the center and the pears are tender, 30 minutes.

322 calories, 4 g protein, 75 g carbohydrates, 6 g fiber, 3 g total fat,
0 g saturated fat, 96 mg sodium

Carrot Cake with Cream Cheese Glaze Desserts 333

Frozen Fruit Mousse Serves 4

Prep Time • 5 minutes

1 cup cold low-fat evaporated milk

2 tablespoons confectioners' sugar

1 teaspoon grated orange zest

2 cups frozen strawberries

Looking for a light, sweet treat? Here's a spoonable way to get all the health benefits of berries when they're out of season.

1. In a measuring cup, combine the milk, sugar, and orange zest.

2. Place the strawberries in a food processor and pulse just until shaved. With the motor running, gradually add the milk mixture just until the ingredients come together. Serve immediately.

88 calories, 5 g protein, 15 g carbohydrates, 2 g fiber, 1 g total fat, 1 g saturated fat, 70 mg sodium

Pomegranate Ice Serves 4

Prep Time • 5 hours

2 cups pomegranate-blueberry juice (100% juice)

1/4 cup lime juice

2 tablespoons sugar

Packed with antioxidants, this delicious dessert is refreshing on a hot summer's night or after a spicy meal. Use any blend of pomegranate juice as long as it's 100% juice.

1. In a 9-inch (23-cm) square metal baking pan, whisk together the pomegranate juice, lime juice, and sugar until the sugar dissolves. Freeze for 1 hour, then stir to blend in any frozen portions. Freeze, stirring every 45 minutes to incorporate frozen portions, until the mixture has a uniform slushy consistency and ice crystals form, about 4 hours.

98 calories, 1 g protein, 25 g carbohydrates, 0 g fiber, 0 g total fat, 0 g saturated fat, 15 mg sodium

Rice Pudding Serves 4

Prep Time • 5 minutes
Cook Time • 1 hour, 35 minutes

3 cups vanilla soy milk

2/3 cup brown rice

1/2 teaspoon ground cinnamon

1/4 teaspoon salt

2 eggs, at room temperature, lightly beaten

1/2 cup raisins

1/2 cup chopped nuts, such as Brazil nuts, almonds, or walnuts

Who doesn't love creamy, comforting rice pudding? This one serves up health benefits that most don't. Soy milk, used here, can easily be substituted for dairy milk in all baked goods.

1. In a medium saucepan over medium heat, combine the soy milk, rice, cinnamon, and salt. Bring to a simmer, then reduce the heat to low, cover, and simmer for 1 1/2 hours. Remove from the heat and let cool for 5 minutes.

2. Stir 1/2 cup of the rice mixture into the eggs, stirring constantly. Gradually stir back into the rice mixture. Cook over low heat, stirring constantly, until thickened, 5 minutes. Stir in the raisins and nuts. Serve warm or refrigerate and serve cold.

354 calories, 13 g protein, 50 g carbohydrates, 4 g fiber, 12 g total fat, 1 g saturated fat, 256 mg sodium

Mixed Berry Tart Serves 12

Prep Time • 2 hours, 35 minutes
Cook Time • 20 minutes

1/4 cup ice water, without ice

3 tablespoons low-fat plain yogurt

1 cup whole-grain pastry flour

1/2 cup all-purpose flour

1 tablespoon + 1/3 cup sugar

1/4 teaspoon ground cinnamon

1/4 teaspoon salt

7 tablespoons butter

5 cups mixed berries, such as
blueberries, raspberries, and
strawberries

2 tablespoons cornstarch

1 tablespoon lemon juice

Confectioners' sugar (optional)

Sweet berries and flaky crust add up to an irresistible dessert rich in anti-oxidants and fiber. Use a blend of berries or just one type. Vary the flavors with lime juice instead of lemon juice and ginger instead of cinnamon.

1. In a measuring cup, whisk together the water and yogurt. In a food processor, combine the pastry and all-purpose flour, 1 tablespoon sugar, cinnamon, and salt. Add the butter and pulse until the mixture resembles coarse crumbs. With the motor running, gradually add the yogurt mixture and process just until the ingredients come together. Gather the dough into a ball. Wrap in plastic and refrigerate for at least 2 hours.

2. Preheat the oven to 350°F. In a large bowl, combine the berries, cornstarch, lemon juice, and 1/3 cup sugar and toss gently.

3. Shape dough into 6 small balls. Roll out each ball on a lightly floured work surface to about a 6-inch (15-cm) circle. Using six 4-inch (10-cm) tartlet pans with removable bottoms, line the pans with the dough. Evenly distribute the fruit mixture into the pans.

4. Bake until the filling is bubbling and crust is browned, 15 to 20 minutes. Transfer to a rack for 15 minutes. Remove from pans and cool completely. Each tartlet is 2 servings. Dust with confectioners' sugar.

165 calories, 3 g protein, 26 g carbohydrates, 3 g fiber, 7 g total fat, 3 g saturated fat, 128 mg sodium

Recipe List

index

B